Past, Present and Future of Protein Kinase CK2 Research

Guest Editors
Mauro Salvi
Department of Biomedical Sciences
University of Padova
Padova
Italy

Maria Ruzzene
Department of Biomedical Sciences
University of Padova
Padova
Italy

Editorial Office
MDPI AG
Grosspeteranlage 5
4052 Basel, Switzerland

This is a reprint of the Special Issue, published open access by the journal *Kinases and Phosphatases* (ISSN), freely accessible at: https://www.mdpi.com/journal/kinasesphosphatases/special_issues/25C1UGVH9W.

For citation purposes, cite each article independently as indicated on the article page online and as indicated below:

Lastname, A.A.; Lastname, B.B. Article Title. *Journal Name* **Year**, *Volume Number*, Page Range.

ISBN 978-3-7258-7222-0 (Hbk)
ISBN 978-3-7258-7223-7 (PDF)
https://doi.org/10.3390/books978-3-7258-7223-7

Contents

About the Editors

Mauro Salvi

Mauro Salvi is an Associate Professor of Biochemistry in the Department of Biomedical Sciences at the University of Padova, Italy. He has authored around 90 scientific publications in international journals, which have been cited over 3,000 times. He is Editor-in-Chief of the journal *Kinases and Phosphatases* (MDPI) and a member of the editorial board of various journals, including the *International Journal of Molecular Sciences* (IJMS), *Current Protein and Peptide Science* (CPPS), and *Molecular Medicine Reports*. The current research interests of his laboratory are focused on post-translational modifications (PTMs), specifically phosphorylation, and acidophilic kinases, particularly protein kinase CK2 and Fam20C. His current research projects aim to investigate PTM-based regulatory mechanisms in various signal transduction pathways. This involves studying enzymes (their function, regulation, and partners) and target protein substrates (their physiological and pathological roles in PTMs), using a combination of in silico, in vitro, and cellular experimental approaches.

Maria Ruzzene

Maria Ruzzene is a Full Professor of Biochemistry in the Department of Biomedical Sciences at the University of Padova, Italy. Her research interests concern phosphorylation signaling in health and disease, biochemical and cellular characterization of different protein kinases and phosphatases, identification of novel pharmacological targets, and the development of specific kinase inhibitors and activators as potential therapeutic drugs. She participated in many international meetings as an invited speaker. She has been PI of several projects granted by national and international organizations and is a member of the editorials boards of several international scientific journals. Career highlights: 116 publications on peer-reviewed international journals; 5 book chapters, Scopus H-index: 42; citations: >6700.

Preface

CK2 (formerly known as casein kinase 2) was the first protein kinase to be discovered in 1954. Since then, a large number of studies have been published to disclose its biochemical properties and physiological and pathological roles. It is now established that CK2 is constitutively active, ubiquitously expressed, and involved in many biological processes, as well as in the pathogenesis of important human diseases, including cancer, neurodegeneration, and inflammation. However, despite extensive time and scientific effort, CK2 remains an enigmatic enzyme, as we are still far from fully understanding its actual pathophysiological roles and the mechanisms that modulate its functions. Moreover, it has long been considered a promising pharmacological target to be inhibited in diverse pathologies, and several inhibitors with increasing efficacy and specificity have been developed over the years. However, the recent discovery of genetic diseases related to mutations in CK2 genes prompts new investigation aimed at identifying and developing strategies to stimulate its activity, which are not available so far.

This Special Issue, on one hand, retraces the main discoveries of CK2 and, on the other, summarizes recent research and presents updates and new advances in the field.

Mauro Salvi and Maria Ruzzene

Guest Editors

kinases and phosphatases

MDPI

Editorial

Past, Present and Future of Protein Kinase CK2 Research

Mauro Salvi * and Maria Ruzzene *

Department of Biomedical Sciences, University of Padova, 35131 Padova, Italy
* Correspondence: mauro.salvi@unipd.it (M.S.); maria.ruzzene@unipd.it (M.R.)

The first described instance of protein kinase activity dates back more than half a century [1] and was later identified as CK2. Since then, this enzyme has attracted enormous scientific interest, with hundreds of studies investigating its structure, function, and physiological and pathological relevance being published each year. We now know that CK2 is a constitutively active, ubiquitously expressed enzyme which is involved in a broad range of functionally diverse biological processes. Therefore, it is not surprising that its dysregulation has been linked to numerous diseases, including cancer, neurodegenerative disorders, and inflammation [2–4]. For this reason, CK2 is considered to be a promising drug target for various diseases, particularly for different forms of cancer. Several CK2-specific inhibitors are available [5–7]. However, despite decades of intensive research, this enzyme remains puzzling. Many aspects of its role in human diseases and the mechanisms that regulate its function are still not fully understood. Moreover, the recent discovery of genetic syndromes linked to mutations in the CK2α and CK2β genes [8] has opened up a new area of investigation.

This Special Issue, "Past, Present and Future of Protein Kinase CK2 Research", comprises eight contributions, some of which are dedicated to reviewing essential features of CK2, while others showcase some of the latest advances in the field.

Niefind and his group focus on the "neglected" α′ catalytic subunit of CK2 [9]. CK2 is a tetrameric enzyme composed of two catalytic (α and/or α′) and two regulatory (β) subunits. While many crystallographic studies have focused on the α subunit, the α′ isoform has been rarely investigated, due to the poor solubility of the recombinant protein. In their work, the authors exploit the Cys336Ser CK2α′ mutant as a crystallographic tool that, along with optimized techniques, allows them to solve the structures of CK2α′ in a complex with various ligands at atomic resolution. In one of these structures, the authors highlight the N-terminal segment site, which is a ligand-binding region with the potential to develop new substrate-competitive CK2 inhibitors.

Dominguez et al. [10] address the largely overlooked issue of the transcriptional regulation of CK2α, marking an important step forward in this field of study. Despite many years of investigation, little has been published on this critical topic since the pioneering studies by Pyerin's group [11]. By focusing on the promoter of the *Csnk2a1* gene (the murine ortholog of human *CSNK2A1* coding for CK2α), the authors demonstrate that the transcription factor NF-κB regulates CK2α expression. Through a combination of promoter deletions, binding assays, and functional analyses, they demonstrate that NF-κB binds to a conserved minimal promoter region. Interestingly, as CK2α itself modulates NF-κB signaling, their findings suggest a positive feedback loop in which CK2α may regulate its own expression via NF-κB.

Cesaro and colleagues [12] review the "rules" of CK2 substrate selection, emphasizing the importance of the CK2 consensus sequence in predicting phosphorylation sites, and analyzing the different experimental approaches used to confirm CK2 involvement in phosphorylation events. The authors also discuss various strategies for modulating CK2 activity, including knockdown, knockout, and inhibition by small molecules, and highlight the strengths and limitations of each method.

Tapia's research group [13] considers the central role that CK2 plays in cancer pathogenesis and the targets involved in the CK2-dependent regulation of cell survival, proliferation, and metastasis. They identify one such target in endothelin-converting enzyme-1 (ECE1), whose isoform ECE1c is frequently overexpressed in cancer. They explore the connections between CK2, ECE1c, and cancer, focusing on the phosphorylation of the ECE1c N-terminus, which appears to protect ECE1c from degradation and activate oncogenic pathways such as Wnt/β-catenin signaling.

Pandit and colleagues [14] explore the role of CK2 in non-oncological diseases, particularly musculoskeletal disorders such as rheumatoid arthritis, osteoarthritis, bone fractures, and osteoporosis. They provide a comprehensive overview of CK2's involvement in these conditions and discuss how targeting CK2 could help to restore biochemical imbalances, offering potential therapeutic benefits.

Quezada Meza and Ruzzene [15] evaluate CK2's role in viral infections, with special reference to SARS-CoV-2 and other coronaviruses. Their review discusses the mechanisms by which CK2 is involved in these infections and the ways in which CK2 inhibitors are repurposed to mitigate their effects. The analysis broadens our understanding of the CK2/virus interplay and discusses how to extrapolate information that could be useful beyond the context of the recent pandemic.

Finally, two reviews provide valuable insights into the diverse strategies used for CK2 inhibition, offering complementary perspectives and highlighting promising avenues for the development of novel therapeutics targeting this kinase.

Axtman and colleagues [16], who recently discovered SGC-CK2-1, the most selective and potent CK2 inhibitor identified so far [17], review various classes of small-molecule inhibitors, including orthosteric, allosteric, and bivalent inhibitors. They also discuss the progress that has been made in developing CK2 chemical probes for in vivo studies.

Spring and coworkers [18] focus on small molecules targeting sites outside the ATP-binding site. This is an innovative strategy that, compared to the more conventional ATP-competitive inhibitors (e.g., CX-4945, SGC-CK2-1), is expected to offer higher selectivity. It includes substrate-competitive inhibitors which block CK2–substrate interactions, bispecific inhibitors binding both ATP and substrate sites, αD site inhibitors exploiting a unique CK2 pocket, and holoenzyme disruptors preventing CK2α/β assembly. PROTACs inducing CK2 degradation are also discussed.

In summary, looking back on seven decades of research into the CK2 field, with hundreds of studies published every year, we can say that "the past" is abundant, and significant progress has been made in unraveling the physio/pathological role of this intriguing enzyme. However, "the present" is still full of surprises, and the journey is far from complete, thus making "the future" an even more exciting promise.

Author Contributions: M.S. and M.R. writing—original draft preparation; M.S. and M.R. writing—review and editing. All authors have read and agreed to the published version of the manuscript.

Funding: This research received no external funding.

Conflicts of Interest: The authors declare no conflicts of interest.

References

1. Burnett, G.; Kennedy, E.P. The Enzymatic Phosphorylation of Proteins. *J. Biol. Chem.* **1954**, *211*, 969–980. [CrossRef] [PubMed]
2. Borgo, C.; D'Amore, C.; Cesaro, L.; Sarno, S.; Pinna, L.A.; Ruzzene, M.; Salvi, M. How Can a Traffic Light Properly Work If It Is Always Green? The Paradox of CK2 Signaling. *Crit. Rev. Biochem. Mol. Biol.* **2021**, *56*, 321–359. [CrossRef] [PubMed]
3. Borgo, C.; D'Amore, C.; Sarno, S.; Salvi, M.; Ruzzene, M. Protein Kinase CK2: A Potential Therapeutic Target for Diverse Human Diseases. *Signal Transduct. Target. Ther.* **2021**, *6*, 183. [CrossRef] [PubMed]
4. St-Denis, N.A.; Litchfield, D.W. Protein Kinase CK2 in Health and Disease: From Birth to Death: The Role of Protein Kinase CK2 in the Regulation of Cell Proliferation and Survival. *Cell. Mol. Life Sci.* **2009**, *66*, 1817–1829. [CrossRef] [PubMed]
5. Strum, S.W.; Gyenis, L.; Litchfield, D.W. CSNK2 in Cancer: Pathophysiology and Translational Applications. *Br. J. Cancer* **2022**, *126*, 994–1003. [CrossRef] [PubMed]
6. Trembley, J.H.; Kren, B.T.; Afzal, M.; Scaria, G.A.; Klein, M.A.; Ahmed, K. Protein Kinase CK2—Diverse Roles in Cancer Cell Biology and Therapeutic Promise. *Mol. Cell. Biochem.* **2023**, *478*, 899–926. [CrossRef] [PubMed]
7. Borgo, C.; Ruzzene, M. Protein Kinase CK2 Inhibition as a Pharmacological Strategy. In *Advances in Protein Chemistry and Structural Biology*; Academic Press: Cambridge, MA, USA, 2021.
8. Ballardin, D.; Cruz-Gamero, J.M.; Bienvenu, T.; Rebholz, H. Comparing Two Neurodevelopmental Disorders Linked to CK2: Okur-Chung Neurodevelopmental Syndrome and Poirier-Bienvenu Neurodevelopmental Syndrome-Two Sides of the Same Coin? *Front. Mol. Biosci.* **2022**, *9*, 850559. [CrossRef] [PubMed]
9. Werner, C.; Lindenblatt, D.; Viht, K.; Uri, A.; Niefind, K. Discovery and Exploration of Protein Kinase CK2 Binding Sites Using CK2α'Cys336Ser as an Exquisite Crystallographic Tool. *Kinases Phosphatases* **2023**, *1*, 306–322. [CrossRef]
10. Imbrie, G.A.; Wilson, N.G.; Seldin, D.C.; Dominguez, I. Regulation of Mouse CK2α (Csnk2a1) Promoter Expression In Vitro and in Cell Lines. *Kinases Phosphatases* **2025**, *3*, 15. [CrossRef]
11. Krehan, A.; Ansuini, H.; Bocher, O.; Grein, S.; Wirkner, U.; Pyerin, W. Transcription Factors Ets1, NF-Kappa B, and Sp1 Are Major Determinants of the Promoter Activity of the Human Protein Kinase CK2alpha Gene. *J. Biol. Chem.* **2000**, *275*, 18327–18336. [CrossRef]
12. Cesaro, L.; Zuliani, A.M.; Bosello Travain, V.; Salvi, M. Exploring Protein Kinase CK2 Substrate Recognition and the Dynamic Response of Substrate Phosphorylation to Kinase Modulation. *Kinases Phosphatases* **2023**, *1*, 251–264. [CrossRef]
13. Villalobos-Nova, K.; Toro, M.d.l.Á.; Pérez-Moreno, P.; Niechi, I.; Tapia, J.C. The CK2/ECE1c Partnership: An Unveiled Pathway to Aggressiveness in Cancer. *Kinases Phosphatases* **2024**, *2*, 1–8. [CrossRef]
14. Pandit, V.; DeGeorge, K.; Nohe, A. Scoping Pleiotropy of CK2 in Musculoskeletal Disorders for a Novel Targeting Approach. *Kinases Phosphatases* **2024**, *2*, 43–66. [CrossRef]
15. Quezada Meza, C.P.; Ruzzene, M. Protein Kinase CK2 and SARS-CoV-2: An Expected Interplay Story. *Kinases Phosphatases* **2023**, *1*, 141–150. [CrossRef]
16. Ong, H.W.; Drewry, D.H.; Axtman, A.D. CK2 Chemical Probes: Past, Present, and Future. *Kinases Phosphatases* **2023**, *1*, 288–305. [CrossRef]
17. Wells, C.I.; Drewry, D.H.; Pickett, J.E.; Tjaden, A.; Krämer, A.; Müller, S.; Gyenis, L.; Menyhart, D.; Litchfield, D.W.; Knapp, S.; et al. Development of a Potent and Selective Chemical Probe for the Pleiotropic Kinase CK2. *Cell Chem. Biol.* **2021**, *28*, 546–558.e10. [CrossRef] [PubMed]
18. Day-Riley, S.; West, R.M.; Brear, P.D.; Hyvönen, M.; Spring, D.R. CK2 Inhibitors Targeting Inside and Outside the Catalytic Box. *Kinases Phosphatases* **2024**, *2*, 110–135. [CrossRef]

kinases and phosphatases

MDPI

Review

Protein Kinase CK2 and SARS-CoV-2: An Expected Interplay Story

Camila Paz Quezada Meza and Maria Ruzzene *

Department of Biomedical Sciences, University of Padova, 35121 Padova, Italy; camilapaz.quezadameza@studenti.unipd.it
* Correspondence: maria.ruzzene@unipd.it

Abstract: Protein kinase CK2 is a Ser/Thr protein kinase that phosphorylates hundreds of substrates mainly related to survival and proliferation pathways. It has long been considered an anti-cancer drug target. However, during the recent COVID-19 pandemic, CK2 inhibitors have been repurposed as anti-SARS-CoV-2 drugs. This was based on the initial finding of CK2 among the proteins of the host cell that interact with the viral proteins and modulate the infection. Since then, several studies have deepened our understanding of the CK2/COVID-19 connection, and we deem it is time to review all the findings. Interestingly, other coronaviruses cross-talk with CK2 as well, with similarities and differences compared to the SARS-CoV-2 case. Therefore, we believe that the analysis of the effects obtained by targeting CK2 in case of coronavirus infections, both at the molecular and phenomenological level, will help in extrapolating information that could be useful not only for COVID-19 (whose pandemic emergency is hopefully turning off) but also for other infections.

Keywords: protein kinase CK2; CSNK2A1; CSNK2A2; CSNK2B; coronaviruses; COVID-19; SARS-CoV-2

1. Introduction

1.1. CK2 General Features, Structure, and Regulation

Protein kinase CK2 is a Ser/Thr kinase expressed in all eukaryotic cells and involved in all cellular processes. It localizes mainly in the nucleus and cytoplasm, but also other sub-cellular compartments [1], such as mitochondria and plasma membrane, where it can be exported to the external side and is therefore considered an ecto-kinase [2]. The acronym CK2 originates from the term "casein kinase 2" since this protein kinase was initially regarded as responsible for the phosphorylation of milk casein [3]. However, it was later clear that casein is physiologically phosphorylated by another kinase (G-CK, or genuine casein kinase, recently identified with Fam20C [3]). At the same time, it is not a physiological substrate of CK2, which in turn phosphorylates hundreds of substrates [4] and is involved in virtually all cellular processes. It is ubiquitously expressed and essential for embryonal development [5], and its levels are particularly high in physiologically and pathologically rapidly proliferating cells [6–8]. Indeed, cancer cells are known to be addicted to CK2 [9], which plays essential roles in potentiating cancer hallmarks and tumorigenic signals [10–12]. Therefore, CK2 is presently considered a cancer drug target [13–17].

CK2 is constitutively active, meaning that it does not require signaling by second messengers or phosphorylation events to be activated, and its functions are roughly regulated by changes in protein expression. However, several mechanisms have been proposed that might contribute to modulating the activity of this enigmatic kinase, ranging from changes in subcellular localization, substrate availability/accessibility, association to other proteins, composition in subunits/isoforms, and supramolecular polymerization of the kinase holoenzyme [18,19].

From a structural point of view, mammalian CK2 is a tetrameric holoenzyme: it is composed of two catalytic subunits (α or α', coded by two different genes, *CSNK2A1* and *CSNK2A2*, respectively) and two regulatory subunits β, coded by the *CSNK2B* gene. Different holoenzyme combinations are possible ($\alpha_2\beta_2$, $\alpha'_2\beta_2$, and $\alpha\alpha'\beta_2$). However, the catalytic subunits are also active as monomers, and the regulatory functions of β are mainly to preserve the enzyme stability and drive the selection of substrates [20]. The actual existence of the isolated CK2 subunits in cells is still uncertain: several pieces of evidence (reviewed in [18]) suggest a role of the monomeric catalytic subunits, not combined with the regulatory ones, in specific pathological conditions, especially in cancer cells. Nevertheless, a direct demonstration of the isolated α or α′ subunits in cells has never been provided.

The two isoforms of the catalytic subunit, α and α′, are supposed to be mainly overlapping in their functions, but a few differential roles have also been reported: they differ mainly for their C-terminal sequences, through which they can bind different partner proteins, what is hypothesized to allow them exerting some isoform-specific functions [21].

1.2. CK2 in Diseases

CK2 activity is implicated in a plethora of diverse human diseases, as recently reviewed [22]. As mentioned above, its pathological functions are mainly documented in cancer. The first connection between CK2 and mammalian tumorigenesis dates back to the late 80s, when Ole-MoiYoi and coworkers, by studying bovine theileriosis (a cattle parasite disease that represents a naturally occurring animal model), provided the earliest evidence of a molecular causative link between CK2 and mammalian lymphoid oncogenesis (as reviewed in [23]). Subsequently, a huge amount of data was collected supporting a tumorigenic role for CK2 in different types of human hematological malignancies and solid cancers, where it is often found overexpressed compared to normal tissues [24,25]. Given the close relationship frequently occurring between viral infections and tumorigenesis, this profound engagement of CK2 in cancer has particular relevance for the topic of this review, as will be discussed below.

For a detailed description of the many other diseases where CK2 has been found involved, we refer the readers to another recent review [22]. Here we can just briefly list the CK2 implication in inflammation and autoimmune disorders [26], diabetes and obesity [27], diverse ophthalmic pathologies [28,29], cardiovascular diseases, such as cardiac ischemia–reperfusion injury, atherosclerosis, and cardiac hypertrophy [30–32]. CK2 is also considered an emerging target for neurological and psychiatric disorders [33] and possibly for cystic fibrosis [34]. Moreover, recently, psychiatric disorders and syndromes due to mutations of the genes for the CK2 subunits have been identified [35]. Specifically, they are called Okur-Chung Neurodevelopmental Syndrome or OC-NDS (mutations of the *CSNK2A1* gene, coding for CK2 α) and Poirier-Benvenu Neurodevelopmental Syndrome or POBINDS (mutations of the *CSNK2B* gene, coding for CK2 β).

Notably, other well-known functions of CK2 are in human infections; given the relevance of the topic of this review, they will be dealt with separately in the next paragraph.

1.3. CK2 in Viral Infections

Protein phosphorylation is a widespread and effective way to modulate protein functions, which even viruses exploit for their replication and life cycle. However, they depend on host protein kinases for the catalysis of this process; consistently, the activation of specific cellular kinases in response to the infection has been frequently observed, with the consequent phosphorylation of viral proteins, but also increased phosphorylation level of host cell proteins [36]. CK2 is among the most pleiotropic kinases, with 25 % of the phospho-proteome depending on its activity [3]. Therefore it makes sense that it could also be crucial for viruses. Indeed, its involvement in the phosphorylation of viral proteins has been known for many years, with 40 cases documented in 2003 [4]. One of the first reported cases is the human papillomavirus E7 protein; interestingly, this is the target of CIGB-300, a clinical-grade drug displaying promising anticancer properties [37,38]. Other notable examples (recently reviewed [8,22]) are the HIV-1 Rev protein, hepatitis C and B virus proteins, NSP1 of rotavirus, the nucleocapsid protein of the Hantaan virus, the matrix M protein of the human respiratory syncytial virus, the leader L protein of the encephalomyocarditis virus, the Kaposi's sarcoma-associated herpesvirus ORF57. Other viruses reported to exploit the activity of CK2 for their infection and propagation are Epstein-Barr Virus (EBV) [39], Herpes Simplex Viruses (HSV), Human Cytomegalovirus (CMV) [8], and the list is continuously increasing, now also including coronaviruses, as described below in more details. In many cases, the infection preludes tumor transformation; therefore, the involvement of CK2, a pro-tumor kinase, is not so unexpected.

The mechanisms by which the phosphorylation by CK2 of viral proteins contributes to the infection are largely unknown. In some cases, the classical antiapoptotic mechanism that CK2 exerts by phosphorylating sites near a caspase site and preventing cleavage [40] might also apply to viral proteins, as reported in the case of ORF57 [41]. For the human papillomavirus E1 protein, it has been demonstrated that the phosphorylation by CK2 stabilizes ATP-dependent DNA helicase activity, which is essential for viral replication [42].

Regardless of the phosphorylated protein and the effect produced, it is worth noting that CK2 targeting has been proposed to stimulate host defence against virus infection by increasing IFN-α and IFN-β response, possibly by regulating the RIG-1 dependent signaling pathway [43,44]. This mechanism would not be limited to a specific viral infection.

2. CK2 and Coronaviruses

Coronaviruses are viruses known for many years, named after the Latin word for crown "corona" due to their peculiar glycoprotein spikes on the virus's surface, visible by electron microscopy, that resemble the solar corona. They are subdivided into four genera, namely α, β, γ, and δ. α and β coronaviruses (β-CoV) infect mammals, while γ and δ primarily infect birds. Until the SARS-CoV outbreak in 2003, coronaviruses were not given much attention by scientists since the ones known to infect humans caused minor symptoms. Presently, three human coronaviruses are known that can produce severe symptoms, all belonging to the β genus: the Severe Acute Respiratory Syndrome Coronavirus (SARS-CoV, identified in 2003), the Middle East Respiratory Syndrome-Related Coronavirus (MERS-CoV, identified in 2012), and the Severe Acute Respiratory Syndrome Coronavirus 2 (SARS-CoV-2, recognised in 2019). They cause diseases called SARS, MERS, and COVID-19, respectively.

The CK2 involvement in coronavirus infection is supported by several observations, as summarized in Figure 1. Firstly, the human β-CoV receptor on the host cell is ACE2 (angiotensin-converting enzyme 2), a known CK2 target [45]. As early as 2010, Chen and coworkers found that the CK2-dependent phosphorylation of ACE2 at the specific site Ser787 is increased upon binding of SARS-CoV; this activates downstream signal transduction pathways, namely ERK1/2 and AP-1, upregulating the fibrosis-associated CCL2 (chemokine C-C motif ligand 2) which mediates lung inflammation and lung fibrosis and facilitates viral invasion into the host cell. Consistently, the dysregulated production of inflammatory cytokines in response to SARS-CoV is reduced by the inhibition of CK2 [46].

The essential role of CK2 in β-CoV replication has been recently demonstrated [47] by developing a β-CoV reporter assay based on mouse hepatitis virus (MHV), a member of the β-CoV genus, frequently used as a model to study the virulence of other β-CoVs, since it does not require restrictive safety facilities. The β-CoV binding to the ACE2 receptor occurs through the spike protein (S protein) present on the surface of the virus [48] and is followed by clathrin-mediated endocytosis [49]. Yang and coworkers used a chemogenomic approach to demonstrate that CK2 inhibitors suppress murine, bat, and human β-CoV replication. They further confirmed the results by the genetic knockdown of the individual CK2 subunits and provided evidence that the effects are due to the reduced endocytosis of the spike protein [47].

A β-coronavirus bovine (BCoV) model was instead exploited by Perea's group [50] to investigate the efficacy of the anti-CK2 peptide CIGB-300 (in ref [50] called CIGB-325) in inhibiting the viral infection. The authors found that CIGB-300 has an antiviral effect in cell-based assays and reduced M (membrane) and N (nucleocapsid) viral protein levels. CIGB-300 is designed to act at the substrate level: it binds to the phospho-acceptor domain and prevents CK2-dependent phosphorylation [51]. Interestingly, in pull-down assays,

CIGB-300 was found to physically interact not only with several cellular CK2 substrates, as expected, but also with the BCoV N protein. The observed CIGB-300/N protein association allows us to speculate that BCoV N protein is a putative CK2 substrate; however, further experiments will be necessary to exclude an indirect binding mediated by other proteins. The results by Perea and coworkers are particularly interesting since BCoV, despite sharing pathogenic properties with other coronaviruses, does not enter host cells by binding to the ACE2 receptor but attaches to N-acetyl-9-O-acetylneuraminic acid (Neu5, 9Ac2) through HE (haemagglutinin esterase) and S proteins [52]. The finding that CK2 targeting reduces the BCoV infection is an additional indication that ACE2 is not the only crossing point between CK2 and coronaviruses and that there are several levels by which CK2 may impact the virus life cycle.

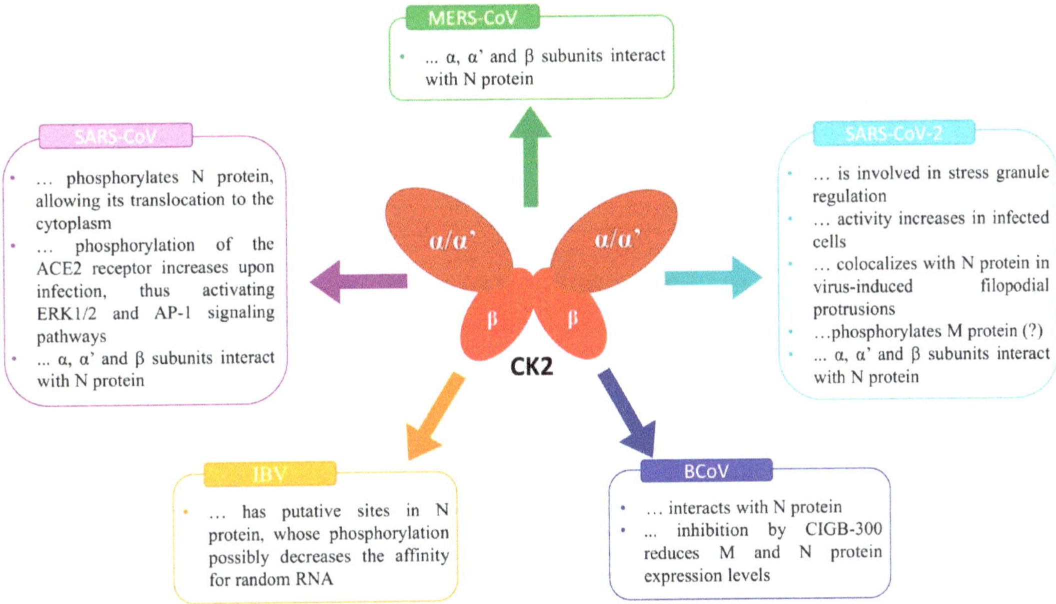

Figure 1. Connections between CK2 and β-CoVs. CK2 is depicted with the typical "butterfly" structure of the tetrameric holoenzyme. The boxes summarise the connections of CK2 to each β-CoV (see the text for references). The question mark (?) indicates still speculative finding.

Indeed, the N protein seems crucial in the CK2 regulation of coronavirus biology. N protein of the Avian infectious bronchitis coronavirus (IBV) was found to display a lower affinity for random RNA, and four phospho-sites were predicted as CK2 sites [53] However, later it was demonstrated that at least two of these sites are not direct targets of CK2 but phosphorylated by ataxia-telangiectasia mutated and Rad3-related (ATR), a kinase activated during IBV replication [54]. In any case, CK2 can be relevant since it can be indirectly stabilized by ATR [55], thus suggesting that phosphorylation of N protein is most likely a dynamic and timely regulated process during the infection cycle.

N protein of SARS-CoV is also regulated by CK2 [56,57]: it was suggested that CK2 is among the multiple kinases that, by phosphorylating SARS-CoV N protein, allow its binding to 14-3-3 proteins and its translocation to the cytoplasm. The functional consequences of this process were not elucidated, but the authors postulated that nuclear localization of the N phosphoprotein might interfere with the cellular machinery and trigger apoptosis; other hypotheses are that phosphorylation may increase the protein stability, or promote its self-association, an essential step for viral assembly, or regulate downstream signaling pathways.

N protein has also been found to be associated with CK2 in MERS and SARS-CoV-2 infection [56], thus pointing to N proteins as a general element exploited by CK2 in β-CoVs-infected cells. The multiple levels of connection between CK2 and SARS-CoV-2 will be described in detail in the following paragraph.

3. CK2 and SARS-CoV-2

SARS-CoV-2, like the other β-CoVs, exploits the ACE receptor, a CK2 substrate [45], raising the interest in CK2 as an anti-COVID-19 target. But regardless of ACE, as early as the first year of the COVID-19 pandemic, two important papers were published that directly correlated CK2 to SARS-CoV-2 infection. Gordon et al. [58] applied an affinity-purification/mass spectrometry approach to identify host proteins exploited by the virus and already targeted by existing drugs. Among the human druggable proteins that physically associate with SARS-CoV-2 proteins, they identified CK2, which was supposed to be involved in stress granule regulation. Consistently, CK2 inhibitors disrupt stress granules. All the CK2 subunits (the α (CSNK2A1) and α′ (CSNK2A2) catalytic isoforms and the β regulatory subunit (CSNK2B)) were found to bind to the N protein [56].

The global phosphorylation landscape of SARS-CoV-2 infection was also published in 2020 [59], reporting that some CK2-dependent phospho-sites (belonging to both viral and host cell proteins) are upregulated in SARS-CoV-2 infected cells. This suggested that SARS-CoV-2 would enhance CK2 activity. They found that CK2 localizes with N protein in filopodia protrusions possessing budding viral particles markedly induced by the infection. Also, employing transcriptome and computational analyses, Shaath and Alajez [60] observed activation of CK2 in Calu-3 infected cells, and Fatoki and coworkers described CK2 as one of the key players in the SARS-CoV-2 lifecycle [61]. As reviewed by Chatterjee and Thakur [36], some of the CK2-dependent phospho-sites found in SARS-CoV-2 infected cells belong to the viral M protein, but the consequences of the phosphorylation remain unknown.

SARS-CoV-2 activates several host cell kinases [36], with the final effect of complex crosstalk between different signaling pathways globally contributing to virus infection and replication. An example of great relevance for this review is the case of the PI3K/Akt pathway: it is deeply interconnected with CK2, which potentiates it by acting at several levels [62]. Since this pathway is instrumental to SARS-CoV-2 biology [63,64], CK2 also contributes to virus replication by boosting it. Another example of the intricate network by which CK2 might sustain the SARS-CoV-2 infection is the ERK1/2 and AP-1 signaling pathway (previously mentioned also for SARS-CoV), in which PAK1, an activator of this pathway and a substrate of CK2, can promote the activation of the transcription nuclear factor-κB (NF-κB) and STAT3 pathways [65]. Both NF-κB and STAT3 are CK2 substrates, involved in the induction of inflammatory cytokine expressions and polarization of M2 macrophages promoting lung fibrosis in response to SARS-CoV-2 infection, respectively [66,67]. An additional crossing point between CK2 and SARS-CoV-2 is the Wnt/β-catenin signaling pathway, which CK2 regulates [68,69] and is crucial in SARS-CoV-2 infection since the treatment of SARS-Cov-2 infected cells with iCRT14t, a specific inhibitor of Wnt/β-catenin, decreased the cytopathic effect (changes in cell morphology caused by the virus) and reduced SARS-CoV-2 N protein level [36].

The multiple levels of connections between CK2 and SARS-CoV-2 are summarized in Figure 2.

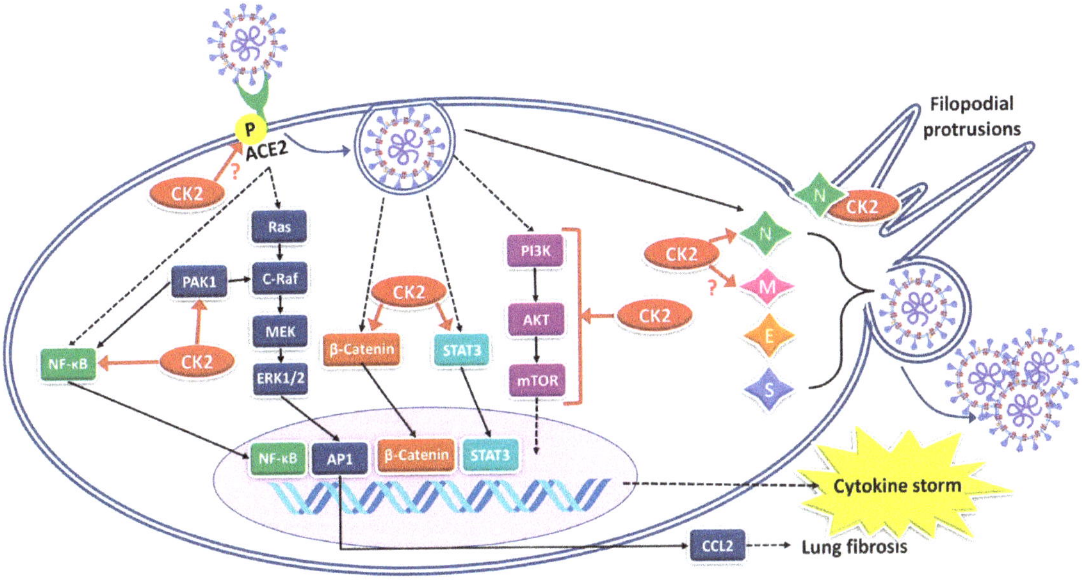

Figure 2. Different levels of CK2 involvement in SARS-CoV-2 infection. CK2 actions are indicated by the red arrows, with a question mark where data are still speculative, or the effects of the phosphorylation are not known. Dashed arrows refer to signaling pathways not defined. See the text for references.

4. CK2 Targeting as Anti-COVID-19 Strategy

The above-described involvement of CK2 in the SARS-CoV-2 biology, its druggability, and the existence of CK2 inhibitors already in human clinical trials as anticancer drugs (CX-4945 or silmitasertib (https://clinicaltrials.gov/ct2/results?cond=&term=CX-4945&cntry=&state=&city=&dist=) (accessed on 15 June 2023) and CIGB-300 (https://clinicaltrials.gov/ct2/results?cond=&term=cigb-300&cntry=&state=&city=&dist=) (accessed on 15 June 2023) have promptly sparked interest in CK2 as a possible target for COVID-19 as well, and the repurposing of the compounds.

Apart from the already quoted study on bovine coronaviruses [50], by a computational biology analysis [70], CIGB-300 has been proposed to interfere with the SARS-CoV-2 life cycle in infected human cells: it might affect the immune response to the infection and perturb the virus hijacking of RNA splicing machinery. An exploratory clinical study with CIGB-300 (now called CIGB-325) has been performed to investigate its safety and putative clinical benefit in COVID-19 patients with pneumonia [71]. Despite the small sample size (twenty patients), and the preliminary level of the study, the results were encouraging since CIGB-300 significantly reduced the median number of pulmonary lesions with mild and/or moderate adverse events.

The CX-4945 repurposing was proposed since the beginning [58] when CK2 was found to interact with SARS-CoV-2 N protein and influence stress granule regulation. CX-4945 is presently in a clinical trial for COVID-19 and coronavirus, besides cancer https://clinicaltrials.gov/ct2/show/NCT04668209?term=CX-4945&draw=2&rank=1 (accessed on 15 June 2023). Other compounds have been investigated as potential anti-COVID-19 drugs. By studying the network of genes expressed in COVID-19-infected patients, Fatoki et al. [61] tried to predict the drug compounds that could interfere with pathologic signaling pathways. They identified CK2 (along with DNA-PK) as playing a crucial role in the SARS-CoV-2 lifecycle, and, by investigating phytochemicals that could represent therapeutic modulators, suggested emodin, ellagic acid, quercetin, and others as CK2 targeting compounds. They are indeed among the already-known inhibitors of CK2 [13].

5. Conclusions

Protein phosphorylation, elicited from the host kinases, is a well-known mechanism viruses exploit for survival. SARS-CoV-2 is no exception: the viral proteins N, M, S, 3a, and 9b were phosphorylated in about 70 different sites, corresponding to the consensus sequences of several kinases. Moreover, in SARS-CoV-2 infected cells, the phosphorylation of many host cell proteins increases (more than 15,000 phosphorylation sites identified) [36,59], and, at least in part, this is achieved through the activation of host kinases induced by the virus. Despite its constitutive activity, CK2 is among the activated enzymes. This could seem counterintuitive: what is the advantage of activating a kinase that is already catalytically competent? However, while the conformation structure of CK2 perfectly explains its constitutive activity [72], this does not exclude regulation events that can further enhance the phosphorylation of its substrates [18]. Since CK2 is very pleiotropic, being responsible for up to 25% of the phosphoproteome [3], its involvement in phosphorylating substrates instrumental for the virus life cycle is not unexpected. Moreover, its peculiar consensus sequence (S/T-x-x-E/D/pX) [73] is very common and present in several virus proteins.

As the Figure 2 summarises, CK2 and SARS-CoV-2 biology signals have several connecting points. Among them, it is worth pointing out the virus receptor ACE2, which is a substrate of CK2. Although the effects of the ACE2 phosphorylation on SARS-CoV-2 infection have never been described, by similarity with what was observed in the case of SARS-CoV [46], they are expected to be essential for the receptor functions. Other crucial levels of SARS-CoV-2/CK2 integration are the several signaling pathways strongly implicated in the infection and regulated by CK2 at multiple levels, such as PI3K/Akt, NF-κB, STAT3, Wnt/β-catenin, ERK1/2, and AP-1. However, the most significant connection is probably represented by the N protein, which can physically interact with each of the CK2 subunits and stimulate its catalytic activity. Indeed, N proteins of different coronaviruses are crucial for the functions played by CK2 in the infected cells (see Figure 1). Future studies will hopefully define the N protein/CK2 interaction at the molecular level, with exciting implications for our knowledge of CK2 biology, and ideally providing hypotheses on possible interventions to regulate its activity.

Although the COVID-19 outbreak is now less scary, it is important to highlight that identifying new antiviral therapies is still desirable to face the continued virus evolution with the possible emergence of new variants. Inevitably, selective pressure can generate drug-resistant mutants: this is frequent with direct antiviral agents, while cellular proteins exploited by the virus are less likely to be circumvented by viral escape mutants [74]. Also, considering the potential emergence of new β-CoVs, a broad-spectrum drug with activity against a wide range of viruses would be advantageous to prevent rapid viral spread. In this view, data reported so far provide strong evidence for CK2 as an ideal target. The wide availability of CK2 inhibitors and the clinical level of some of them complete the rationale for considering this kinase as a valuable target.

Author Contributions: M.R. conceptualized the manuscript. C.P.Q.M. and M.R. contributed to researching the content for the review, discussing the content, and writing the review. C.P.Q.M. perceived and designed the figures. M.R. critically reviewed the manuscript. C.P.Q.M. edited the manuscript before submission. All authors have read and agreed to the published version of the manuscript.

Funding: The work performed in the Authors' laboratory was supported by Institutional Funding (DOR and SID) to MR.

Institutional Review Board Statement: Not applicable.

Informed Consent Statement: Not applicable.

Data Availability Statement: Not applicable.

Acknowledgments: The Authors thank all the members of their laboratory for the helpful discussion.

Conflicts of Interest: The authors declare no conflict of interest.

References

1. Filhol, O.; Cochet, C. Protein Kinase CK2 in Health and Disease: Cellular Functions of Protein Ki-nase CK2: A Dynamic Affair. *Cell. Mol. Life Sci. CMLS* **2009**, *66*, 1830–1839. [CrossRef] [PubMed]
2. Rodríguez, F.; Allende, C.C.; Allende, J.E. Protein Kinase Casein Kinase 2 Holoenzyme Produced Ectopi-cally in Human Cells Can Be Exported to the External Side of the Cellular Membrane. *Proc. Natl. Acad. Sci. USA* **2005**, *102*, 4718–4723. [CrossRef] [PubMed]
3. Venerando, A.; Ruzzene, M.; Pinna, L.A. Casein Kinase: The Triple Meaning of a Misnomer. *Biochem. J.* **2014**, *460*, 141–156. [CrossRef]
4. Meggio, F.; Pinna, L.A. One-Thousand-and-One Substrates of Protein Kinase CK2? *FASEB J. Off. Publ. Fed. Am. Soc. Exp. Biol.* **2003**, *17*, 349–368. [CrossRef]
5. Dominguez, I.; Degano, I.R.; Chea, K.; Cha, J.; Toselli, P.; Seldin, D.C. CK2α Is Essential for Embryonic Morphogenesis. *Mol. Cell. Biochem.* **2011**, *356*, 209–216. [CrossRef]
6. Guerra, B.; Issinger, O.G. Protein Kinase CK2 and Its Role in Cellular Proliferation, Development and Pathology. *Electrophoresis* **1999**, *20*, 391–408. [CrossRef]
7. Issinger, O.G. Casein Kinases: Pleiotropic Mediators of Cellular Regulation. *Pharmacol. Ther.* **1993**, *59*, 1–30. [CrossRef]
8. St-Denis, N.A.; Litchfield, D.W. Protein Kinase CK2 in Health and Disease: From Birth to Death: The Role of Protein Kinase CK2 in the Regulation of Cell Proliferation and Survival. *Cell. Mol. Life Sci. CMLS* **2009**, *66*, 1817–1829. [CrossRef]
9. Ruzzene, M.; Pinna, L.A. Addiction to Protein Kinase CK2: A Common Denominator of Diverse Cancer Cells? *Biochim. Biophys. Acta* **2010**, *1804*, 499–504. [CrossRef] [PubMed]
10. Firnau, M.-B.; Brieger, A. CK2 and the Hallmarks of Cancer. *Biomedicines* **2022**, *10*, 1987. [CrossRef] [PubMed]
11. Strum, S.W.; Gyenis, L.; Litchfield, D.W. CSNK2 in Cancer: Pathophysiology and Translational Applications. *Br. J. Cancer* **2022**, *126*, 994–1003. [CrossRef] [PubMed]
12. Trembley, J.H.; Kren, B.T.; Afzal, M.; Scaria, G.A.; Klein, M.A.; Ahmed, K. Protein Kinase CK2—Diverse Roles in Cancer Cell Biology and Therapeutic Promise. *Mol. Cell. Biochem.* **2022**, *478*, 899–926. [CrossRef]
13. Borgo, C.; Ruzzene, M. Protein Kinase CK2 Inhibition as a Pharmacological Strategy. In *Advances in Protein Chemistry and Structural Biology*; Academic Press: Cambridge, MA, USA, 2021.
14. Borgo, C.; Ruzzene, M. Role of Protein Kinase CK2 in Antitumor Drug Resistance. *J. Exp. Clin. Cancer Res. CR* **2019**, *38*, 287. [CrossRef] [PubMed]
15. Buontempo, F.; McCubrey, J.A.; Orsini, E.; Ruzzene, M.; Cappellini, A.; Lonetti, A.; Evangelisti, C.; Chiarini, F.; Evangelisti, C.; Barata, J.T.; et al. Therapeutic Targeting of CK2 in Acute and Chronic Leukemias. *Leukemia* **2018**, *32*, 1–10. [CrossRef]
16. Gowda, C.; Sachdev, M.; Muthusami, S.; Kapadia, M.; Petrovic-Dovat, L.; Hartman, M.; Ding, Y.; Song, C.; Payne, J.L.; Tan, B.-H.; et al. Casein Kinase II (CK2) as a Therapeutic Target for Hematological Malignancies. *Curr. Pharm. Des.* **2017**, *23*, 95–107. [CrossRef]
17. Trembley, J.H.; Chen, Z.; Unger, G.; Slaton, J.; Kren, B.T.; Van Waes, C.; Ahmed, K. Emergence of Protein Kinase CK2 as a Key Target in Cancer Therapy. *BioFactors Oxf. Engl.* **2010**, *36*, 187–195. [CrossRef] [PubMed]
18. Borgo, C.; D'Amore, C.; Cesaro, L.; Sarno, S.; Pinna, L.A.; Ruzzene, M.; Salvi, M. How Can a Traffic Light Properly Work If It Is Always Green? The Paradox of CK2 Signaling. *Crit. Rev. Biochem. Mol. Biol.* **2021**, *56*, 321–359. [CrossRef]
19. Roffey, S.E.; Litchfield, D.W. CK2 Regulation: Perspectives in 2021. *Biomedicines* **2021**, *9*, 1361. [CrossRef]
20. Pinna, L.A. Protein Kinase CK2: A Challenge to Canons. *J. Cell Sci.* **2002**, *115*, 3873–3878. [CrossRef]
21. Litchfield, D.W.; Bosc, D.G.; Canton, D.A.; Saulnier, R.B.; Vilk, G.; Zhang, C. Functional Specialization of CK2 Isoforms and Characterization of Isoform-Specific Binding Partners. *Mol. Cell. Biochem.* **2001**, *227*, 21–29. [CrossRef]
22. Borgo, C.; D'Amore, C.; Sarno, S.; Salvi, M.; Ruzzene, M. Protein Kinase CK2: A Potential Therapeutic Target for Diverse Human Diseases. *Signal Transduct. Target. Ther.* **2021**, *6*, 183. [CrossRef]
23. ole-MoiYoi, O.K. Casein Kinase II in Theileriosis. *Science* **1995**, *267*, 834–836. [CrossRef] [PubMed]
24. Ortega, C.E.; Seidner, Y.; Dominguez, I. Mining CK2 in Cancer. *PLoS ONE* **2014**, *9*, e115609. [CrossRef]
25. Chua, M.M.J.; Lee, M.; Dominguez, I. Cancer-Type Dependent Expression of CK2 Transcripts. *PLoS ONE* **2017**, *12*, e0188854. [CrossRef]
26. Hong, H.; Benveniste, E.N. The Immune Regulatory Role of Protein Kinase CK2 and Its Implications for Treatment of Cancer. *Biomedicines* **2021**, *9*, 1932. [CrossRef] [PubMed]
27. Ampofo, E.; Nalbach, L.; Menger, M.D.; Montenarh, M.; Götz, C. Protein Kinase CK2-A Putative Target for the Therapy of Diabetes Mellitus? *Int. J. Mol. Sci.* **2019**, *20*, 4398. [CrossRef] [PubMed]
28. Ljubimov, A.V.; Caballero, S.; Aoki, A.M.; Pinna, L.A.; Grant, M.B.; Castellon, R. Involvement of Protein Kinase CK2 in Angiogenesis and Retinal Neovascularization. *Investig. Ophthalmol. Vis. Sci.* **2004**, *45*, 4583–4591. [CrossRef]

29. Morooka, S.; Hoshina, M.; Kii, I.; Okabe, T.; Kojima, H.; Inoue, N.; Okuno, Y.; Denawa, M.; Yoshida, S.; Fukuhara, J.; et al. Identification of a Dual Inhibitor of SRPK1 and CK2 That Attenuates Pathological Angiogenesis of Macular Degeneration in Mice. *Mol. Pharmacol.* **2015**, *88*, 316–325. [CrossRef]
30. Hauck, L.; Harms, C.; An, J.; Rohne, J.; Gertz, K.; Dietz, R.; Endres, M.; von Harsdorf, R. Protein Kinase CK2 Links Extracellular Growth Factor Signaling with the Control of P27 Kip1 Stability in the Heart. *Nat. Med.* **2008**, *14*, 315–324. [CrossRef]
31. Wadey, K.S.; Brown, B.A.; Sala-Newby, G.B.; Jayaraman, P.-S.; Gaston, K.; George, S.J. Protein Kinase CK2 Inhibition Suppresses Neointima Formation via a Proline-Rich Homeodomain-Dependent Mechanism. *Vascul. Pharmacol.* **2017**, *99*, 34–44. [CrossRef]
32. Zhou, H.; Zhu, P.; Wang, J.; Zhu, H.; Ren, J.; Chen, Y. Pathogenesis of Cardiac Ischemia-Reperfusion Injury Is Associated with CK2α-Disturbed Mitochondrial Homeostasis via Suppression of FUNDC1-Related Mitophagy. *Cell Death Differ.* **2018**, *25*, 1080–1093. [CrossRef] [PubMed]
33. Castello, J.; Ragnauth, A.; Friedman, E.; Rebholz, H. CK2-An Emerging Target for Neurological and Psychiatric Disorders. *Pharmaceuticals* **2017**, *10*, 7. [CrossRef]
34. Mehta, A. Cystic Fibrosis as a Bowel Cancer Syndrome, and the Potential Role of CK2. *Mol. Cell. Biochem.* **2008**, *316*, 169–175. [CrossRef]
35. Ballardin, D.; Cruz-Gamero, J.M.; Bienvenu, T.; Rebholz, H. Comparing Two Neurodevelopmental Disorders Linked to CK2: Okur-Chung Neurodevelopmental Syndrome and Poirier-Bienvenu Neurodevelopmental Syndrome-Two Sides of the Same Coin? *Front. Mol. Biosci.* **2022**, *9*, 850559. [CrossRef]
36. Chatterjee, B.; Thakur, S.S. SARS-CoV-2 Infection Triggers Phosphorylation: Potential Target for Anti-COVID-19 Therapeutics. *Front. Immunol.* **2022**, *13*, 829474. [CrossRef]
37. Gottardo, M.F.; Capobianco, C.S.; Sidabra, J.E.; Garona, J.; Perera, Y.; Perea, S.E.; Alonso, D.F.; Farina, H.G. Preclinical Efficacy of CIGB-300, an Anti-CK2 Peptide, on Breast Cancer Metastasic Colonization. *Sci. Rep.* **2020**, *10*, 14689. [CrossRef] [PubMed]
38. Perea, S.E.; Reyes, O.; Baladron, I.; Perera, Y.; Farina, H.; Gil, J.; Rodriguez, A.; Bacardi, D.; Marcelo, J.L.; Cosme, K.; et al. CIGB-300, a Novel Proapoptotic Peptide That Impairs the CK2 Phosphorylation and Exhibits Anticancer Properties Both in Vitro and Vivo. *Mol. Cell. Biochem.* **2008**, *316*, 163–167. [CrossRef]
39. Montenarh, M.; Grässer, F.A.; Götz, C. Protein Kinase CK2 and Epstein-Barr Virus. *Biomedicines* **2023**, *11*, 358. [CrossRef] [PubMed]
40. Duncan, J.S.; Turowec, J.P.; Vilk, G.; Li, S.S.C.; Gloor, G.B.; Litchfield, D.W. Regulation of Cell Proliferation and Survival: Convergence of Protein Kinases and Caspases. *Biochim. Biophys. Acta* **2010**, *1804*, 505–510. [CrossRef]
41. Majerciak, V.; Pripuzova, N.; Chan, C.; Temkin, N.; Specht, S.I.; Zheng, Z.-M. The Stability of Structured Kaposi's Sarcoma-Associated Herpesvirus ORF57 Protein Is Regulated by Protein Phosphorylation and Homodimerization. *J. Virol.* **2015**, *89*, 3256–3274. [CrossRef]
42. Piirsoo, A.; Piirsoo, M.; Kala, M.; Sankovski, E.; Lototskaja, E.; Levin, V.; Salvi, M.; Ustav, M. Activity of CK2alpha Protein Kinase Is Required for Efficient Replication of Some HPV Types. *PLoS Pathog.* **2019**, *15*, e1007788. [CrossRef]
43. Du, M.; Liu, J.; Chen, X.; Xie, Y.; Yuan, C.; Xiang, Y.; Sun, B.; Lan, K.; Chen, M.; James, S.J.; et al. Casein Kinase II Controls TBK1/IRF3 Activation in IFN Response against Viral Infection. *J. Immunol.* **2015**, *194*, 4477–4488. [CrossRef]
44. Sun, Z.; Ren, H.; Liu, Y.; Teeling, J.L.; Gu, J. Phosphorylation of RIG-I by Casein Kinase II Inhibits Its Antiviral Response. *J. Virol.* **2011**, *85*, 1036–1047. [CrossRef]
45. Kohlstedt, K.; Shoghi, F.; Müller-Esterl, W.; Busse, R.; Fleming, I. CK2 Phosphorylates the Angiotensin-Converting Enzyme and Regulates Its Retention in the Endothelial Cell Plasma Membrane. *Circ. Res.* **2002**, *91*, 749–756. [CrossRef] [PubMed]
46. Chen, I.-Y.; Chang, S.C.; Wu, H.-Y.; Yu, T.-C.; Wei, W.-C.; Lin, S.; Chien, C.-L.; Chang, M.-F. Upregulation of the Chemokine (C-C Motif) Ligand 2 via a Severe Acute Respiratory Syndrome Coronavirus Spike-ACE2 Signaling Pathway. *J. Virol.* **2010**, *84*, 7703–7712. [CrossRef] [PubMed]
47. Yang, X.; Dickmander, R.J.; Bayati, A.; Taft-Benz, S.A.; Smith, J.L.; Wells, C.I.; Madden, E.A.; Brown, J.W.; Lenarcic, E.M.; Yount, B.L.; et al. Host Kinase CSNK2 Is a Target for Inhibition of Pathogenic SARS-like β-Coronaviruses. *ACS Chem. Biol.* **2022**, *17*, 1937–1950. [CrossRef] [PubMed]
48. Lan, J.; Ge, J.; Yu, J.; Shan, S.; Zhou, H.; Fan, S.; Zhang, Q.; Shi, X.; Wang, Q.; Zhang, L.; et al. Structure of the SARS-CoV-2 Spike Receptor-Binding Domain Bound to the ACE2 Receptor. *Nature* **2020**, *581*, 215–220. [CrossRef]
49. Burkard, C.; Verheije, M.H.; Wicht, O.; van Kasteren, S.I.; van Kuppeveld, F.J.; Haagmans, B.L.; Pelkmans, L.; Rottier, P.J.M.; Bosch, B.J.; Haan, C.A.M. de Coronavirus Cell Entry Occurs through the Endo-/Lysosomal Pathway in a Proteolysis-Dependent Manner. *PLoS Pathog.* **2014**, *10*, e1004502. [CrossRef]
50. Ramón, A.C.; Pérez, G.V.; Caballero, E.; Rosales, M.; Aguilar, D.; Vázquez-Blomquist, D.; Ramos, Y.; Rodríguez-Ulloa, A.; Falcón, V.; Rodríguez-Moltó, M.P.; et al. Targeting of Protein Kinase CK2 Elicits Antiviral Activity on Bovine Coronavirus Infection. *Viruses* **2022**, *14*, 552. [CrossRef]
51. Perea, S.E.; Reyes, O.; Puchades, Y.; Mendoza, O.; Vispo, N.S.; Torrens, I.; Santos, A.; Silva, R.; Acevedo, B.; López, E.; et al. Antitumor Effect of a Novel Proapoptotic Peptide That Impairs the Phosphorylation by the Protein Kinase 2 (Casein Kinase 2). *Cancer Res.* **2004**, *64*, 7127–7129. [CrossRef]
52. Vlasova, A.N.; Saif, L.J. Bovine Coronavirus and the Associated Diseases. *Front. Vet. Sci.* **2021**, *8*, 643220. [CrossRef] [PubMed]
53. Chen, H.; Gill, A.; Dove, B.K.; Emmett, S.R.; Kemp, C.F.; Ritchie, M.A.; Dee, M.; Hiscox, J.A. Mass Spectroscopic Characterization of the Coronavirus Infectious Bronchitis Virus Nucleoprotein and Elucidation of the Role of Phosphorylation in RNA Binding by Using Surface Plasmon Resonance. *J. Virol.* **2005**, *79*, 1164–1179. [CrossRef] [PubMed]

54. Fang, S.; Xu, L.; Huang, M.; Qisheng Li, F.; Liu, D.X. Identification of Two ATR-Dependent Phosphorylation Sites on Coronavirus Nucleocapsid Protein with Nonessential Functions in Viral Replication and Infectivity in Cultured Cells. *Virology* **2013**, *444*, 225–232. [CrossRef] [PubMed]
55. Martin, S.A.; Ouchi, T. Cellular Commitment to Reentry into the Cell Cycle after Stalled DNA Is Determined by Site-Specific Phosphorylation of Chk1 and PTEN. *Mol. Cancer Ther.* **2008**, *7*, 2509–2516. [CrossRef]
56. Gordon, D.E.; Hiatt, J.; Bouhaddou, M.; Rezelj, V.V.; Ulferts, S.; Braberg, H.; Jureka, A.S.; Obernier, K.; Guo, J.Z.; Batra, J.; et al. Comparative Host-Coronavirus Protein Interaction Networks Reveal Pan-Viral Disease Mechanisms. *Science* **2020**, *370*, eabe9403. [CrossRef]
57. Surjit, M.; Kumar, R.; Mishra, R.N.; Reddy, M.K.; Chow, V.T.K.; Lal, S.K. The Severe Acute Respiratory Syndrome Coronavirus Nucleocapsid Protein Is Phosphorylated and Localizes in the Cytoplasm by 14-3-3-Mediated Translocation. *J. Virol.* **2005**, *79*, 11476–11486. [CrossRef]
58. Gordon, D.E.; Jang, G.M.; Bouhaddou, M.; Xu, J.; Obernier, K.; White, K.M.; O'Meara, M.J.; Rezelj, V.V.; Guo, J.Z.; Swaney, D.L.; et al. A SARS-CoV-2 Protein Interaction Map Reveals Targets for Drug Repurposing. *Nature* **2020**, *583*, 459–468. [CrossRef] [PubMed]
59. Bouhaddou, M.; Memon, D.; Meyer, B.; White, K.M.; Rezelj, V.V.; Correa Marrero, M.; Polacco, B.J.; Melnyk, J.E.; Ulferts, S.; Kaake, R.M.; et al. The Global Phosphorylation Landscape of SARS-CoV-2 Infection. *Cell* **2020**, *182*, 685–712.e19. [CrossRef]
60. Shaath, H.; Alajez, N.M. Computational and Transcriptome Analyses Revealed Preferential Induction of Chemotaxis and Lipid Synthesis by SARS-CoV-2. *Biology* **2020**, *9*, 260. [CrossRef]
61. Fatoki, T.H.; Ibraheem, O.; Ogunyemi, I.O.; Akinmoladun, A.C.; Ugboko, H.U.; Adeseko, C.J.; Awofisayo, O.A.; Olusegun, S.J.; Enibukun, J.M. Network Analysis, Sequence and Structure Dynamics of Key Proteins of Coronavirus and Human Host, and Molecular Docking of Selected Phytochemicals of Nine Medicinal Plants. *J. Biomol. Struct. Dyn.* **2020**, *39*, 6195–6217. [CrossRef]
62. Ruzzene, M.; Bertacchini, J.; Toker, A.; Marmiroli, S. Cross-Talk between the CK2 and AKT Signaling Pathways in Cancer. *Adv. Biol. Regul.* **2017**, *64*, 1–8. [CrossRef]
63. Basile, M.S.; Cavalli, E.; McCubrey, J.; Hernández-Bello, J.; Muñoz-Valle, J.F.; Fagone, P.; Nicoletti, F. The PI3K/Akt/mTOR Pathway: A Potential Pharmacological Target in COVID-19. *Drug Discov. Today* **2022**, *27*, 848–856. [CrossRef] [PubMed]
64. Klann, K.; Bojkova, D.; Tascher, G.; Ciesek, S.; Münch, C.; Cinatl, J. Growth Factor Receptor Signaling Inhibition Prevents SARS-CoV-2 Replication. *Mol. Cell* **2020**, *80*, 164–174.e4. [CrossRef] [PubMed]
65. Berretta, A.A.; Silveira, M.A.D.; Cóndor Captcha, J.M.; De Jong, D. Propolis and Its Potential against SARS-CoV-2 Infection Mechanisms and COVID-19 Disease: Running Title: Propolis against SARS-CoV-2 Infection and COVID-19. *Biomed. Pharmacother.* **2020**, *131*, 110622. [CrossRef]
66. Su, C.-M.; Wang, L.; Yoo, D. Activation of NF-KB and Induction of Proinflammatory Cytokines Expressions Mediated by ORF7a Protein of SARS-CoV-2. *Sci. Rep.* **2021**, *11*, 13464. [CrossRef] [PubMed]
67. Jafarzadeh, A.; Nemati, M.; Jafarzadeh, S. Contribution of STAT3 to the Pathogenesis of COVID-19. *Microb. Pathog.* **2021**, *154*, 104836. [CrossRef]
68. Ponce, D.P.; Yefi, R.; Cabello, P.; Maturana, J.L.; Niechi, I.; Silva, E.; Galindo, M.; Antonelli, M.; Marcelain, K.; Armisen, R.; et al. CK2 Functionally Interacts with AKT/PKB to Promote the β-Catenin-Dependent Expression of Survivin and Enhance Cell Survival. *Mol. Cell. Biochem.* **2011**, *356*, 127–132. [CrossRef] [PubMed]
69. Song, D.H.; Sussman, D.J.; Seldin, D.C. Endogenous Protein Kinase CK2 Participates in Wnt Signaling in Mammary Epithelial Cells. *J. Biol. Chem.* **2000**, *275*, 23790–23797. [CrossRef]
70. Miranda, J.; Bringas, R.; Fernandez-de-Cossio, J.; Perera-Negrin, Y. Targeting CK2 Mediated Signaling to Impair/Tackle SARS-CoV-2 Infection: A Computational Biology Approach. *Mol. Med.* **2021**, *27*, 161. [CrossRef]
71. Cruz, L.R.; Baladrón, I.; Rittoles, A.; Díaz, P.A.; Valenzuela, C.; Santana, R.; Vázquez, M.M.; García, A.; Chacón, D.; Thompson, D.; et al. Treatment with an Anti-CK2 Synthetic Peptide Improves Clinical Response in COVID-19 Patients with Pneumonia. A Randomized and Controlled Clinical Trial. *ACS Pharmacol. Transl. Sci.* **2021**, *4*, 206–212. [CrossRef]
72. Niefind, K.; Guerra, B.; Ermakowa, I.; Issinger, O.G. Crystal Structure of Human Protein Kinase CK2: Insights into Basic Properties of the CK2 Holoenzyme. *EMBO J.* **2001**, *20*, 5320–5331. [CrossRef] [PubMed]
73. Meggio, F.; Marin, O.; Pinna, L.A. Substrate Specificity of Protein Kinase CK2. *Cell. Mol. Biol. Res.* **1994**, *40*, 401–409. [PubMed]
74. Chitalia, V.C.; Munawar, A.H. A Painful Lesson from the COVID-19 Pandemic: The Need for Broad-Spectrum, Host-Directed Antivirals. *J. Transl. Med.* **2020**, *18*, 390. [CrossRef] [PubMed]

kinases and phosphatases

MDPI

Review

Exploring Protein Kinase CK2 Substrate Recognition and the Dynamic Response of Substrate Phosphorylation to Kinase Modulation

Luca Cesaro [1], Angelica Maria Zuliani [1], Valentina Bosello Travain [2] and Mauro Salvi [1,*]

1 Department of Biomedical Sciences, University of Padova, 35131 Padova, Italy
2 Department of Molecular Medicine, University of Padova, 35131 Padova, Italy
* Correspondence: mauro.salvi@unipd.it

Abstract: Protein kinase CK2 (formerly known as casein kinase 2 or II), a ubiquitous and constitutively active enzyme, is widely recognized as one of the most pleiotropic serine/threonine kinases. It plays a critical role in numerous signaling pathways, with hundreds of bona fide substrates. However, despite considerable research efforts, our understanding of the entire CK2 substratome and its functional associations with the majority of these substrates is far from being completely deciphered. In this context, we aim to provide an overview of how CK2 recognizes its substrates. We will discuss the pros and cons of the existing methods to manipulate CK2 activity in cells, as well as exploring the dynamic response of substrate phosphorylation to CK2 modulation.

Keywords: protein kinase CK2; casein kinase 2; protein phosphorylation; kinase consensus sequence; kinase inhibitors; kinase activity

1. Introduction

PhosphoSitePlus, the most up-to-date and most comprehensive database of post-translational modifications, collects nearly 300,000 non-redundant Ser/Thr/Tyr phosphosites [1]. The majority of these phosphosites have been identified by large-scale mass spectrometry analysis, but the kinases responsible for their generation have been determined only for a few of them. Protein kinase CK2 is one of the most pleiotropic kinases (767 human bona fide phosphosite substrates identified to date according to the PhosphoSitePlus database—https://www.phosphosite.org, accessed on 1 May 2023). CK2's ubiquity and constitutive activity contribute to its versatility, allowing it to participate in a wide range of cellular signaling events [2–9]. Consequently, CK2 has attracted significant attention as a potential therapeutic target for various human pathologies [10–20]. In a previous study, we proposed that CK2 might be responsible for generating at least 20% of the total human phosphoproteome [21]. However, it is important to acknowledge that this percentage may have been overestimated due to the promiscuity of the CK2 consensus sequence, which may affect the accuracy of substrate prediction [22]. Nevertheless, it is widely recognized that a significant number of CK2 substrates remain unidentified, highlighting the fact that our understanding of CK2 functions is still incomplete.

CK2 is the acronym for casein kinase to denote its ability to efficiently phosphorylate casein in vitro, but the true physiological kinase has been lately identified as Fam20C, the kinase responsible for generating the majority of Ser/Thr phosphosites in secreted proteins [23,24]. The term CK2 does not refer to a single enzyme but rather to a heterotetrameric complex composed of two catalytic subunits (α and/or α') and two regulatory subunits (β). The two catalytic subunits α and α' (encoded by the two different genes, *CSNK2A1* and *CSNK2A2*, respectively) may differ in tissue distribution but share a high structural homology. These two isoforms share approximately 90% identity within their catalytic domains differing mainly in the C-terminal domain. However, there is evidence that in addition to the tetrameric form, CK2 can also exist as monomeric catalytic enzymes and regulatory proteins. Crystallographic analysis and cell experiments have suggested that CK2 complex formation is a dynamic process, allowing for the presence of both tetrameric and monomeric forms [25,26]. Furthermore, the expression levels of CK2 subunits may not always be balanced [27–29], further supporting the existence of monomeric CK2 catalytic and regulatory subunits. In addition, it has been proposed that the CK2β regulatory subunit may have CK2-independent functions by acting as a partner of other kinases, potentially contributing to diverse signaling pathways beyond CK2-mediated phosphorylation [30,31].

2. CK2 Consensus Sequence

The recognition mechanism by which kinases identify their substrates has been extensively examined and discussed in previous reviews [32–34]. Briefly, successful phosphorylation depends on some key factors. First, the kinase and its substrate must come into contact, which is only possible if they share the same subcellular localization. In addition, the proximity of kinase and substrate can be facilitated by kinase docking motifs outside the catalytic domain functioning by tethering enzyme and substrate. Secondly, the target site on the substrate must interact with the catalytic domain of the kinase. This interaction requires the presence of specific determinants surrounding the target site, which vary depending on the structural characteristics of the catalytic fold. These specific determinants are commonly referred to as "kinase consensus sequences". Recent research has shown that approximately 60% of the Ser/Thr kinases can be classified into three distinct motif classes: proline-directed (requiring a Pro in the +1 position), basophilic and acidophilic kinases [35]. The importance of specific determinants surrounding the target site varies between different kinases, with serine/threonine kinases placing greater emphasis on these determinants compared to tyrosine kinases. Indeed, for tyrosine kinases the presence of docking sites that facilitate proximity between the substrate and the kinase is generally considered to be the most critical factor [36].

How does CK2 recognize its substrates? CK2 localizes in a variety of subcellular compartments, including the nucleus, cytosol, and plasma membrane. The two β-regulatory subunits present in the tetrameric CK2 complex play an important role in substrate recruitment and phosphorylation. As the catalytic subunits of CK2 are constitutively active, as mentioned above, the β-subunits do not function to switch the activity on/off. Instead, the primary function of the β-subunits is to act as a docking protein, facilitating the interaction between the kinase and its substrate [37]. Based on the dependence on the β-subunit, a classification of CK2 substrates as β-dependent or β-independent has been proposed [38]. For example, the downregulation or knockout of the β-subunit is sufficient to completely inhibit the endogenous phosphorylation of S129 Akt and a wide range of other CK2 substrates [39].

CK2 is widely recognized as an acidophilic kinase, indicating a preference for phosphorylation sites surrounded by acidic residues at both the N- and C-termini. The crystal structure of protein kinase CK2α shown in Figure 1A highlights its substrate-binding region, which is characterized by a positively charged electrostatic surface (blue zone). Interestingly, the presence of a proline residue in the +1 position, typically associated with proline-directed kinases, inhibits CK2 activity [33]. In general, a detailed analysis of the kinase consensus sequence can be obtained by analyzing the phosphorylation sites of a peptide library or, better still, by analyzing the bona fide substrates of the kinase once a sufficient number has been identified. In the case of CK2, 767 substrates have been identified in humans according to the PhosphoSitePlus database (https://www.phosphosite.org, accessed on 1 May 2023). Online tools such as WebLogo [40] or Two-Sample Logo [41] can help analyze the primary structure of peptide substrates and identify the most recurrent residues around the target amino acid. These tools are graphical representations of an amino acid multiple sequence alignment that provide an informative representation of sequence motifs, where the height of the stack represents the degree of sequence conservation, and the height of the individual residue within the stack represents its relative frequency at that position. The Weblogo analysis of CK2 phosphosites presented in Figure 1B is the graphical representation of the amino acids surrounding 767 CK2 phosphorylation sites. A closer examination of the selected frame (+7, −7) reveals that acidic residues are favored at all positions, with particular significance at position +3 (69% of substrates containing it) and at position +1 (51% of substrates containing it), confirming the general CK2 consensus sequence as S/T[E/D]x[E/D]. The CK2 substrate logo generated in 2009 [21] with a lower number of substrates (433) shows significant similarity to the logo generated in this study. In fact, the most frequent residues are the same in all positions between −7 and +7 in the two logos. This similarity suggests that the identified sequence motifs and conservation patterns are robust and consistent, and the generated logo represents the definitive fingerprint of the CK2 kinase. How useful are these considerations? In our work from 2009 [21], by analyzing the entire human phosphoproteome we assigned a certain number of substrates to CK2 only according to this CK2 fingerprint. We also demonstrated in vitro and, in some cases, in cell phosphorylation by CK2 for some of these putative substrates, confirming the reliability of the approach. Based on this observation, we proposed that approximately 20% of the phosphoproteome could be attributed to CK2 [21]. However, a more recent analysis suggests that a significative proportion of the phosphopeptides that have the CK2 consensus sequence also have consensus sequences for other kinases, suggesting that these sites could be phosphorylated by multiple kinases or by kinases other than CK2, thus revising the conclusion of our previous analysis [22].

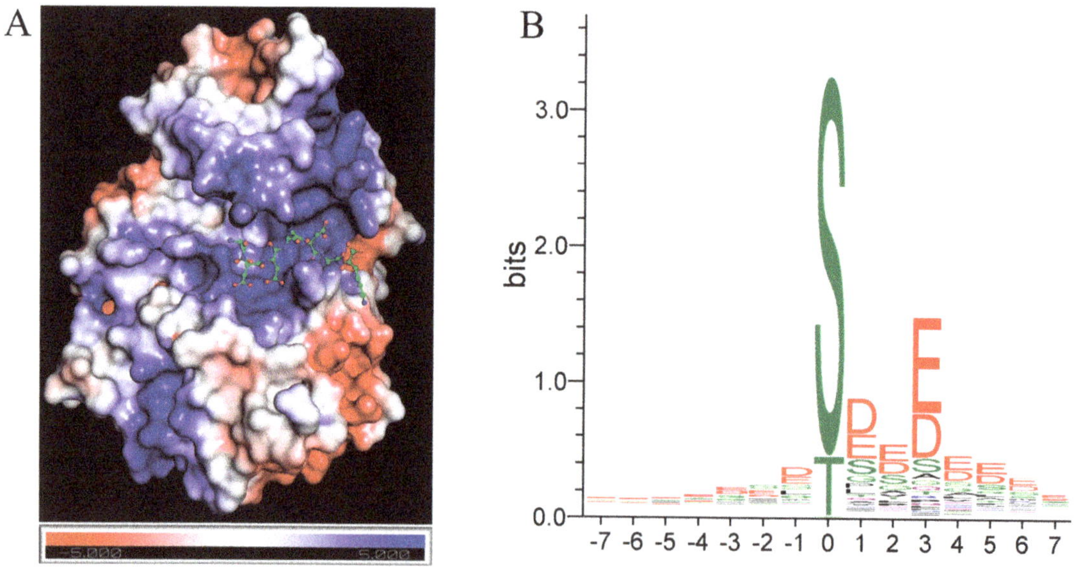

Figure 1. CK2 substrate recognition. (**A**) Electrostatic potential mapped onto the molecular surface of CK2α (PDB ID: 6SPW) and the binding of a peptide substrate (D_6K derived from ARC3140 inhibitor). The image was generated with PyMol 2.5 Software (Schrodinger, LLC., New York, NY, USA). The electrostatic surface has been calculated with APBS [42]. (**B**) Web logo analysis of CK2-validated phosphosites. A total of 767 non-redundant phosphosites have been collected from the PhosphoSitePlus database (https://www.phosphosite.org, accessed on 1 May 2023) and analyzed. Weblogo was generated using WebLogo 3: Public Beta.

Despite this, the identification of the CK2 consensus sequence in a substrate remains the first approach to understanding whether a site could be a direct substrate of CK2.

3. Is a Phosphopeptide Containing the CK2 Consensus Sequence a True CK2 Substrate?

While the consensus sequence is important for substrate recognition by CK2, experimental verification of CK2 phosphorylation is necessary. The first step in verifying direct CK2 phosphorylation of a substrate is to perform in vitro phosphorylation. In vitro phosphorylation is usually performed with the single recombinant catalytic subunit. However, the outcome of in vitro phosphorylation could differ in the presence or absence of the regulatory CK2β subunits, which play an important role in facilitating the correct binding of the substrate to the catalytic domain. The requirement for the β-subunit is not universal and previous studies have classified CK2 substrates into β-dependent and β-independent categories based on their reliance on CK2β for efficient phosphorylation (see [38] for details).

Identifying CK2 as the kinase responsible for phosphorylating a specific site on a protein in the cell and understanding the functional significance of this phosphorylation event require the ability to detect the phosphorylation site and assess the changes following manipulation of CK2 activity in the cell. The assessment of site-specific phosphorylation in a protein in cells typically requires the development of specific tools. One potential approach to detecting and quantifying the phosphorylation state of the protein is to generate phosphospecific antibodies that specifically recognize and bind to the phosphorylated site of interest for use in immunoblotting and/or immunofluorescence. Another method involves the use of Phos-tag, a chemical compound that binds selectively to phosphorylated residues and can be incorporated into polyacrylamide gels allowing the visualization of the phosphorylation states of a protein by Western blotting [43], the reliability of which, however, appears to be substrate-specific. In some cases, radioactive orthophosphate incorporation or phosphostaining molecules such as ProQdiamond [44] can be used to study the changes in phosphorylation of the whole protein after immunoprecipitation and Western blotting. In addition to these approaches, mass spectrometry plays a crucial role in the identification and quantification of phosphorylation sites in a single protein or in whole-cell lysate after phosphosite enrichment [45]. However, a comprehensive discussion of these techniques and their applications is beyond the scope of this review.

Here, we will describe and critically discuss the methods available to modulate the activity of protein kinase CK2 in the cell.

4. CK2 Knockdown, Knockout and Inhibition: Advantages and Disadvantages

Modulating CK2 activity in cells is crucial to establish the link between CK2 and the regulation of physiological functions of a target protein. Transient overexpression of the catalytic or regulatory subunits is readily achievable, subject to limitations in transfection efficiency that depend on the cell line. However, as CK2 is constitutively active [37], reducing its activity is likely to be the most effective approach to identify the functional consequences of protein phosphorylation. Furthermore, although transient kinase overexpression provides some information, it can be misleading as it generally results in the expression of a large amount of kinases, which may be mislocalized and phosphorylate substrates that are not typically phosphorylated at physiological levels.

Two different and complementary approaches can be used to reduce kinase activity: inhibition of the catalytic activity or knockdown/knockout of the protein kinase expression. Although both lead to a reduction in total kinase activity in the cell, these approaches are not equivalent and can give different results, as in the second case kinase-independent effects are still possible due to the binding interactions of the inactive kinase.

Inhibition of CK2 using small chemical molecules is the simplest and most efficient method of reducing CK2 activity in cells. Several inhibitors targeting CK2 have been identified over the years and Table 1 lists the most important compounds with their K_i/IC_{50} (for a comprehensive list of CK2 inhibitors please refer to [46,47]). The most commonly used inhibitors in the past, such as 4,5,6,7-tetrabromobenzotriazole (TBB) or 2-dimethylamino-4,5,6,7-tetrabromo-benzimidazole (DMAT), exhibited numerous off-target effects and have largely been discarded. The discovery of CX-4945 [48] (also known as Silmitasertib) has represented a breakthrough for its potency and specificity compared to previous molecules and has until recently been considered the inhibitor of choice for targeting CK2 in cells. However, over the years it has been shown that this molecule also inhibits other kinases with high potency including PIM-1 [49], GSK3β [50] and DYRK1A [50,51]. It is also worth mentioning other off-target effects of CX4945: it acts as a splicing regulator [52] and as an inducer of methuosis [53,54], which are two phenomena independent of CK2 activity.

Table 1. Most commonly used CK2 inhibitors. For a comprehensive list of CK2 inhibitors please refer to [46,47].

	ATP-Competitive Inhibitors	K_i or IC_{50}	References
Polyhalogenated benzimidazole and benzotriazole derivates	**DRB**	K_i = 23 μM	[55]
	TBB	IC_{50} = 1.6 μM	[56]
	TDB	IC_{50} = 0.032 μM	[57]
	TBI	IC_{50} = 0.5 μM	[58]
	DMAT	IC_{50} = 0.14 μM	[58]
Flavonoids	**Quercetin**	IC_{50} = 0.55 μM	[59]
	Apigenin	IC_{50} = 0.8 μM	[59]
	Fisetin	IC_{50} = 0.35 μM	[59]
Coumarins	**Ellagic acid**	IC_{50} = 40 nM	[60]
Antraquinones	**Emodin**	K_i = 1.85 μM	[61]
	MNX	K_i = 0.8 μM	[62]
	MNA	K_i = 0.78 μM	[62]
	Quinalizarin	K_i = 0.06 μM	[63]
Pyrazolo[1,5-a]pyrimidine derivatives	**SGC-CK2-1**	IC_{50} = 36 nM (CK2α) IC_{50} = 16 nM (CK2α′)	[64]
Carboxyl acid derivatives	**IQA**	IC_{50} = 0.39 μM	[65]
	TBCA	IC_{50} = 110 nM	[66]
	CX-5011	IC_{50} = 2.3 nM	[67]
	CX-4945	IC_{50} = 1 nM	[48]
Other compounds	**GO289**	IC_{50} = 7 nM	[68]

Recently, new specific CK2 inhibitors have been developed, such as GO289 [68] and SGC-CK2-1 [64]. The latter is the most specific CK2 inhibitor to date and the compound of choice for dissecting the cellular functions of CK2. The superior efficacy of SGC-CK2-1 compared to CX4945 has been highlighted in a recent comparative phosphoproteomic analysis [69]. However, it should be emphasized that no inhibitor is completely free of off-target effects. Therefore, the use of at least two different structurally unrelated inhibitors is always recommended [70]. The use of the two inhibitors CX-4945 and GO289, in addition to SGC-CK2-1, seems to be one of the best options. These three inhibitors are structurally unrelated (see structure in Figure 2A), and even if they bind to the same regions of CK2 (the catalytic pocket), they interact with different residues (Figure 2A). Another general consideration supporting the use of different inhibitors is that despite their in vitro efficacy, the inhibitors may have different subcellular distributions, preferentially affecting specific pools of the kinase (see, for example, the recent study in ref. [71]), suggesting that the potency of each inhibitor may differ depending on the type of substrate.

How do we know when treatment with a small molecule inhibitor has reached its effect in the cell? Determining the endpoint of small molecule inhibitor treatment depends on the desired outcome, such as inhibition efficiency of kinase activity or downstream signaling events.

The degree of CK2 inhibition can be measured by incubating the cell lysate with radioactive ATP and a specific peptide substrate (such as R3AD2SD5, which is phosphorylated by both the tetrameric and monomeric forms of CK2 [72]) or a protein substrate (such as casein). This assay has also been used for non-covalent inhibitors demonstrating the persistence of inhibition in diluted cell extracts [73]. However, a successful inhibition of most of the kinase's activity in cells does not necessarily reflect an immediate effect on the phosphorylation of specific substrates. Indeed, it should be emphasized that CK2 is a constitutively active kinase [37] and its signaling involves both phosphorylation and dephosphorylation events. The dephosphorylation rate at a given phosphosite is not constant. Some phosphosites may have a rapid turnover, while others may have a longer half-life, resulting in variable rates of dephosphorylation when CK2 activity is reduced.

In addition, different phosphosites may respond differently to the same level of CK2 inhibition. Some phosphosites may be more sensitive to changes in CK2 activity, while others may require a stronger inhibition. For example, in lymphoblastic cells, treatment with the CK2 inhibitor CX-5011 can lead to a more pronounced dephosphorylation of pS129Akt compared to pS13 Cdc37 [74]. Furthermore, the same concentration of a CK2 inhibitor, CX-4945 or GO289, can differentially affect the phosphorylation of CK2 substrates in C2C12 cells, as demonstrated using an antibody specific for p-CK2 substrates [75]. Similarly, in genetically engineered C2C12 cells with less than 10% of total CK2 activity [76, 77], the phosphorylation of S529 NF-kBp65 and S129 Akt is reduced to a much greater extent than the phosphorylation of pS13 Cdc37 [78]. This phenomenon is further illustrated in Figure 2B,C, which display a similar scenario in human bronchial 16-HBE cells that were treated with increasing doses of the CK2 inhibitor SGC-CK2-1 (Figure 2B). p-S129 Akt, disappears completely at the lower concentration of the inhibitor, whereas S13 Cdc-37 phosphorylation [79] is more resistant to CK2 inhibition exhibiting a dose-dependent response. This observation can also be applied to other substrates. Indeed, it is possible to detect phosphosites that display different responses to the same concentration of CK2 inhibitor by using a mixture of phospho-CK2 substrate-specific antibodies that recognize endogenous proteins containing the CK2 pS/pTDXE motif (Figure 2C). These findings imply that the optimal dosage of inhibitor is substrate-specific and not uniform within the same cellular context.

The second approach to reducing CK2 activity is to target the expression of the protein. Two methods can be used to modulate CK2 protein expression: RNA interference (RNAi) (gene knockdown) or CRISPR tools (gene knockout). RNAi for gene silencing can be achieved using several RNAi platforms, including small interfering RNA (siRNA), short hairpin RNA (shRNA), miRNA, and antisense oligonucleotides (ASO).

Several miRNAs have been identified that target the mRNA of CK2 subunits and may provide insight into the mechanisms behind altered CK2 expression in conditions including cancer [80], ischemia [81] and cell senescence [82,83]. For a comprehensive list of all identified miRNAs that affect CK2 subunits, please refer to [37]. A recent study revealed that the long non-coding RNA *KCNQ1OT1* regulates CK2α expression in senescence and caloric restriction by targeting miR-760 [84]. Manipulation of miRNA expression could theoretically be an approach to modulate cellular CK2 expression. However, the limitations of this approach are as follows: (i) this type of regulation is cell-specific, (ii) each miRNA generally has several different targets [85], and (iii) a single mRNA can be targeted by a variety of miRNAs [85], indicating that a single miRNA often has a limited effect on a specific target. For instance, a 50% downregulation of CK2α in colon cancer cells requires the simultaneous transfection of four different miRNAs [86].

The most common method for gene silencing is the transient transfection of specific siRNA oligo targeting the mRNA of one of the three subunits. Downregulation of CK2α, α', β is easily achieved, and several siRNAs that effectively work have been described in the literature. The advantage of this method is its ease of use, adaptability to different cell types, and efficacy even in hard-to-transfect cells (as siRNAs are smaller and easier to transfect than plasmids). This method leads to a reduction in mRNA expression or a block in its translation, so the effect of a siRNA on the cellular amount of protein is closely linked to its stability.

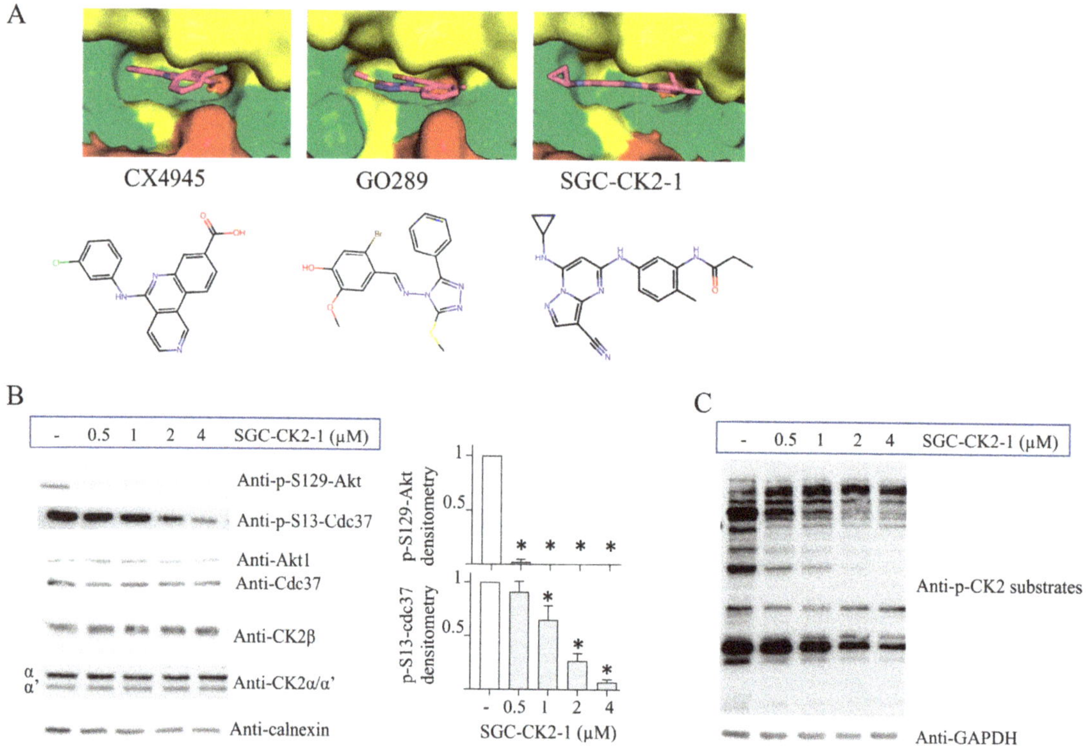

Figure 2. Recent CK2-specific inhibitors. (**A**) Molecular structure of the latest CK2-specific inhibitors and their binding to the CK2 ATP-binding pocket. (**B**,**C**) Effect of increasing doses of SGC-CK2-1 on CK2 substrates. 16-HBE cells have been treated with crescent doses of SGC-CK2-1 or with vehicle (DMSO) for 24 h. Cells have been lysed as described in [87] and loaded in SDS-PAGE. The phosphorylation of CK2 substrates (S129-Akt and S13-Cdc37 in panel (**B**), proteins containing the CK2 S/TDXE motif in panel (**C**)) have been assessed using Western blotting. The following antibodies have been used: anti-p-S129-Akt (ab133458), anti-Akt (sc-5298), anti-p-S13-Cdc37 (ab108360), anti-cdc-37 (sc-13129), anti-CK2β (ab76025), anti-CK2α/α′ (MCA3031Z), anti CK2-p-substrates (CS# 8738). Calnexin (sc-46669) and GAPDH (ABS16) are the loading controls. The graph in panel (**B**) represents the densitometric quantification of the immunostained bands p-S129-Akt and p-S13-Cdc37 (mean ± SD, n = 3; * $p < 0.05$).

The choice of which subunit to target depends on the specific research question and the desired outcome. siRNA could be designed to target one or both catalytic subunits and the β-regulatory subunit. Downregulation of a single catalytic subunit typically abolishes no more than 40–60% of the total CK2 activity [28,88]. It is worth noting that CK2 catalytic subunits may be highly redundant, and knockdown of a single catalytic subunit may do not guarantee the inhibition of the phosphorylation of the protein of interest. The situation is different when a substrate is specifically recognized by one or the other catalytic subunit (see below). The downregulation of the only β-regulatory subunit could instead have a dramatic effect on the phosphorylation of the substrate, but again the effect is substrate-dependent.

Despite the potential efficacy of siRNA downregulation, it is important to note that the downregulation is never complete, and a variable residual amount of the targeted protein is still present.

Complete abolition of protein expression is possible by gene editing (CRISPR tools). We generated for the first time CK2 knockout clonal cells [76]. However, although knockout of the single CK2 subunit is generally achievable in different cell types [76,88–91], to our knowledge, a double knockout of the catalytic subunits has never been achieved. Despite our efforts, we have only been able to obtain clones with minimal CK2 activity (less than 10% of the total) in C2C12 cells expressing a truncated form of CK2α′ and without CK2α [77]. We have hypothesized that a minimal level of activity is required for cell viability [77,87], meaning that it may not be possible to generate clones that are completely devoid of CK2 activity.

Even though CRISPR tools allow the complete abolition of the protein expression, there are two major drawbacks to this approach. First, it is more labor-intensive, because it requires the selection of the gene-edited clones, which takes about 1–3 months depending on the cell proliferation rate. Another important limitation is that a clonal cell population is generated, and not all clones show the same phenotype. This variability is due to the clonal selection starting from a single cell and the potential impact of the selection procedures, especially when the kinase the expression of which has been knocked out has key roles in cell functions. Cells can overcome the lack of protein in a stochastic manner. Therefore, it is necessary to test different clones to validate the involvement of the knocked-out protein in a specific biological phenomenon.

The advantage of the knockdown/knockout methods over inhibitor treatments is the ability to uncover the distinct biological roles of each CK2 subunit. Indeed, if in some cases CK2 catalytic subunits are highly redundant, as discussed above, isoform-specific roles have also been described [92–94]. It has also been shown that knockout of a specific subunit may have a greater effect on the phosphorylation level of some CK2 substrates [76,88]. The same is observed with siRNA downregulation of individual CK2 subunits, as shown in Figure 3. Indeed, the phosphorylation level of CK2 substrates changes not as a consequence of the overall reduction in the kinase but depending on which subunit is downregulated (Figure 3). For example, p-S129-AKT is reduced by CK2α or CK2β downregulation, but it is not affected by CK2α′ downregulation. On the contrary, p-S13-Cdc37 is only reduced by CK2β downregulation (Figure 3A). Moreover, the Western blotting experiments performed on the p-CK2 substrates provide compelling evidence that the phosphorylation of specific phosphosites is generated by different CK2 isoforms (Figure 3B). However, it is important to consider the interrelated expression of individual CK2 subunits, as shown in Figure 3A. In the context of 16-HBE cells, the knockdown of CK2α leads to the downregulation of CK2β expression, and conversely, the downregulation of CK2β leads to the downregulation of CK2α′. This interdependence between CK2 subunits has been observed in different cell types, both with knockdown and knockout experiments [76,88]. Interestingly, some of the effects are cell-specific. For example, in C2C12 cells, the downregulation of CK2β increases the expression of CK2α [76]. These findings highlight the complexity of CK2 regulation and of the interactions between subunits, which can vary depending on the cellular context.

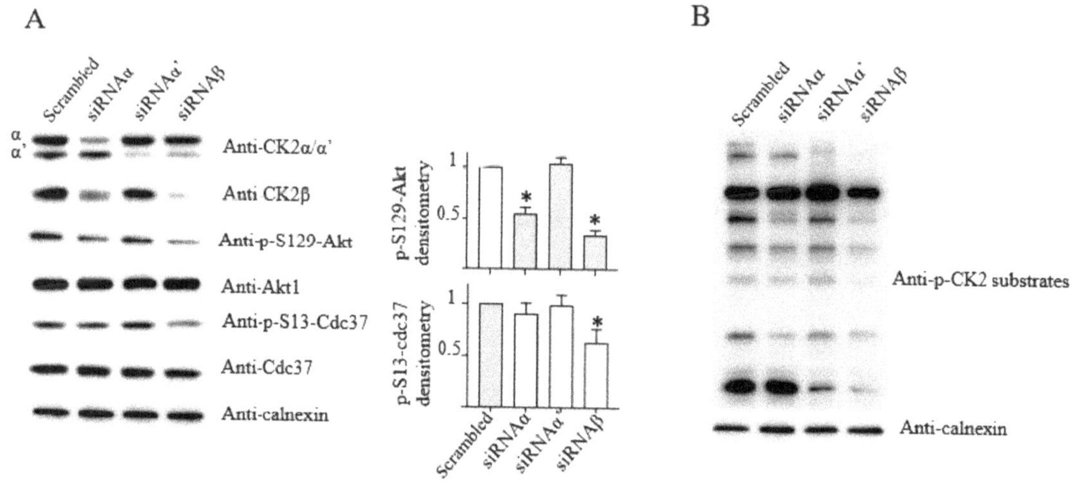

Figure 3. Silencing of CK2 subunits. 16-HBE cells have been treated for 72h with siRNA targeting CK2α, CK2α′, CK2β or scramble siRNA as control (siRNA sequences are reported in [88]). After incubation, cells have been lysed as described in [87] and loaded in SDS-PAGE. The CK2 protein amount and the phosphorylation of CK2 substrates have been assessed by Western blotting. The antibodies have been described in Figure 2. The graph in panel (**A**) represents the densitometric quantification of the immunostained bands p-S129-Akt and p-S13-Cdc37 (mean ± SD, n = 3; * $p < 0.05$). Calnexin (sc-46669) are the loading controls.

5. Conclusions

The exploration of the entire CK2 substratome and the functional implications of CK2 phosphorylation events remains an active area of research. Several tools have been developed to establish the relationship between substrates and CK2, which is crucial for unraveling the physiological functions of this kinase. The use of CK2-specific inhibitors is probably the most feasible approach to improve our understanding of the functions of this kinase. Recently, the use of specific inhibitors in combination with the expression of inhibitor-resistant CK2 mutants has been shown to be a valuable tool for the identification of CK2 substrates [69]. Ongoing research and development efforts are focused on improving the potency and specificity of CK2 inhibitors. Currently the most effective inhibitors are ATP-competitive molecules, with SGC-CK2-1 being the most specific one available to date. An intensive line of research is also working on the development of inhibitors targeting different domains of CK2, including allosteric inhibitors [95,96]. Nevertheless, we emphasize the need for cautious interpretation when using kinase inhibitors. It is important to note that the dephosphorylation of different substrates may have different time courses and/or require different inhibitor concentrations. Simply demonstrating that a kinase inhibitor reduces the phosphorylation of a single substrate may not be sufficient to suggest the block of the entire CK2 signaling.

Furthermore, knockdown/knockout tools serve as valuable complementary approaches that offer significant advantages in elucidating the isoform-specific effects of the catalytic isoforms (CK2α and CK2α′) and the regulatory CK2β on the phosphorylation of CK2 substrates. Although some evidence has been generated over the years, a clear understanding of the redundancy and specificity of each catalytic isoform and the definition of the entire CK2β-dependent substratome still remain elusive. This aspect becomes even more critical in light of the recent discovery of specific mutations in the *CSNK2A1* gene associated with Okur–Chung Neurodevelopmental Syndrome (OCNDS) and mutations in the *CSNK2B* gene associated with Poirier–Bienvenu Neurodevelopmental Syndrome (POBINDS) [19,97]. A predictive analysis of OCNDS and POBINDS variants suggests that mutations in CK2α and CK2β have functional and structural implications [68]. Fifteen distinct OCNDS missense mutations in CK2α result in varying degrees of loss of kinase activity when expressed as recombinant purified proteins [98], while the most common mutation (K198R) is responsible for altered substrate specificity of CK2α [99,100]. To gain deeper insights into disease mechanisms, further investigations are warranted to comprehensively characterize the CK2 subunit-specific effects and their implications in these neurodevelopmental syndromes.

Funding: This research received no external funding.

Institutional Review Board Statement: Not applicable.

Informed Consent Statement: Not applicable.

Data Availability Statement: Not applicable.

Conflicts of Interest: The authors declare no conflict of interest.

References

1. Hornbeck, P.V.; Zhang, B.; Murray, B.; Kornhauser, J.M.; Latham, V.; Skrzypek, E. PhosphoSitePlus, 2014: Mutations, PTMs and Recalibrations. *Nucleic Acids Res.* **2015**, *43*, D512–D520. [CrossRef] [PubMed]
2. D'Amore, C.; Salizzato, V.; Borgo, C.; Cesaro, L.; Pinna, L.A.; Salvi, M. A Journey through the Cytoskeleton with Protein Kinase CK2. *Curr. Protein Pept. Sci.* **2019**, *20*, 547–562. [CrossRef] [PubMed]
3. Hashemolhosseini, S. The Role of Protein Kinase CK2 in Skeletal Muscle: Myogenesis, Neuromuscular Junctions, and Rhabdomyosarcoma. *Neurosci. Lett.* **2020**, *729*, 135001. [CrossRef]
4. Montenarh, M. Protein Kinase CK2 and Angiogenesis. *Adv. Clin. Exp. Med.* **2014**, *23*, 153–158. [CrossRef] [PubMed]
5. Nuñez de Villavicencio-Diaz, T.; Rabalski, A.J.; Litchfield, D.W. Protein Kinase CK2: Intricate Relationships within Regulatory Cellular Networks. *Pharmaceuticals* **2017**, *10*, 27. [CrossRef]
6. Montenarh, M.; Götz, C. Protein Kinase CK2 and Ion Channels (Review). *Biomed. Rep.* **2020**, *13*, 55. [CrossRef]
7. St-Denis, N.A.; Litchfield, D.W. Protein Kinase CK2 in Health and Disease: From Birth to Death: The Role of Protein Kinase CK2 in the Regulation of Cell Proliferation and Survival. *Cell. Mol. Life Sci.* **2009**, *66*, 1817–1829. [CrossRef] [PubMed]
8. Götz, C.; Montenarh, M. Protein Kinase CK2 in Development and Differentiation. *Biomed. Rep.* **2017**, *6*, 127–133. [CrossRef] [PubMed]
9. Kanki, T.; Kurihara, Y.; Jin, X.; Goda, T.; Ono, Y.; Aihara, M.; Hirota, Y.; Saigusa, T.; Aoki, Y.; Uchiumi, T.; et al. Casein Kinase 2 Is Essential for Mitophagy. *EMBO Rep.* **2013**, *14*, 788–794. [CrossRef]
10. Borgo, C.; D'Amore, C.; Sarno, S.; Salvi, M.; Ruzzene, M. Protein Kinase CK2: A Potential Therapeutic Target for Diverse Human Diseases. *Signal Transduct. Target. Ther.* **2021**, *6*, 183. [CrossRef] [PubMed]
11. Quezada Meza, C.P.; Ruzzene, M. Protein Kinase CK2 and SARS-CoV-2: An Expected Interplay Story. *Kinases Phosphatases* **2023**, *1*, 141–150. [CrossRef]
12. Baier, A.; Szyszka, R. CK2 and Protein Kinases of the CK1 Superfamily as Targets for Neurodegenerative Disorders. *Front. Mol. Biosci.* **2022**, *9*, 916063. [CrossRef] [PubMed]
13. White, A.; McGlone, A.; Gomez-Pastor, R. Protein Kinase CK2 and Its Potential Role as a Therapeutic Target in Huntington's Disease. *Biomedicines* **2022**, *10*, 1979. [CrossRef] [PubMed]
14. Halloran, D.; Pandit, V.; Nohe, A. The Role of Protein Kinase CK2 in Development and Disease Progression: A Critical Review. *J. Dev. Biol.* **2022**, *10*, 31. [CrossRef]
15. Ampofo, E.; Nalbach, L.; Menger, M.D.; Montenarh, M.; Götz, C. Protein Kinase CK2-A Putative Target for the Therapy of Diabetes Mellitus? *Int. J. Mol. Sci.* **2019**, *20*, 4398. [CrossRef]
16. Trembley, J.H.; Kren, B.T.; Afzal, M.; Scaria, G.A.; Klein, M.A.; Ahmed, K. Protein Kinase CK2—Diverse Roles in Cancer Cell Biology and Therapeutic Promise. *Mol. Cell. Biochem.* **2023**, *478*, 899–926. [CrossRef] [PubMed]
17. Strum, S.W.; Gyenis, L.; Litchfield, D.W. CSNK2 in Cancer: Pathophysiology and Translational Applications. *Br. J. Cancer* **2022**, *126*, 994–1003. [CrossRef] [PubMed]
18. Castello, J.; Ragnauth, A.; Friedman, E.; Rebholz, H. CK2-An Emerging Target for Neurological and Psychiatric Disorders. *Pharmaceuticals* **2017**, *10*, 7. [CrossRef]
19. Unni, P.; Friend, J.; Weinberg, J.; Okur, V.; Hochscherf, J.; Dominguez, I. Predictive Functional, Statistical and Structural Analysis of CSNK2A1 and CSNK2B Variants Linked to Neurodevelopmental Diseases. *Front. Mol. Biosci.* **2022**, *9*, 851547. [CrossRef]
20. Hong, H.; Benveniste, E.N. The Immune Regulatory Role of Protein Kinase CK2 and Its Implications for Treatment of Cancer. *Biomedicines* **2021**, *9*, 1932. [CrossRef] [PubMed]
21. Salvi, M.; Sarno, S.; Cesaro, L.; Nakamura, H.; Pinna, L.A. Extraordinary Pleiotropy of Protein Kinase CK2 Revealed by Weblogo Phosphoproteome Analysis. *Biochim. Biophys. Acta* **2009**, *1793*, 847–859. [CrossRef] [PubMed]

22. Cesaro, L.; Pinna, L.A. Prevalence and Significance of the Commonest Phosphorylated Motifs in the Human Proteome: A Global Analysis. *Cell Mol. Life Sci.* **2020**, *77*, 5281–5298. [CrossRef] [PubMed]
23. Salvi, M.; Cesaro, L.; Tibaldi, E.; Pinna, L.A. Motif Analysis of Phosphosites Discloses a Potential Prominent Role of the Golgi Casein Kinase (GCK) in the Generation of Human Plasma Phospho-Proteome. *J. Proteome Res.* **2010**, *9*, 3335–3338. [CrossRef] [PubMed]
24. Tagliabracci, V.S.; Wiley, S.E.; Guo, X.; Kinch, L.N.; Durrant, E.; Wen, J.; Xiao, J.; Cui, J.; Nguyen, K.B.; Engel, J.L.; et al. A Single Kinase Generates the Majority of the Secreted Phosphoproteome. *Cell* **2015**, *161*, 1619–1632. [CrossRef]
25. Filhol, O.; Nueda, A.; Martel, V.; Gerber-Scokaert, D.; Benitez, M.J.; Souchier, C.; Saoudi, Y.; Cochet, C. Live-Cell Fluorescence Imaging Reveals the Dynamics of Protein Kinase CK2 Individual Subunits. *Mol. Cell. Biol.* **2003**, *23*, 975–987. [CrossRef]
26. Niefind, K.; Guerra, B.; Ermakowa, I.; Issinger, O.G. Crystal Structure of Human Protein Kinase CK2: Insights into Basic Properties of the CK2 Holoenzyme. *EMBO J.* **2001**, *20*, 5320–5331. [CrossRef]
27. Chua, M.M.J.; Lee, M.; Dominguez, I. Cancer-Type Dependent Expression of CK2 Transcripts. *PLoS ONE* **2017**, *12*, e0188854. [CrossRef]
28. Salizzato, V.; Zanin, S.; Borgo, C.; Lidron, E.; Salvi, M.; Rizzuto, R.; Pallafacchina, G.; Donella-Deana, A. Protein Kinase CK2 Subunits Exert Specific and Coordinated Functions in Skeletal Muscle Differentiation and Fusogenic Activity. *FASEB J.* **2019**, *33*, 10648–10667. [CrossRef]
29. Guerra, B.; Siemer, S.; Boldyreff, B.; Issinger, O.-G. Protein Kinase CK2: Evidence for a Protein Kinase CK2β Subunit Fraction, Devoid of the Catalytic CK2α Subunit, in Mouse Brain and Testicles. *FEBS Lett.* **1999**, *462*, 353–357. [CrossRef]
30. Bibby, A.C.; Litchfield, D.W. The Multiple Personalities of the Regulatory Subunit of Protein Kinase CK2: CK2 Dependent and CK2 Independent Roles Reveal a Secret Identity for CK2β. *Int. J. Biol. Sci.* **2005**, *1*, 67–79. [CrossRef]
31. Guerra, B.; Issinger, O.-G.; Wang, J.Y.J. Modulation of Human Checkpoint Kinase Chk1 by the Regulatory Beta-Subunit of Protein Kinase CK2. *Oncogene* **2003**, *22*, 4933–4942. [CrossRef]
32. Ubersax, J.A.; Ferrell, J.E. Mechanisms of Specificity in Protein Phosphorylation. *Nat. Rev. Mol. Cell. Biol.* **2007**, *8*, 530–541. [CrossRef]
33. Pinna, L.A.; Ruzzene, M. How Do Protein Kinases Recognize Their Substrates? *Biochim. Biophys. Acta* **1996**, *1314*, 191–225. [CrossRef] [PubMed]
34. de Oliveira, P.S.L.; Ferraz, F.A.N.; Pena, D.A.; Pramio, D.T.; Morais, F.A.; Schechtman, D. Revisiting Protein Kinase–Substrate Interactions: Toward Therapeutic Development. *Sci. Signal.* **2016**, *9*, re3. [CrossRef] [PubMed]
35. Johnson, J.L.; Yaron, T.M.; Huntsman, E.M.; Kerelsky, A.; Song, J.; Regev, A.; Lin, T.-Y.; Liberatore, K.; Cizin, D.M.; Cohen, B.M.; et al. An Atlas of Substrate Specificities for the Human Serine/Threonine Kinome. *Nature* **2023**, *613*, 759–766. [CrossRef] [PubMed]
36. Salvi, M.; Cesaro, L.; Pinna, L.A. Variable Contribution of Protein Kinases to the Generation of the Human Phosphoproteome: A Global Weblogo Analysis. *Biomol. Concepts* **2010**, *1*, 185–195. [CrossRef] [PubMed]
37. Borgo, C.; D'Amore, C.; Cesaro, L.; Sarno, S.; Pinna, L.A.; Ruzzene, M.; Salvi, M. How Can a Traffic Light Properly Work If It Is Always Green? The Paradox of CK2 Signaling. *Crit. Rev. Biochem. Mol. Biol.* **2021**, *56*, 321–359. [CrossRef] [PubMed]
38. Pinna, L.A. Protein Kinase CK2: A Challenge to Canons. *J. Cell Sci.* **2002**, *115*, 3873–3878. [CrossRef]
39. Borgo, C.; Franchin, C.; Cesaro, L.; Zaramella, S.; Arrigoni, G.; Salvi, M.; Pinna, L.A. A Proteomics Analysis of CK2β(-/-) C2C12 Cells Provides Novel Insights into the Biological Functions of the Non-Catalytic β Subunit. *FEBS J.* **2019**, *286*, 1561–1575. [CrossRef]
40. Schneider, T.D.; Stephens, R.M. Sequence Logos: A New Way to Display Consensus Sequences. *Nucleic Acids Res.* **1990**, *18*, 6097–6100. [CrossRef]
41. Vacic, V.; Iakoucheva, L.M.; Radivojac, P. Two Sample Logo: A Graphical Representation of the Differences between Two Sets of Sequence Alignments. *Bioinformatics* **2006**, *22*, 1536–1537. [CrossRef] [PubMed]
42. Jurrus, E.; Engel, D.; Star, K.; Monson, K.; Brandi, J.; Felberg, L.E.; Brookes, D.H.; Wilson, L.; Chen, J.; Liles, K.; et al. Improvements to the APBS Biomolecular Solvation Software Suite. *Protein Sci.* **2018**, *27*, 112–128. [CrossRef] [PubMed]
43. Kinoshita, E.; Kinoshita-Kikuta, E.; Takiyama, K.; Koike, T. Phosphate-Binding Tag, a New Tool to Visualize Phosphorylated Proteins. *Mol. Cell. Proteom.* **2006**, *5*, 749–757. [CrossRef] [PubMed]
44. Martin, K.; Steinberg, T.H.; Cooley, L.A.; Gee, K.R.; Beechem, J.M.; Patton, W.F. Quantitative Analysis of Protein Phosphorylation Status and Protein Kinase Activity on Microarrays Using a Novel Fluorescent Phosphorylation Sensor Dye. *Proteomics* **2003**, *3*, 1244–1255. [CrossRef]
45. Urban, J. A Review on Recent Trends in the Phosphoproteomics Workflow. From Sample Preparation to Data Analysis. *Anal. Chim. Acta* **2022**, *1199*, 338857. [CrossRef]
46. Borgo, C.; Ruzzene, M. Protein Kinase CK2 Inhibition as a Pharmacological Strategy. *Adv. Protein Chem. Struct. Biol.* **2021**, *124*, 23–46. [CrossRef]
47. Chen, Y.; Wang, Y.; Wang, J.; Zhou, Z.; Cao, S.; Zhang, J. Strategies of Targeting CK2 in Drug Discovery: Challenges, Opportunities, and Emerging Prospects. *J. Med. Chem.* **2023**, *66*, 2257–2281. [CrossRef]
48. Pierre, F.; Chua, P.C.; O'Brien, S.E.; Siddiqui-Jain, A.; Bourbon, P.; Haddach, M.; Michaux, J.; Nagasawa, J.; Schwaebe, M.K.; Stefan, E.; et al. Discovery and SAR of 5-(3-Chlorophenylamino)Benzo[c][2,6]Naphthyridine-8-Carboxylic Acid (CX-4945), the First Clinical Stage Inhibitor of Protein Kinase CK2 for the Treatment of Cancer. *J. Med. Chem.* **2011**, *54*, 635–654. [CrossRef]

49. Bogusz, J.; Zrubek, K.; Rembacz, K.P.; Grudnik, P.; Golik, P.; Romanowska, M.; Wladyka, B.; Dubin, G. Structural Analysis of PIM1 Kinase Complexes with ATP-Competitive Inhibitors. *Sci. Rep.* **2017**, *7*, 13399. [CrossRef]
50. Grygier, P.; Pustelny, K.; Nowak, J.; Golik, P.; Popowicz, G.M.; Plettenburg, O.; Dubin, G.; Menezes, F.; Czarna, A. Silmitasertib (CX-4945), a Clinically Used CK2-Kinase Inhibitor with Additional Effects on GSK3β and DYRK1A Kinases: A Structural Perspective. *J. Med. Chem.* **2023**, *66*, 4009–4024. [CrossRef]
51. Kim, H.; Lee, K.-S.; Kim, A.-K.; Choi, M.; Choi, K.; Kang, M.; Chi, S.-W.; Lee, M.-S.; Lee, J.-S.; Lee, S.-Y.; et al. A Chemical with Proven Clinical Safety Rescues Down-Syndrome-Related Phenotypes in through DYRK1A Inhibition. *Dis. Model Mech.* **2016**, *9*, 839–848. [CrossRef]
52. Kim, H.; Choi, K.; Kang, H.; Lee, S.-Y.; Chi, S.-W.; Lee, M.-S.; Song, J.; Im, D.; Choi, Y.; Cho, S. Identification of a Novel Function of CX-4945 as a Splicing Regulator. *PLoS ONE* **2014**, *9*, e94978. [CrossRef]
53. Lertsuwan, J.; Lertsuwan, K.; Sawasdichai, A.; Tasnawijitwong, N.; Lee, K.Y.; Kitchen, P.; Afford, S.; Gaston, K.; Jayaraman, P.-S.; Satayavivad, J. CX-4945 Induces Methuosis in Cholangiocarcinoma Cell Lines by a CK2-Independent Mechanism. *Cancers* **2018**, *10*, 283. [CrossRef]
54. D'Amore, C.; Moro, E.; Borgo, C.; Itami, K.; Hirota, T.; Pinna, L.A.; Salvi, M. "Janus" Efficacy of CX-5011: CK2 Inhibition and Methuosis Induction by Independent Mechanisms. *Biochim. Biophys. Acta BBA Mol. Cell Res.* **2020**, *1867*, 118807. [CrossRef]
55. Zandomeni, R.O. Kinetics of Inhibition by 5,6-Dichloro-1-β-d-Ribofuranosylbenzimidazole on Calf Thymus Casein Kinase II. *Biochem. J.* **1989**, *262*, 469–473. [CrossRef]
56. Andrzejewska, M.; Pagano, M.A.; Meggio, F.; Brunati, A.M.; Kazimierczuk, Z. Polyhalogenobenzimidazoles: Synthesis and Their Inhibitory Activity against Casein Kinases. *Bioorganic Med. Chem.* **2003**, *11*, 3997–4002. [CrossRef]
57. Cozza, G.; Girardi, C.; Ranchio, A.; Lolli, G.; Sarno, S.; Orzeszko, A.; Kazimierczuk, Z.; Battistutta, R.; Ruzzene, M.; Pinna, L.A. Cell-Permeable Dual Inhibitors of Protein Kinases CK2 and PIM-1: Structural Features and Pharmacological Potential. *Cell. Mol. Life Sci.* **2014**, *71*, 3173–3185. [CrossRef]
58. Pagano, M.A.; Andrzejewska, M.; Ruzzene, M.; Sarno, S.; Cesaro, L.; Bain, J.; Elliott, M.; Meggio, F.; Kazimierczuk, Z.; Pinna, L.A. Optimization of Protein Kinase CK2 Inhibitors Derived from 4,5,6,7-Tetrabromobenzimidazole. *J. Med. Chem.* **2004**, *47*, 6239–6247. [CrossRef]
59. McCarty, M.F.; Assanga, S.I.; Lujan, L.L. Flavones and Flavonols May Have Clinical Potential as CK2 Inhibitors in Cancer Therapy. *Med. Hypotheses* **2020**, *141*, 109723. [CrossRef]
60. Urolithin as a Converging Scaffold Linking Ellagic Acid and Coumarin Analogues: Design of Potent Protein Kinase CK2 Inhibitors—Cozza—2011—ChemMedChem—Wiley Online Library. Available online: https://chemistry-europe.onlinelibrary.wiley.com/doi/10.1002/cmdc.201100338 (accessed on 20 September 2023).
61. Yim, H.; Lee, Y.H.; Lee, C.H.; Lee, S.K. Emodin, an Anthraquinone Derivative Isolated from the Rhizomes of Rheum Palmatum, Selectively Inhibits the Activity of Casein Kinase II as a Competitive Inhibitor. *Planta Medica* **1999**, *65*, 9–13. [CrossRef]
62. Meggio, F.; Pagano, M.A.; Moro, S.; Zagotto, G.; Ruzzene, M.; Sarno, S.; Cozza, G.; Bain, J.; Elliott, M.; Deana, A.D.; et al. Inhibition of Protein Kinase CK2 by Condensed Polyphenolic Derivatives. An in Vitro and in Vivo Study. *Biochemistry* **2004**, *43*, 12931–12936. [CrossRef]
63. Cozza, G.; Mazzorana, M.; Papinutto, E.; Bain, J.; Elliott, M.; di Maira, G.; Gianoncelli, A.; Pagano, M.A.; Sarno, S.; Ruzzene, M.; et al. Quinalizarin as a Potent, Selective and Cell-Permeable Inhibitor of Protein Kinase CK2. *Biochem. J.* **2009**, *421*, 387–395. [CrossRef]
64. Wells, C.I.; Drewry, D.H.; Pickett, J.E.; Tjaden, A.; Krämer, A.; Müller, S.; Gyenis, L.; Menyhart, D.; Litchfield, D.W.; Knapp, S.; et al. Development of a Potent and Selective Chemical Probe for the Pleiotropic Kinase CK2. *Cell Chem. Biol.* **2021**, *28*, 546–558. [CrossRef]
65. Vangrevelinghe, E.; Zimmermann, K.; Schoepfer, J.; Portmann, R.; Fabbro, D.; Furet, P. Discovery of a Potent and Selective Protein Kinase CK2 Inhibitor by High-Throughput Docking. *J. Med. Chem.* **2003**, *46*, 2656–2662. [CrossRef]
66. Pagano, M.A.; Poletto, G.; Di Maira, G.; Cozza, G.; Ruzzene, M.; Sarno, S.; Bain, J.; Elliott, M.; Moro, S.; Zagotto, G.; et al. Tetrabromocinnamic Acid (TBCA) and Related Compounds Represent a New Class of Specific Protein Kinase CK2 Inhibitors. *Chembiochem* **2007**, *8*, 129–139. [CrossRef]
67. Battistutta, R.; Cozza, G.; Pierre, F.; Papinutto, E.; Lolli, G.; Sarno, S.; O'Brien, S.E.; Siddiqui-Jain, A.; Haddach, M.; Anderes, K.; et al. Unprecedented Selectivity and Structural Determinants of a New Class of Protein Kinase CK2 Inhibitors in Clinical Trials for the Treatment of Cancer. *Biochemistry* **2011**, *50*, 8478–8488. [CrossRef]
68. Oshima, T.; Niwa, Y.; Kuwata, K.; Srivastava, A.; Hyoda, T.; Tsuchiya, Y.; Kumagai, M.; Tsuyuguchi, M.; Tamaru, T.; Sugiyama, A.; et al. Cell-Based Screen Identifies a New Potent and Highly Selective CK2 Inhibitor for Modulation of Circadian Rhythms and Cancer Cell Growth. *Sci. Adv.* **2019**, *5*, eaau9060. [CrossRef]
69. Menyhart, D.; Gyenis, L.; Jurcic, K.; Roffey, S.E.; Puri, A.; Jovanovic, P.; Szkop, K.J.; Pittock, P.; Lajoie, G.; Axtman, A.D.; et al. Comparison of CX-4945 and SGC-CK2-1 as Inhibitors of CSNK2 Using Quantitative Phosphoproteomics: Triple SILAC in Combination with Inhibitor-Resistant CSNK2. *Curr. Res. Chem. Biol.* **2023**, *3*, 100041. [CrossRef]
70. Cohen, P. Guidelines for the Effective Use of Chemical Inhibitors of Protein Function to Understand Their Roles in Cell Regulation. *Biochem. J.* **2009**, *425*, 53–54. [CrossRef]

71. Birus, R.; El-Awaad, E.; Ballentin, L.; Alchab, F.; Aichele, D.; Ettouati, L.; Götz, C.; Le Borgne, M.; Jose, J. 4,5,7-Trisubstituted Indeno[1,2-b]Indole Inhibits CK2 Activity in Tumor Cells Equivalent to CX-4945 and Shows Strong Anti-Migratory Effects. *FEBS Open Bio* **2022**, *12*, 394–411. [CrossRef]
72. Marin, O.; Meggio, F.; Pinna, L.A. Design and Synthesis of Two New Peptide Substrates for the Specific and Sensitive Monitoring of Casein Kinases-1 and -2. *Biochem. Biophys. Res. Commun.* **1994**, *198*, 898–905. [CrossRef] [PubMed]
73. Ruzzene, M.; Penzo, D.; Pinna, L.A. Protein Kinase CK2 Inhibitor 4,5,6,7-Tetrabromobenzotriazole (TBB) Induces Apoptosis and Caspase-Dependent Degradation of Haematopoietic Lineage Cell-Specific Protein 1 (HS1) in Jurkat Cells. *Biochem. J.* **2002**, *364*, 41–47. [CrossRef] [PubMed]
74. Zanin, S.; Borgo, C.; Girardi, C.; O'Brien, S.E.; Miyata, Y.; Pinna, L.A.; Donella-Deana, A.; Ruzzene, M. Effects of the CK2 Inhibitors CX-4945 and CX-5011 on Drug-Resistant Cells. *PLoS ONE* **2012**, *7*, e49193. [CrossRef] [PubMed]
75. Borgo, C.; Cesaro, L.; Hirota, T.; Kuwata, K.; D'Amore, C.; Ruppert, T.; Blatnik, R.; Salvi, M.; Pinna, L.A. Comparing the Efficacy and Selectivity of Ck2 Inhibitors. A Phosphoproteomics Approach. *Eur. J. Med. Chem.* **2021**, *214*, 113217. [CrossRef]
76. Borgo, C.; Franchin, C.; Scalco, S.; Bosello-Travain, V.; Donella-Deana, A.; Arrigoni, G.; Salvi, M.; Pinna, L.A. Generation and Quantitative Proteomics Analysis of CK2α/α'(-/-) Cells. *Sci. Rep.* **2017**, *7*, 42409. [CrossRef] [PubMed]
77. Borgo, C.; D'Amore, C.; Cesaro, L.; Itami, K.; Hirota, T.; Salvi, M.; Pinna, L.A. A N-Terminally Deleted Form of the CK2α' Catalytic Subunit Is Sufficient to Support Cell Viability. *Biochem. Biophys. Res. Commun.* **2020**, *531*, 409–415. [CrossRef] [PubMed]
78. Franchin, C.; Borgo, C.; Cesaro, L.; Zaramella, S.; Vilardell, J.; Salvi, M.; Arrigoni, G.; Pinna, L.A. Re-Evaluation of Protein Kinase CK2 Pleiotropy: New Insights Provided by a Phosphoproteomics Analysis of CK2 Knockout Cells. *Cell. Mol. Life Sci.* **2018**, *75*, 2011–2026. [CrossRef]
79. Miyata, Y.; Nishida, E. CK2 Binds, Phosphorylates, and Regulates Its Pivotal Substrate Cdc37, an Hsp90-Cochaperone. *Mol. Cell. Biochem.* **2005**, *274*, 171–179. [CrossRef]
80. Feliciano, A.; Castellvi, J.; Artero-Castro, A.; Leal, J.A.; Romagosa, C.; Hernández-Losa, J.; Peg, V.; Fabra, A.; Vidal, F.; Kondoh, H.; et al. MiR-125b Acts as a Tumor Suppressor in Breast Tumorigenesis via Its Novel Direct Targets ENPEP, CK2-α, CCNJ, and MEGF9. *PLoS ONE* **2013**, *8*, e76247. [CrossRef]
81. Liang, Y.; Xu, J.; Wang, Y.; Tang, J.-Y.; Yang, S.-L.; Xiang, H.-G.; Wu, S.-X.; Li, X.-J. Inhibition of MiRNA-125b Decreases Cerebral Ischemia/Reperfusion Injury by Targeting CK2α/NADPH Oxidase Signaling. *Cell. Physiol. Biochem.* **2018**, *45*, 1818–1826. [CrossRef]
82. Lee, Y.-H.; Kim, S.Y.; Bae, Y.-S. Upregulation of MiR-760 and MiR-186 Is Associated with Replicative Senescence in Human Lung Fibroblast Cells. *Mol. Cells* **2014**, *37*, 620–627. [CrossRef]
83. Song, J.; Bae, Y.-S. CK2 Down-Regulation Increases the Expression of Senescence-Associated Secretory Phenotype Factors through NF-KB Activation. *Int. J. Mol. Sci.* **2021**, *22*, 406. [CrossRef] [PubMed]
84. Lee, Y.; Bae, Y.-S. Long Non-Coding RNA KCNQ1OT1 Regulates Protein Kinase CK2 Via MiR-760 in Senescence and Calorie Restriction. *Int. J. Mol. Sci.* **2022**, *23*, 1888. [CrossRef] [PubMed]
85. Naeli, P.; Winter, T.; Hackett, A.P.; Alboushi, L.; Jafarnejad, S.M. The Intricate Balance between MicroRNA-Induced MRNA Decay and Translational Repression. *FEBS J.* **2023**, *290*, 2508–2524. [CrossRef] [PubMed]
86. Kim, S.Y.; Lee, Y.-H.; Bae, Y.-S. MiR-186, MiR-216b, MiR-337-3p, and MiR-760 Cooperatively Induce Cellular Senescence by Targeting α Subunit of Protein Kinase CKII in Human Colorectal Cancer Cells. *Biochem. Biophys. Res. Commun.* **2012**, *429*, 173–179. [CrossRef]
87. Borgo, C.; Cesaro, L.; Hirota, T.; Kuwata, K.; D'Amore, C.; Ruppert, T.; Blatnik, R.; Salvi, M.; Pinna, L.A. Analysis of the Phosphoproteome of CK2α(-/-)/$\Delta\alpha$' C2C12 Myoblasts Compared to the Wild-Type Cells. *Open Biol.* **2023**, *13*, 220220. [CrossRef]
88. Lettieri, A.; Borgo, C.; Zanieri, L.; D'Amore, C.; Oleari, R.; Paganoni, A.; Pinna, L.A.; Cariboni, A.; Salvi, M. Protein Kinase CK2 Subunits Differentially Perturb the Adhesion and Migration of GN11 Cells: A Model of Immature Migrating Neurons. *Int. J. Mol. Sci.* **2019**, *20*, 5951. [CrossRef]
89. Di Maira, G.; Gentilini, A.; Pastore, M.; Caligiuri, A.; Piombanti, B.; Raggi, C.; Rovida, E.; Lewinska, M.; Andersen, J.B.; Borgo, C.; et al. The Protein Kinase CK2 Contributes to the Malignant Phenotype of Cholangiocarcinoma Cells. *Oncogenesis* **2019**, *8*, 61. [CrossRef]
90. D'Amore, C.; Borgo, C.; Bosello-Travain, V.; Vilardell, J.; Salizzato, V.; Pinna, L.A.; Venerando, A.; Salvi, M. Deciphering the Role of Protein Kinase CK2 in the Maturation/Stability of F508del-CFTR. *Biochim. Biophys. Acta BBA Mol. Basis Dis.* **2020**, *1866*, 165611. [CrossRef]
91. Schmitt, B.M.; Boewe, A.S.; Götz, C.; Philipp, S.E.; Urbschat, S.; Oertel, J.; Menger, M.D.; Laschke, M.W.; Ampofo, E. CK2 Activity Mediates the Aggressive Molecular Signature of Glioblastoma Multiforme by Inducing Nerve/Glial Antigen (NG)2 Expression. *Cancers* **2021**, *13*, 1678. [CrossRef]
92. Vilk, G.; Saulnier, R.B.; St Pierre, R.; Litchfield, D.W. Inducible Expression of Protein Kinase CK2 in Mammalian Cells. Evidence for Functional Specialization of CK2 Isoforms. *J. Biol. Chem.* **1999**, *274*, 14406–14414. [CrossRef] [PubMed]
93. Xu, X.; Toselli, P.A.; Russell, L.D.; Seldin, D.C. Globozoospermia in Mice Lacking the Casein Kinase II Alpha' Catalytic Subunit. *Nat. Genet.* **1999**, *23*, 118–121. [CrossRef]
94. Lou, D.Y.; Dominguez, I.; Toselli, P.; Landesman-Bollag, E.; O'Brien, C.; Seldin, D.C. The Alpha Catalytic Subunit of Protein Kinase CK2 Is Required for Mouse Embryonic Development. *Mol. Cell. Biol.* **2008**, *28*, 131–139. [CrossRef] [PubMed]

95. Prudent, R.; Cochet, C. New Protein Kinase CK2 Inhibitors: Jumping out of the Catalytic Box. *Chem. Biol.* **2009**, *16*, 112–120. [CrossRef] [PubMed]
96. Iegre, J.; Atkinson, E.L.; Brear, P.D.; Cooper, B.M.; Hyvönen, M.; Spring, D.R. Chemical Probes Targeting the Kinase CK2: A Journey Outside the Catalytic Box. *Org. Biomol. Chem.* **2021**, *19*, 4380–4396. [CrossRef]
97. Ballardin, D.; Cruz-Gamero, J.M.; Bienvenu, T.; Rebholz, H. Comparing Two Neurodevelopmental Disorders Linked to CK2: Okur-Chung Neurodevelopmental Syndrome and Poirier-Bienvenu Neurodevelopmental Syndrome-Two Sides of the Same Coin? *Front. Mol. Biosci.* **2022**, *9*, 850559. [CrossRef]
98. Dominguez, I.; Cruz-Gamero, J.M.; Corasolla, V.; Dacher, N.; Rangasamy, S.; Urbani, A.; Narayanan, V.; Rebholz, H. Okur-Chung Neurodevelopmental Syndrome-Linked CK2α Variants Have Reduced Kinase Activity. *Hum. Genet.* **2021**, *140*, 1077–1096. [CrossRef]
99. Caefer, D.M.; Phan, N.Q.; Liddle, J.C.; Balsbaugh, J.L.; O'Shea, J.P.; Tzingounis, A.V.; Schwartz, D. The Okur-Chung Neurodevelopmental Syndrome Mutation CK2K198R Leads to a Rewiring of Kinase Specificity. *Front. Mol. Biosci.* **2022**, *9*, 850661. [CrossRef]
100. Werner, C.; Gast, A.; Lindenblatt, D.; Nickelsen, A.; Niefind, K.; Jose, J.; Hochscherf, J. Structural and Enzymological Evidence for an Altered Substrate Specificity in Okur-Chung Neurodevelopmental Syndrome Mutant CK2αLys198Arg. *Front. Mol. Biosci.* **2022**, *9*, 831693. [CrossRef]

kinases and phosphatases

MDPI

Review

CK2 Chemical Probes: Past, Present, and Future

Han Wee Ong [1], David H. Drewry [1,2] and Alison D. Axtman [1,*]

1 Structural Genomics Consortium, UNC Eshelman School of Pharmacy, University of North Carolina at Chapel Hill, Chapel Hill, NC 27599, USA; onghw@live.unc.edu (H.W.O.); david.drewry@unc.edu (D.H.D.)

2 UNC Lineberger Comprehensive Cancer Center, UNC School of Medicine, University of North Carolina at Chapel Hill, Chapel Hill, NC 27599, USA

* Correspondence: alison.axtman@unc.edu

Abstract: Protein kinase casein kinase 2 (CK2/CSNK2) is a pleiotropic kinase involved in many cellular processes and, accordingly, has been identified as a potential target for therapeutic intervention for multiple indications. Significant research effort has been invested into identifying CK2 inhibitors as potential drug candidates and potent and selective CK2 chemical probes to interrogate CK2 function. Here, we review the small molecule inhibitors reported for CK2 and discuss various orthosteric, allosteric, and bivalent inhibitors of CK2. We focus on the pyrazolo[1,5-*a*]pyrimidines and naphthyridines, two chemotypes that have been extensively explored for chemical probe development. We highlight the uptake and demonstrated utility of the pyrazolo[1,5-*a*]pyrimidine chemical probe **SGC-CK2-1** by the scientific community in cellular studies. Finally, we propose criteria for an ideal in vivo chemical probe for investigating CK2 function in a living organism. While no compound currently meets these metrics, we discuss ongoing and future directions in the development of in vivo chemical probes for CK2.

Keywords: protein kinase CK2; CSNK2A1; CSNK2A2; chemical probe; pyrazolopyrimidine; naphthyridine; orthosteric; allosteric; bivalent

1. Introduction

1.1. CK2 General Structure and Small Molecule Binding Sites

Protein kinase casein kinase 2 (CK2/CSNK2) is a constitutively active, ubiquitously expressed Ser/Thr kinase with hundreds of reported substrates [1,2]. Accordingly, CK2 plays regulatory roles in most cellular processes, and it has been identified as a potential therapeutic target for diverse diseases, including cancer, viral infections, neurodegenerative disorders, and many others [3–10]. Structurally, CK2 is a tetrameric holoenzyme composed of two catalytic subunits (α and α') and two regulatory subunits (β, Figure 1). The catalytic and regulatory subunits can assemble to make different CK2 holoenzyme combinations: $\alpha_2\beta_2$, $\alpha'_2\beta_2$, and $\alpha\alpha'\beta_2$. CK2α (CSNK2A1) and CK2α' (CSNK2A2) share high sequence similarity within their catalytic domains. However, due to differences within their C-terminal sequences, the two isoforms demonstrate some differences in their partner proteins and thus exert selected isoform-specific functions [11].

While the dimeric CK2β regulatory subunits reinforce the stability of the intact holoenzyme, drive selection of substrates, and influence CK2 localization, there is no small molecule binding site in this domain [12–14]. Both CK2α and CK2α' have an ATP-binding site that accommodates small molecule ligands. Due to their extensive sequence identity, this orthosteric site on CK2α and CK2α' binds the same ligands with similar affinity. Many different scaffolds have been exemplified as ATP-competitive CK2 inhibitors, though they vary in potency for CK2 and kinome-wide selectivity [14–20]. Through methods such as X-ray crystallography fragment screening and virtual screening, allosteric sites on CK2 capable of binding a small molecule have been identified [14,21]. These sites include the CK2α/CK2β interface [21–24] and the αD pocket [25–28], which is located near the αD helix of the C-terminal domain of CK2α and CK2α′ [14]. The development of bivalent compounds capable of simultaneously binding the CK2 ATP-binding pocket and αD pocket has been a major focus for several groups [25–28]. In addition to small molecules, peptides have also been exemplified that bind to the CK2 substrate channel as well as at the CK2α/CK2β interface [14,29,30]. Finally, bi-specific compounds that simultaneously bind to the CK2α ATP site and CK2α substrate-binding channel have been reported, but these compounds have a peptidic component and thus suffer from physicochemical limitations [28,31–34]. The various binding sites and positions within those pockets of example orthosteric, allosteric, and bivalent small molecules have been highlighted in Figure 1, with corresponding PDB codes included.

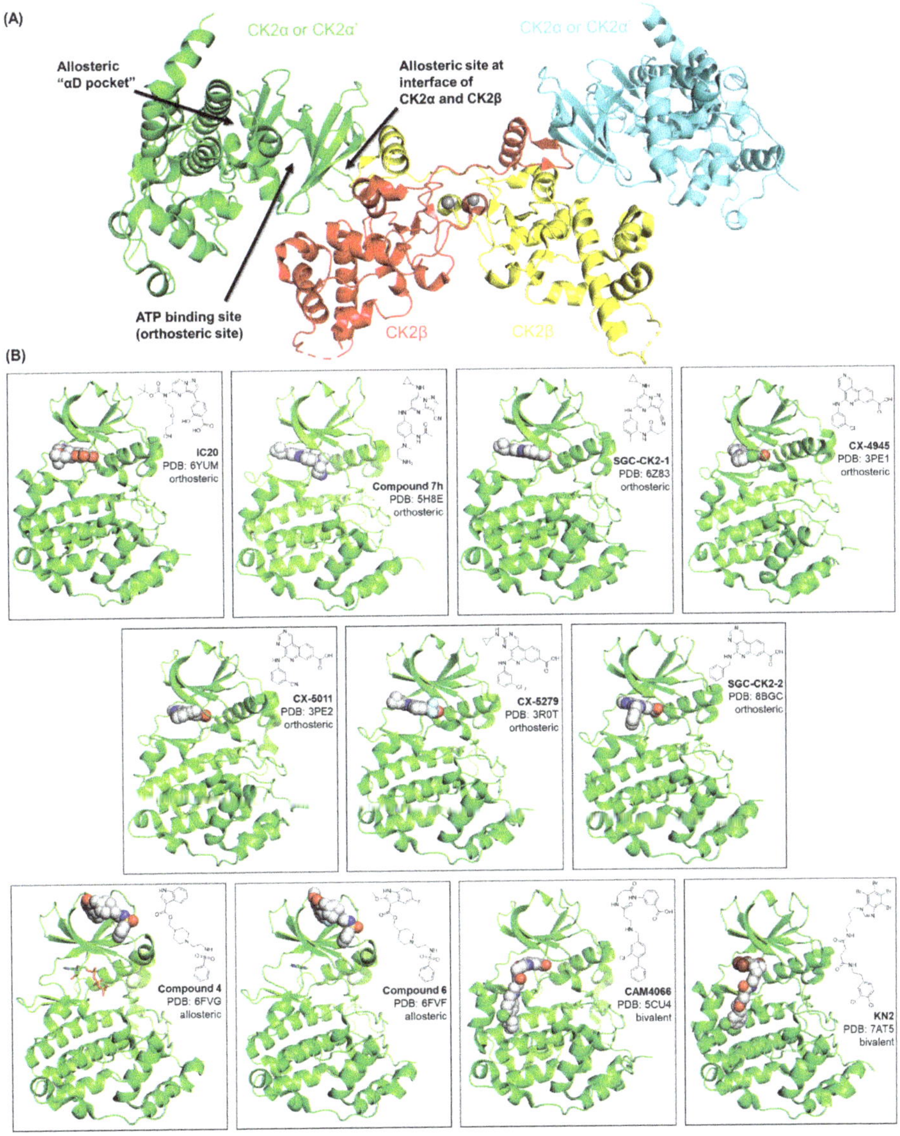

Figure 1. (**A**) Cartoon representation of human CK2 holoenzyme (PDB: 4MD7) with approximate positions of small molecule binding sites labeled. The holoenzyme is crystallized with two units of

CK2α (green and cyan) and two units of CK2β (red and yellow). CK2α may be substituted by CK2α′ in physiological conditions. Zn^{2+} ions are shown as grey spheres. (**B**) Binding sites of small molecule inhibitors (in spheres, colored by elements with carbon as white, oxygen as red, nitrogen as blue, fluorine as cyan, chlorine as green, and bromine as brown) to CK2α (green ribbon). ATP is present in the structures of compound **4** and compound **6**, shown in sticks, colored by elements with carbon as green. The binding mode and PDB code corresponding to the crystal structures are provided for each inhibitor.

1.2. Chemical Probe Definition

Recent emphasis has been placed on the development of inhibitors that interact selectively with CK2. This aligns with the notion that a potent and selective molecule that targets a single protein is a high-quality tool for interrogating the biological pathways regulated by that protein. A chemical probe fits these criteria and has been defined by the Structural Genomics Consortium (SGC) as meeting the metrics included in Table 1. To be approved as an SGC chemical probe, a kinase inhibitor must demonstrate a potency of <100 nM in a biochemical or biophysical assay (Table 1, #1). Enzymatic, surface plasmon resonance (SPR), isothermal calorimetry (ITC), and active site-directed competition binding assays are examples of methodologies that can and have been used to determine the cell-free potency of a putative chemical probe. Kinome-wide selectivity must be ascertained using a large human kinase panel, preferably comprising more than half of the screenable kinome (>200 kinases, Table 1, #2) [35]. The SGC kinase chemical probe selectivity goal requires that a compound demonstrates high affinity binding (percent of control <10) to <4% of the kinases within the panel when screening at a single concentration, typically 1 μM or greater [35]. Kinase chemical probes have historically exhibited better kinome-wide selectivity scores than those listed in Table 1. A deeper examination of selectivity is required, and any kinases that are inhibited and/or bind within 30-fold of the biochemical IC_{50}/K_D of the primary target are considered additional targets of the chemical probe (Table 1, #3). Often near neighbor kinases, including kinases within the same kinase subfamily, fall into this category, such as AP2-associated kinase 1 (AAK1) and BMP-2-inducible kinase (BMP2K, also known as BIKE) for **SGC-AAK1-1** [36]. A kinase chemical probe typically inhibits ≤5 kinases.

Many proteins bind ATP and thus profiling against at least one other ATP-binding protein class is expected for kinase chemical probes (Table 1, #4). These compounds are sent for profiling in the PDSP GPCR panel of ~46 primary binding assays, and secondary follow-up assays are run in dose–response, where appropriate [37–39]. These data, especially for potent binders, are made available to the community as part of the data package for SGC chemical probes. For SGC kinase chemical probes, demonstration of potent cellular target engagement is required (Table 1, #5). The NanoBRET assay is typically employed to determine a cellular target engagement IC_{50} value in HEK293 cells [40]. Finally, once a compound has met criteria 1–5 in Table 1, a suitable negative control is identified. This negative control must be structurally similar to the chemical probe but lack biochemical and cellular activity on the protein target(s) inhibited by the chemical probe. The use of a negative control compound alongside the chemical probe in experiments allows for ruling out chemotype-specific effects and results in the most robust science.

Table 1. Kinase chemical probe metrics standardized by the Structural Genomics Consortium (SGC) [41].

SGC Kinase Chemical Probe Criteria
1. Inhibitor/agonist cell-free potency: <100 nM IC_{50} or K_D;
2. Excellent kinome-wide selectivity: S_{10} (1 μM) < 0.04;
3. Selectivity within kinase family: >30-fold excluding near neighbor kinases;
4. Selectivity outside kinase family: describe the off-target proteins;
5. On target activity in cells: <1 μM IC_{50} or EC_{50};
6. Negative control: in vitro potency 100× less; cellular activity 100× less.

2. Small Molecule Inhibitors of CK2 and Chemical Probe Development

2.1. Selected Orthosteric CK2 Inhibitors and Chemical Probes

Two chemotypes have received a lot of attention in the pursuit of orthosteric CK2 chemical probes: pyrazolo[1,5-*a*]pyrimidines (referred to as pyrazolopyrimidines from here forth) and naphthyridines. AstraZeneca was the first to publish a series of papers and patents summarizing their efforts to tune the pyrazolopyrimidine scaffold to improve CK2 potency [42–45]. Examples of lead compounds from the AstraZeneca efforts are compounds **7b** and **7h** in Table 2 and Figure 2 [43,44]. While these pyrazolopyrimidines were found to be potent inhibitors of the enzymatic activity of CK2α and later potently engage CK2α and CK2α′ in cells [17], their suboptimal kinome-wide selectivity would need to be improved to furnish a pyrazolopyrimidine-based CK2 chemical probe [17,43,44]. Next, a team at SGC Frankfurt developed a series of acyclic/macrocyclic pyrazolopyrimidines. Macrocyclization was pursued as a strategy to deliver a selective CK2 chemical probe. While the lead compound **IC20** (Figure 2 and Table 2) proved to be a potent and selective CK2 inhibitor and outperformed its acyclic counterpart **IC19** (Figure 2 and Table 2) in both of these categories, the series suffered from poor cellular penetrance that precluded the advancement of **IC20** as a CK2 chemical probe [18]. Building on the work of AstraZeneca, SGC-UNC pursued optimization of the pyrazolopyrimidine scaffold toward a CK2 chemical probe. The best available CK2 chemical probe to date was delivered from these efforts: **SGC-CK2-1** (Figure 2). This compound demonstrates potent CK2 inhibition as well as the sub-micromolar engagement of CK2 in cells (Table 2). Broad profiling revealed that **SGC-CK2-1** is exquisitely selective (Table 2): it only inhibits CK2α and CK2α′ and has a 100-fold selectivity window over the next most potently inhibited kinase (DYRK2). Screening of **SGC-CK2-1** against nearly 180 cancer cell lines challenged the essentiality of CK2 for cancer cell proliferation [17], a notion that was challenged by others in responsive publications [3,15]. Finally, **SGC-CK2-1N** (Figure 2) was released alongside **SGC-CK2-1** as a structurally related negative control compound [17].

The naphthyridine scaffold gave rise to the most clinically advanced CK2 inhibitor: **CX-4945** (Figure 2). This compound, despite its suboptimal selectivity (Table 2), has advanced into clinical trials for several oncological indications as well as for the treatment of COVID-19 [19,46–48]. Efforts have been made to improve the selectivity of naphthyridine-based CK2 inhibitors. Collaborative work between members of the University of Padova and Cylene Pharmaceuticals led to the development of **CX-5011**, **CX-5033**, and **CX-5279** (Figure 2), which retained potent biochemical inhibition of CK2 (Table 2). Selectivity profiling of these compounds versus **CX-4945** in assay panels comprising 102–235 kinases established that the more recently generated analogs are more selective than **CX-4945** [20]. Kinome-wide profiling (468 kinase panel) of **CX-4945** and **CX-5033** confirmed that these compounds do not have the selectivity exhibited by **SGC-CK2-1** (Table 2) [16,17]. Finally, when **CX-5011**, **CX-5033**, and **CX-4945** were evaluated for CK2 cellular target engagement, only **CX-4945** and **CX-5011** demonstrated sub-micromolar CK2 cellular target engagement (Table 2). Building on the structure–activity relationships developed by these efforts, the SGC-UNC team identified **SGC-CK2-2**, a naphthyridine-based CK2 chemical probe (Figure 2). Like the previously discussed naphthyridines, **SGC-CK2-2** is a potent inhibitor of CK2 in cell-free enzymatic assays (Table 2). It also demonstrates sub-micromolar CK2 cellular target engagement in the corresponding NanoBRET assays (Table 2). An important distinction from its predecessors is the kinome-wide selectivity of **SGC-CK2-2**. This compound is exquisitely selective (Table 2) and inhibits only CK2α and CK2α′, with a 200-fold selectivity window over the next most potently inhibited kinase (HIPK2). Like **SGC-CK2-1**, **SGC-CK2-2** was not broadly antiproliferative when evaluated in panels of different cancer cell lines [16]. Finally, **SGC-CK2-2N** (Figure 2) was designed as a structurally related negative control compound to be used alongside **SGC-CK2-2** [16].

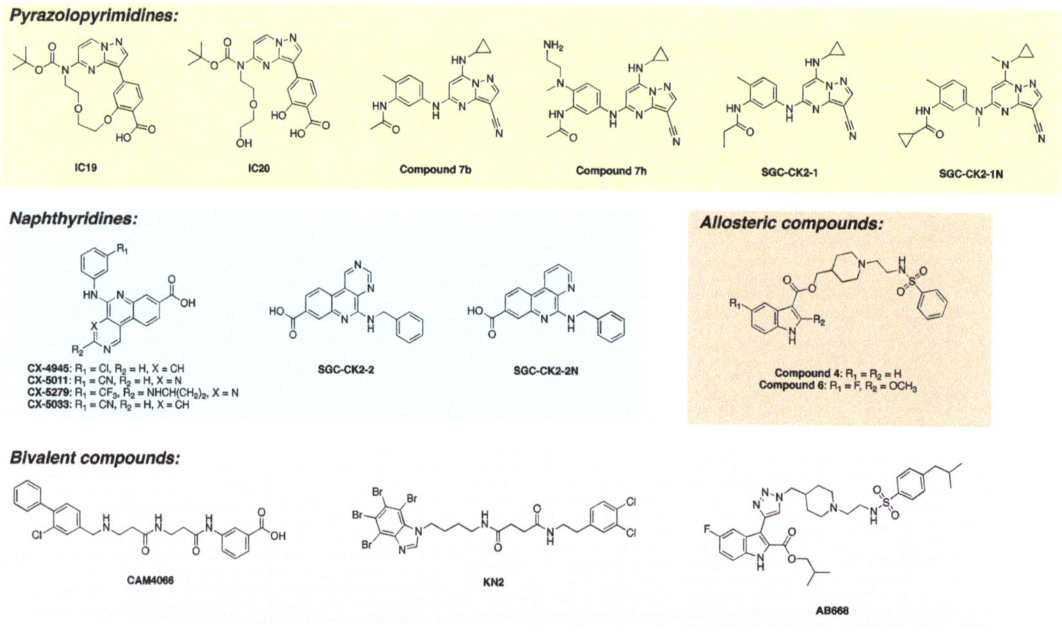

Figure 2. Structures of selected orthosteric, allosteric, and bivalent CK2 inhibitors discussed herein. The pyrazolopyrimidines and naphthyridines represent two chemotypes that have been extensively explored as orthosteric CK2 inhibitors.

Where possible, it is best practice to interrogate a phenotype using chemical probes built upon orthogonal chemotypes. When comparing the in vitro properties of **SGC-CK2-1** and **SGC-CK2-2** (Table 3), some advantages and disadvantages to using each in cell-based studies arise. While the two chemical probes have very similar cell-free enzymatic potency, **SGC-CK2-1** is much more potent in cells. The low nanomolar CK2 cellular target engagement IC_{50} values for **SGC-CK2-1** translate to a much lower concentration needed for efficacy in cell-based studies compared with **SGC-CK2-2**. The aqueous kinetic solubility of **SGC-CK2-2**, however, is much better than that observed for **SGC-CK2-1**. Both compounds are exquisitely selective and, when used at a proper concentration, can be used to deduce that an observed phenotype is driven by the inhibition of CK2. Both CK2 chemical probes were evaluated in cell-based systems only, and thus it has been stressed that their use is limited to in vitro studies.

Table 2. Summary of data for selected orthosteric, allosteric, and bivalent CK2 inhibitors. Details on the binding site and the core scaffold of each inhibitor are specified, together with their biochemical and cellular affinity, if reported. Kinome-wide selectivity data are also summarized, specifying the size of the kinase panel used for selectivity screening and the results. An S_X (Y μM) score indicates the proportion of the kinase panel that binds with <X percent of control remaining when dosed at a concentration of Y μM. The Gini coefficient is a score describing kinase selectivity, with perfect selectivity (inhibiting only a single target, and zero inhibition of all other targets) achieving a score of 1 and equal inhibition of all kinases achieving a score of 0. Negative controls designed to pair with identified chemical probes are also indicated, where available. One or more PDB codes for co-crystal structures with CK2 are also provided, if available. Finally, key references that describe the discovery and characterization of the inhibitor and were used to populate the table are provided as PMID or DOI identifiers.

CK2 Inhibitor	Binding Site	Core Scaffold	Biochemical CK2 Affinity	Cellular CK2 Affinity	Selectivity	Negative Control	PDB Entries	PMIDs/DOI
IC19	Orthosteric	Pyrazolopyrimidine	CK2α ITC K_D = 82 nM	CK2α NB [1] IC_{50} = 1.5 μM; CK2α′ NB IC_{50} = 7.4 μM	469 kinase DiscoverX KINOMEscan S_{35} (1 μM) = 0.07	-	-	32883634
IC20	Orthosteric	Pyrazolopyrimidine	CK2α ITC K_D = 12 nM	CK2α NB IC_{50} = 1.5 μM; CK2α′ NB IC_{50} = 7.6 μM	469 kinase DiscoverX KINOMEscan S_{35} (1 μM) = 0.02	-	6YUM	32883634
Compound 7b	Orthosteric	Pyrazolopyrimidine	CK2α enzymatic IC_{50} < 3.0 nM	CK2α NB IC_{50} = 3.2 nM; CK2α′ NB IC_{50} = 1.8 nM	402 kinase DiscoverX KINOMEscan S_{40} (0.1 μM) = 0.025; 469 kinase DiscoverX KINOMEscan S_{10} (1 μM) = 0.032	-	-	24900749, 33484635
Compound 7h	Orthosteric	Pyrazolopyrimidine	CK2α enzymatic IC_{50} < 3.0 nM; CK2α SPR K_D = 6.3 pM	CK2α NB IC_{50} = 5.3 nM; CK2α′ NB IC_{50} = 4.4 nM	402 kinase DiscoverX KINOMEscan S_{50} (0.1 μM) = 0.03; 469 kinase DiscoverX KINOMEscan S_{10} (1 μM) = 0.042	-	5H8E	26985319, 33484635
SGC-CK2-1	Orthosteric	Pyrazolopyrimidine	CK2α enzymatic IC_{50} = 4.2 nM; CK2α′ enzymatic IC_{50} = 2.3 nM	CK2α NB IC_{50} = 36 nM; CK2α′ NB IC_{50} = 16 nM	468 kinase DiscoverX KINOMEscan S_{10} (1 μM) = 0.007	SGC-CK2-1N	6Z83	33484635
CX-4945	Orthosteric	Naphthyridine	CK2α enzymatic IC_{50} = 1 nM; CK2α′ enzymatic IC_{50} = 1 nM	CK2α NB IC_{50} = 240 nM; CK2α′ NB IC_{50} = 180 nM	468 kinase DiscoverX KINOMEscan S_{10} (1 μM) = 0.069; 235 kinases at 0.5 μM; Gini coefficient = 0.667	-	3NGA, 3PE1	33484635, 21174434, 21870818, 37077385

Table 2. *Cont.*

CK2 Inhibitor	Binding Site	Core Scaffold	Biochemical CK2 Affinity	Cellular CK2 Affinity	Selectivity	Negative Control	PDB Entries	PMIDs/DOI
CX-5011	Orthosteric	Naphthyridine	CK2α enzymatic IC_{50} = 2.3 nM	CK2α NB IC_{50} = 350 nM; CK2α′ NB IC_{50} = 66 nM	235 kinases at 0.5 μM; Gini coefficient = 0.794	-	3PE2	21870818, 37077385
CX-5033	Orthosteric	Naphthyridine	CK2 holoenzyme enzymatic IC_{50} = 4.0 nM	CK2α NB IC_{50} = 4300 nM; CK2α′ NB IC_{50} = 1900 nM	468 kinase DiscoverX KINOMEscan S_{10} (1 μM) = 0.079; 103 kinases at 0.5 μM; Gini coefficient = 0.570	-	-	21174434, 21870818, 37077385
CX-5279	Orthosteric	Naphthyridine	CK2α enzymatic IC_{50} = 0.91 nM	-	102 kinases at 0.5 μM; Gini coefficient = 0.755	-	3R0T	21870818
SGC-CK2-2	Orthosteric	Naphthyridine	CK2α enzymatic IC_{50} = 3.0 nM; CK2α′ enzymatic IC_{50} < 1.0 nM	CK2α NB IC_{50} = 920 nM; CK2α′ NB IC_{50} = 200 nM	468 kinase DiscoverX KINOMEscan S_{10} (1 μM) = 0.007	SGC-CK2-2N	8BGC	37077385
Compound 4	Allosteric	Indole-3-carboxylate	CK2β-dependent enzymatic IC_{50} = 45 μM; CK2α K_D = 41 μM	-	-	-	6FVG	31685885
Compound 6	Allosteric	Indole-3-carboxylate	CK2β-dependent enzymatic IC_{50} = 22 μM; CK2α K_D = 30 μM	-	-	-	6FVF	31685885
CAM4066	Bivalent	Biphenylmethylamine	CK2α ITC K_D = 320 nM; CK2α enzymatic IC_{50} = 370 nM	-	52 kinases at 2 μM; Gini coefficient = 0.82	-	5CU3, 5CU4, 5MO8	28451126

Table 2. *Cont.*

CK2 Inhibitor	Binding Site	Core Scaffold	Biochemical CK2 Affinity	Cellular CK2 Affinity	Selectivity	Negative Control	PDB Entries	PMIDs/DOI
KN2	Bivalent	Benzoimidazole	$CK2\alpha_2\beta_2$ holoenzyme enzymatic IC_{50} = 19 nM and K_i = 6.1 nM; $CK2\alpha'_2\beta_2$ holoenzyme enzymatic IC_{50} = 16 nM and K_i = 4.0 nM	-	83 kinases at 3 µM; Gini coefficient = 0.76	-	7AT5	34323071
AB668	Bivalent	Indole-2-carboxylate	CK2α binding assay K_D = 86 nM; CK2β-dependent enzymatic K_i = 41 nM	-	468 kinase DiscoverX KINOMEscan S_{10} (2 µM) = 0.007	-	-	10.1101/2022.12.16.520736

[1] NB = NanoBRET.

Table 3. Comparison of SGC-CK2-1 and SGC-CK2-2 in terms of potency, selectivity, and solubility.

	SGC-CK2-1	SGC-CK2-2
CK2α enzymatic IC_{50}	4.2 nM	3.0 nM
CK2α′ enzymatic IC_{50}	2.3 nM	<1.0 nM
Selectivity: S_{10} (1 μM)	0.007	0.007
Selectivity window	100-fold over DYRK2	200-fold over HIPK2
CK2α NanoBRET IC_{50}	36 nM	920 nM
CK2α′ NanoBRET IC_{50}	19 nM	200 nM
Kinetic solubility	3.7 μM	211 μM

2.2. Selected Allosteric and Bivalent CK2 Inhibitors in Development

As a strategy to achieve selectivity for CK2, several groups have pursued the identification of CK2 inhibitors that bind outside of the ATP-binding site. Compounds **4** and **6** (Figure 2), which were developed from a parent compound discovered via virtual screening, are reported to bind to the CK2α/CK2β interface. SPR, crystallographic, and nMR experiments were used to confirm binding to CK2α and inhibition of CK2β-dependent enzymatic activity, albeit with mid-micromolar K_D/IC_{50} values (Table 2). While inhibition of cancer cell growth and downstream signaling was demonstrated in response to treatment with compound **6**, CK2 cellular target engagement was not demonstrated, and a lack of selectivity data makes it difficult to interpret the results as CK2-specific [21].

CAM4066 is a bivalent CK2 inhibitor that binds to the αD pocket on CK2α and also occupies the CK2α ATP site. This compound is an elaborated version of the original fragment hit, which was identified via a high-concentration crystallographic screen. **CAM4066** was shown to bind to CK2α via ITC with a K_D = 320 nM and, correspondingly, to inhibit the enzymatic activity of CK2α with an IC_{50} = 370 nM (Table 2). In a small, 52-member selectivity screen, **CAM4066** exhibited improved selectivity versus **CX-4945** (Table 2). The ability of **CAM4066** to inhibit the growth of three different cancer cell lines was examined but its cellular penetrance was questioned when no effect on cellular viability was observed [25,27]. No experiments that would provide evidence of cellular target engagement with CK2 by **CAM4066** have been provided.

Like **CAM4066**, **KN2** is a bivalent CK2 inhibitor that occupies the αD pocket and ATP site as well. **KN2**, however, was designed to bind to the CK2α′, rather than the CK2α, αD pocket and ATP site. 3,4-Dichlorophenethylamine (DPA) was used to anchor the bivalent ligand in the CK2α′ αD pocket, while a derivative of 4,5,6,7-tetrabromo-1*H*-benzo[*d*]imidazole (TBI) called TBIa engaged the CK2α′ ATP site. The two were covalently linked via succinic acid through the formation of amide bonds. **KN2** was found to bind and inhibit the CK2 holoenzymes comprising $CK2\alpha_2\beta_2$ or $CK2\alpha'_2\beta_2$ with low nanomolar K_i/IC_{50} values, respectively (Table 2). The CK2 binding affinity of **KN2** was between that of **CX-4945** and **CAM4066**. Selectivity profiling of **KN2** versus 83 kinases revealed it to demonstrate a selectivity score between that of **CAM4066** (more selective) and **CX-4945** (less selective), albeit kinase panels of variable sizes and different concentrations of the inhibitor were employed in each screen (Table 2). While cell-based toxicity assays demonstrated that **KN2** is cytotoxic and, therefore, cell-permeable, CK2 cellular target engagement has not been assessed for this compound. Western blots of CK2 substrates have been used to demonstrate the inhibition of downstream CK2 signaling by **KN2** [26].

A final bivalent compound that has recently been disclosed is **AB668**. Like **CAM4066** and **KN2**, **AB668** binds both at the CK2 ATP site and the allosteric αD pocket. A thermal shift assay and X-ray crystallography were used to confirm binding to CK2α, which was then quantified using a CK2α active site-directed competition binding assay, revealing a K_D = 86 nM (Table 2). **AB668** demonstrated inhibition of the CK2 holoenzyme with K_i = 41 nM. The kinome-wide selectivity of **AB668** was profiled using the largest commercial panel and was found to be exquisitely selective, matching the selectivity of **SGC-CK2-1** and **SGC-CK2-2**. **AB668** was found to induce caspase-3 activation in clear cell renal cell carcinoma, elicit significant cell proliferation arrest in two cancer cell lines, and reduce cell viability in an ex vivo culture model of renal carcinoma. Assaying the CK2 activity in treated cell extracts has been used to indirectly assess the CK2 cellular target engagement of **AB668** [28].

3. Use of SGC-CK2-1 by the Community in Cell-Based Studies

SGC-CK2-1 was developed to be a useful CK2-targeting chemical probe in cells. The seminal paper on this probe did not evaluate its utility in vivo. This compound was made immediately available to all interested investigators via request from the original authors, through the SGC, and by multiple chemical vendors. Additional attention was drawn to **SGC-CK2-1** by a spotlight in *Trends in Pharmacological Sciences* [49]. Follow-up studies have been carried out with **SGC-CK2-1**, both in collaboration with the original authors and independently.

The development and validation of an assay in microglia derived from human-induced stem cells (hiPSCs) enabled side-by-side evaluation of the ability of **SGC-CK2-1** and **CX-4945** to blunt an inflammatory response. Briefly, to define the role of CK2 in microglia, wild type hiPSC-derived microglial-like cells (MGLs) and those homozygous for an autosomal dominant mutation in presenilin-1 (PSEN1ΔE9), which is causative for early-onset familial Alzheimer's disease (AD), were stimulated with lipopolysaccharides for 24 h in the absence or presence of either **SGC-CK2-1** or **CX-4945** [50]. Both mRNA and protein for IL-6 and IL1-β, two pro-inflammatory cytokines that are increased in AD patients and, when increased, correlate with cognitive impairments, were examined [50–56]. A dose–dependent and significant inhibition of the inflammatory response without associated toxicity was observed in both wild type and PSEN1ΔE9 MGLs in response to low nanomolar **SGC-CK2-1** treatment. Furthermore, **SGC-CK2-1** much more efficiently suppressed inflammatory cytokine expression than **CX-4945,** and the data suggested a difference in the effectiveness of CK2 inhibition in the wild type versus PSEN1ΔE9 MGLs [50].

SGC-CK2-1 was also employed in a study that characterized the role of CK2 in β-coronavirus replication and entry. Alongside other pyrazolopyrimidines, the efficiency of **SGC-CK2-1** and **CX-4945** to block the replication of pathogenic human, bat, and murine β-coronaviruses was explored and confirmed. The potency of CK2α cellular target engagement by CK2 inhibitors from divergent chemical series was found to correlate with antiviral activity. Furthermore, the essential role of the CK2 holoenzyme in β-coronavirus replication was corroborated via genetic knockdown. Through the use of a spike protein endocytosis assay, **SGC-CK2-1** was also shown to suppress viral entry [4].

In a study aimed at refining the list of bona fide CK2 substrates, **SGC-CK2-1** and **CX-4945** were once again used side-by-side and compared. Using triple stable isotope labeling by amino acids in cell culture (SILAC) in combination with inhibitor-resistant CK2, a reliable method was established for the identification and validation of CK2 substrates [57]. This methodology was employed to evaluate the selectivity of **CX-4945** versus **SGC-CK2-1**. It was determined that only a minority of phosphosites that were significantly downregulated in response to **CX-4945** treatment were CSNK2A1-dependent. In comparison, the majority of phosphosites that were significantly downregulated in response to **SGC-CK2-1** treatment were CSNK2A1-dependent. The authors concluded based on their data that **SGC-CK2-1** demonstrates significantly enhanced selectivity toward CSNK2A1 compared to **CX-4945**. Through the use of inhibitor-resistant CK2 cells in tandem with **SGC-CK2-1**, more than 300 CSNK2A1-dependent phosphosites were identified [2,10].

SGC-CK2-1 and **CX-4945** were used in parallel to evaluate the importance of CK2 in promoting insulin production and secretion from pancreatic β-cells. Without associated toxicity, both compounds downregulated the endogenous CK2 activity to a similar extent. In addition, both **SGC-CK2-1** and **CX-4945** increased the message for insulin and amplified insulin secretion from storage vesicles. The use of **SGC-CK2-1** in their experiments allowed the authors to unambiguously attribute the observed responses to inhibition of CK2 [58].

A known role of CK2 in the regulation of NG2 gene expression and the connection of NG2 expression with juvenile angiofibroma (JA) motivated the exploration of whether

CK2 inhibition could be a therapeutical avenue for JA patients. For this study, the authors explored whether CK2 inhibition suppressed NG2-dependent JA cell proliferation and migration. Via Western blot, immunohistochemistry, flow cytometry, and quantitative real-time PCR, NG2, and CK2 were found to be expressed in JA patient-derived tissue samples and JA patient-derived cells. The treatment of JA patient-derived cells with either **SGC-CK2-1** or **CX-4945** resulted in a significant reduction in the NG2 gene and protein expression, which was accompanied by reduced proliferation and migration of these cells. The use of **SGC-CK2-1** enabled the interrogation of a promising new therapeutic approach for a cohort of JA patients [59].

4. Development of an In Vivo CK2 Probe

4.1. Definition of an In Vivo Chemical Probe

While the abovementioned chemical probes are validated in vitro, it is also of interest to develop chemical probes that can be used to interrogate CK2 function in vivo. While there has not been a consensus on the properties of an in vivo chemical probe, we propose the following criteria (Table 4) in addition to the criteria required for an in vitro chemical probe (Table 1).

Table 4. Proposed parameters to benchmark an in vivo chemical probe.

Proposed In Vivo Chemical Probe Criteria
1. For at least one animal model, detailed characterization is provided for pharmacokinetic parameters: bioavailability (F), half-life ($t_{1/2}$), intrinsic clearance (CL_{int}), the volume of distribution (V_d), maximum concentration (C_{max}) and the time taken to reach it (t_{max});
2. Dosing regimen optimized: dose amount, frequency of dose, route of administration, and formulation;
3. Maintain a concentration $\geq 3\times$ the in vitro cellular IC_{50}/EC_{50} in the plasma or relevant tissue compartment;
4. Demonstrate in vivo target engagement or target inhibition in the plasma or relevant tissue compartment.

Firstly, a detailed pharmacokinetic study would be required to investigate key pharmacokinetic parameters relevant to drug dosing in an appropriate animal model. These parameters include the bioavailability (F) of an oral (p.o.) or intraperitoneal (i.p.) route of administration. The compound concentration over time in the plasma, as well as in any relevant tissue compartments, should be characterized to determine the half-life ($t_{1/2}$), intrinsic clearance (CL_{int}), and maximum concentration (C_{max}) and the time taken to reach it (t_{max}). The volume of distribution (V_d) would also provide information about the distribution of the compound within the animal. We do not propose specific criteria or cut-offs for any of these parameters, as we recognize that these parameters are primarily relevant for the optimization of the dosing regimen, including the dose amount, frequency of dose, route of administration, and formulation. While the oral route of administration is preferred for drugs, for chemical probes intended to interrogate the effects of target inhibition in vivo, the intraperitoneal route of administration is acceptable and offers benefits to bypass absorption challenges [60]. It is crucial to note that the pharmacokinetic parameters will likely differ by animal species and strain. However, given the diversity of animal models used for different studies, it would be cost- and time-prohibitive to characterize such parameters and optimize dosing regimens across multiple animal models. Therefore, we emphasize that the prudent use of in vivo chemical probes across different animal models would require measuring the pharmacokinetic parameters and adjusting the dosing regimen in each case. However, the data provided in one animal model would ideally provide a clear starting point to enable optimization of the dosing regimen for different models. For this reason, we recommend detailed characterization and reporting of pharmacokinetic parameters as a criterion for an in vivo chemical probe (Table 4).

An optimal dosing regimen should maintain the compound concentration at least 3-fold higher than the cellular IC_{50}/EC_{50} in the plasma or the relevant tissue compartment. The duration of which the necessary compound concentration is maintained should be taken into account when optimizing dosing frequency. Finally, for an in vivo chemical probe, it is also important to demonstrate either target engagement or target inhibition in plasma or a relevant tissue compartment and relate this with concentration measured for a pharmacokinetic–pharmacodynamic (PK–PD) analysis [61]. This could be performed by measuring a biochemical effect of inhibiting the target (e.g., downstream phosphorylation of a phosphosite specific to the kinase inhibited), or through other target engagement techniques, such as the cellular thermal shift assay (CETSA) [62,63]. We summarize a general workflow that aligns with our above proposal to arrive at an in vivo chemical probe (Figure 3).

4.2. Progress toward an In Vivo Chemical Probe

Efforts have been made to develop an in vivo chemical probe using the pyrazolopyrimidine scaffold. AstraZeneca reported the inhibition of in vivo downstream phosphorylation of AKT^{S129} by compounds **7b** and **7h** in mouse xenografts [43,44]. These compounds, however, demonstrate suboptimal selectivity, and their pharmacokinetic parameters are not reported, precluding characterization of their suitability as in vivo chemical probes. As mentioned previously, **SGC-CK2-1** is a great cellular tool but is recognized only as an in vitro chemical probe. Efforts to optimize **SGC-CK2-1** for in vivo use were hindered by its moderate aqueous solubility and rapid metabolism, where 60% of the compound was degraded in vitro in mouse liver microsomes with 30 min of incubation [64]. Even after successful medicinal chemistry optimization to reduce metabolism in mouse liver microsomes, the SGC-UNC team found that Phase II metabolism in mouse hepatocytes in vitro and in mice (in vivo) contributed significantly to the rapid metabolism of compounds of the pyrazolopyrimidine scaffold [64]. While it was possible to improve the exposure of pyrazolopyrimidines in vivo by co-dosing with CYP450 inhibitor 1-aminobenzotriazole and GST inhibitor ethacrynic acid, co-dosing with these broad metabolic inhibitors would likely affect other physiological processes unrelated to CK2 inhibition, and is thus unsuitable for the study of CK2 in vivo [64]. Further work is still ongoing to optimize the pyrazolopyrimidines for use in vivo without the need to co-dose with metabolic inhibitors.

Relative to the pyrazolopyrimidines, the naphthyridine series has been used in vivo more frequently. Of the naphthyridines, **CX-4945** is the frontrunner as a drug candidate under clinical investigation [47,65]. **CX-4945** demonstrated an excellent pharmacokinetic profile, with 20–51% oral bioavailability and long half-lives of 5.0–11.6 h in mice, rats, and dogs. This outstanding pharmacokinetic profile also extends to other naphthyridines, such as **CX-5011**, which demonstrates 44% oral bioavailability and 3.3–6.4 h half-life in rats and dogs [66]. When dosed in vivo, **CX-4945** also demonstrated tumor growth inhibition in mouse xenograft models with oral dosing [19,67], concurrent with a decrease in phosphorylation of $p21^{T145}$ in the tumor xenografts [67,68]. **CX-4945** also demonstrated permeability through the blood–brain barrier, which was reflected by the inhibition of CK2 substrates in intracranial xenograft models [6]. This is especially exciting as CK2 is a key player in neurodevelopment and in multiple neurological disorders [8,69], including Alzheimer's disease [5,7,70–73], and having a potent and selective, brain-penetrant in vivo tool molecule for CK2 inhibition would be extremely valuable. The limited selectivity of **CX-4945** must be acknowledged, and its application as an in vivo tool to attribute phenotypic effects to CK2 inhibition must be considered with caution. For example, DYRK1A is one of the potent off-targets of **CX-4945** [17,74]. Consequently, the in vivo inhibition of Tau^{T212}, a substrate of DYRK1A, was confirmed in mice, and **CX-4945** rescued neurological defects from overexpression of *mnb*, the ortholog of DYRK1A, in *Drosophila* [74]. It is important to note that the strain of mice and the doses of **CX-4945** used in this study were similar to those for the aforementioned in vivo studies. As such, both the inhibition of CK2 in this study and the inhibition of DYRK1A in the other in vivo studies are expected, and any phenotypic effect cannot be solely attributed to the inhibition of either CK2 or DYRK1A. This accentuates the need for selectivity in the criteria for a chemical probe and highlights the importance of utilizing orthogonal chemical probes when possible. As the naphthyridine compounds have better pharmacokinetic properties than the pyrazolopyrimidines, optimization based on a selective starting point, such as **SGC-CK2-2,** is a promising path forward toward an in vivo chemical probe for this chemical series.

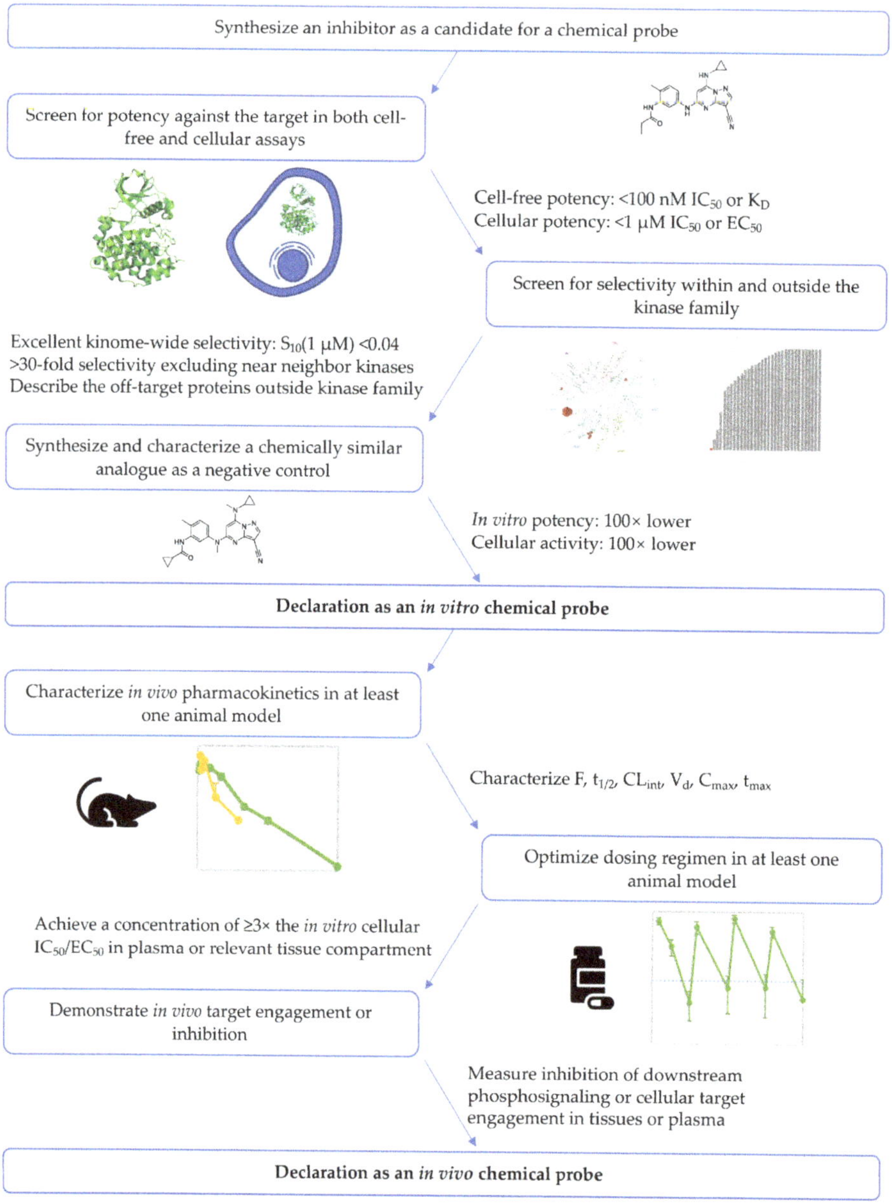

Figure 3. A proposed workflow for the development of an in vivo chemical probe, starting from a candidate compound. Characterization as an in vitro chemical probe and then in vivo characterization as an in vivo chemical probe are the next steps in the process.

Another CK2 inhibitor under clinical investigation is **CIGB-300** (also known as **CIGB-325**), a cell-permeable peptide that binds to CK2 substrates [29,75] and to CK2 directly [76,77] to prevent CK2-induced phosphorylation. **CIGB-300** demonstrated the inhibition of tumor growth in multiple cancer cell lines in vitro and also in vivo when administered via intratumor injections [29]. A follow-up study showed that **CIGB-300** may also be administered via intraperitoneal or intravenous routes and accumulates in tumors [78]. **CIGB-300** demonstrated preliminary efficacy in clinical investigations [79–82], lending support for its tolerability and efficacy in vivo. Because of the unique mechanism of action of **CIGB-300**, it offers an orthogonal approach to interrogate CK2 activity in vivo. If efforts are made to fully characterize the binding partners and mechanism of action of **CIGB-300**, it may demonstrate utility as a chemical probe.

5. Conclusions

The two clinically investigated inhibitors, **CX-4945** and **CIGB-300,** are the culmination of the extensive research invested in the development of CK2 inhibitors as drugs with a focus on oncology. The inhibition of tumor growth in response to CK2 inhibitors is often attributed to CK2 inhibition. Yet, full characterization of the kinome-wide inhibitory profile of traditional CK2 inhibitors reveals that some, including **CX-4945**, are not sufficiently selective to allow attribution of a phenotype to CK2. A more selective chemical probe is thus required for investigating CK2 function. The development of **SGC-CK2-1** and **SGC-CK2-2**, two highly selective CK2 chemical probes from distinct chemotypes, addresses this need and helps to deconvolute responses driven by CK2 inhibition. In particular, the lack of broad-spectrum antitumor activity of **SGC-CK2-1** calls into question if the antitumor effects of **CX-4945** are indeed caused by the on-target inhibition of CK2 alone [17]. The adoption of **SGC-CK2-1** as a CK2 chemical probe by the scientific community for use in cell-based studies is a positive step forward. We emphasize that the best practice of using a chemical probe is in parallel with its associated negative control, and/or the use of two orthogonal chemical probes [83]. Both options are currently enabled for CK2.

CK2 chemical probes can still be further improved. Of the allosteric and bivalent inhibitors reported, **AB668** demonstrates the best selectivity profile. This represents a promising direction toward the development of a third CK2 chemical probe, with an orthogonal scaffold to the two currently established chemical probes and differential binding mode. The peptidic inhibitor **CIGB-300** is also a potential candidate orthogonal chemical probe for CK2, but further characterization of its binding partners is required due to its unique mechanism of action. It is also of interest to develop probes for in vivo study of CK2 function, and much work still needs to be performed in this area. While optimization of pyrazolopyrimidines was met with challenges due to metabolic instability, the naphthyridines have demonstrated an improved pharmacokinetic profile. Further optimization of their in vivo potency would potentially lead to a suitable chemical probe from the naphthyridine series for use in living organisms.

The use of CK2 chemical probes has shed much light on the function of this pleiotropic kinase. Two chemical probes have been vetted and embraced so far, but the development of additional chemical probes would allow the scientific community to perform better experiments, in vitro or in vivo. These basic science experiments with high-quality probes will enable the community to determine which diseases are candidates for treatment with selective CK2 inhibitors.

Author Contributions: Conceptualization, D.H.D. and A.D.A.; methodology, H.W.O. and D.H.D.; investigation, H.W.O. and A.D.A.; writing—original draft preparation, H.W.O. and A.D.A.; writing—review and editing, all authors.; visualization, H.W.O. and A.D.A.; supervision, D.H.D. and A.D.A.; project administration, D.H.D. and A.D.A.; funding acquisition, D.H.D. and A.D.A. All authors have read and agreed to the published version of the manuscript.

Funding: The Structural Genomics Consortium (SGC) is a registered charity (number 1097737) that receives funds from Bayer AG, Boehringer Ingelheim, the Canada Foundation for Innovation, the Eshelman Institute for Innovation, Genentech, Genome Canada through the Ontario Genomics Institute, EU/EFPIA/OICR/McGill/KTH/Diamond, Innovative Medicines Initiative 2 Joint Undertaking, Janssen, Merck KGaA (aka EMD in Canada and USA), Pfizer, the São Paulo Research Foundation-FAPESP, and Takeda. Research reported in this publication was supported in part by NIH U24DK116204 and DoD ALSRP award AL190107. The North Carolina Policy Collaboratory at the University of North Carolina at Chapel Hill with funding from the North Carolina Coronavirus Relief Fund established and appropriated by the North Carolina General Assembly and a grant from Takeda contributed to work reviewed herein.

Institutional Review Board Statement: Not applicable.

Informed Consent Statement: Not applicable.

Data Availability Statement: Not applicable.

Conflicts of Interest: The authors declare no conflict of interest.

References

1. Meggio, F.; Pinna, L.A. One-thousand-and-one substrates of protein kinase CK2? *FASEB J. Off. Publ. Fed. Am. Soc. Exp. Biol.* **2003**, *17*, 349–368. [CrossRef] [PubMed]
2. Menyhart, D.; Gyenis, L.; Jurcic, K.; Roffey, S.E.; Puri, A.; Jovanovic, P.; Szkop, K.J.; Pittock, P.; Lajoie, G.; Axtman, A.D.; et al. Comparison of CX-4945 and SGC-CK2-1 as inhibitors of CSNK2 using quantitative phosphoproteomics: Triple SILAC in combination with inhibitor-resistant CSNK2. *Curr. Res. Chem. Biol.* **2023**, *3*, 100041. [CrossRef]
3. Salvi, M.; Borgo, C.; Pinna, L.A.; Ruzzene, M. Targeting CK2 in cancer: A valuable strategy or a waste of time? *Cell Death Discov.* **2021**, *7*, 325. [CrossRef] [PubMed]
4. Yang, X.; Dickmander, R.J.; Bayati, A.; Taft-Benz, S.A.; Smith, J.L.; Wells, C.I.; Madden, E.A.; Brown, J.W.; Lenarcic, E.M.; Yount, B.L.; et al. Host Kinase CSNK2 is a Target for Inhibition of Pathogenic SARS-like β-Coronaviruses. *ACS Chem. Biol.* **2022**, *17*, 1937–1950. [CrossRef] [PubMed]
5. Zhang, Q.; Xia, Y.; Wang, Y.; Shentu, Y.; Zeng, K.; Mahaman, Y.A.R.; Huang, F.; Wu, M.; Ke, D.; Wang, Q.; et al. CK2 Phosphorylating I2PP2A/SET Mediates Tau Pathology and Cognitive Impairment. *Front. Mol. Neurosci.* **2018**, *11*, 146. [CrossRef] [PubMed]
6. Zheng, Y.; McFarland, B.C.; Drygin, D.; Yu, H.; Bellis, S.L.; Kim, H.; Bredel, M.; Benveniste, E.N. Targeting Protein Kinase CK2 Suppresses Prosurvival Signaling Pathways and Growth of Glioblastoma. *Clin. Cancer Res.* **2013**, *19*, 6484–6494. [CrossRef]
7. Rosenberger, A.F.N.; Morrema, T.H.J.; Gerritsen, W.H.; van Haastert, E.S.; Snkhchyan, H.; Hilhorst, R.; Rozemuller, A.J.M.; Scheltens, P.; van der Vies, S.M.; Hoozemans, J.J.M. Increased occurrence of protein kinase CK2 in astrocytes in Alzheimer's disease pathology. *J. Neuroinflamm.* **2016**, *13*, 4. [CrossRef]
8. Perez, D.I.; Gil, C.; Martinez, A. Protein kinases CK1 and CK2 as new targets for neurodegenerative diseases. *Med. Res. Rev.* **2011**, *31*, 924–954. [CrossRef] [PubMed]
9. Borgo, C.; D'Amore, C.; Sarno, S.; Salvi, M.; Ruzzene, M. Protein kinase CK2: A potential therapeutic target for diverse human diseases. *Signal Transduct. Target. Ther.* **2021**, *6*, 183. [CrossRef]
10. Litchfield, D.W.; Gyenis, L.; Menyhart, D.; Roffey, S.E. Towards the CSNK2 phosphoproteome—With lessons from the COVID-19 pandemic to revealing the secrets of CSNK2 and its promise as a therapeutic target. *Biochim. Biophys. Acta (BBA)—Gen. Subj.* **2023**, *1867*, 130441. [CrossRef]
11. Litchfield, D.W.; Bosc, D.G.; Canton, D.A.; Saulnier, R.B.; Vilk, G.; Zhang, C. Functional specialization of CK2 isoforms and characterization of isoform-specific binding partners. *Mol. Cell. Biochem.* **2001**, *227*, 21–29. [CrossRef] [PubMed]
12. Pinna, L.A. Protein kinase CK2: A challenge to canons. *J. Cell Sci.* **2002**, *115*, 3873–3878. [CrossRef] [PubMed]
13. Bibby, A.C.; Litchfield, D.W. The multiple personalities of the regulatory subunit of protein kinase CK2: CK2 dependent and CK2 independent roles reveal a secret identity for CK2beta. *Int. J. Biol. Sci.* **2005**, *1*, 67–79. [CrossRef] [PubMed]
14. Iegre, J.; Atkinson, E.L.; Brear, P.D.; Cooper, B.M.; Hyvönen, M.; Spring, D.R. Chemical probes targeting the kinase CK2: A journey outside the catalytic box. *Org. Biomol. Chem.* **2021**, *19*, 4380–4396. [CrossRef]
15. Atkinson, E.L.; Iegre, J.; Brear, P.D.; Zhabina, E.A.; Hyvönen, M.; Spring, D.R. Downfalls of Chemical Probes Acting at the Kinase ATP-Site: CK2 as a Case Study. *Molecules* **2021**, *26*, 1977. [CrossRef]
16. Davis-Gilbert, Z.W.; Krämer, A.; Dunford, J.E.; Howell, S.; Senbabaoglu, F.; Wells, C.I.; Bashore, F.M.; Havener, T.M.; Smith, J.L.; Hossain, M.A.; et al. Discovery of a Potent and Selective Naphthyridine-Based Chemical Probe for Casein Kinase 2. *ACS Med. Chem. Lett.* **2023**, *14*, 432–441. [CrossRef]
17. Wells, C.I.; Drewry, D.H.; Pickett, J.E.; Tjaden, A.; Krämer, A.; Müller, S.; Gyenis, L.; Menyhart, D.; Litchfield, D.W.; Knapp, S.; et al. Development of a Potent and Selective Chemical Probe for the Pleiotropic Kinase CK2. *Cell Chem. Biol.* **2021**, *28*, 546–558.e10. [CrossRef]

18. Krämer, A.; Kurz, C.G.; Berger, B.-T.; Celik, I.E.; Tjaden, A.; Greco, F.A.; Knapp, S.; Hanke, T. Optimization of pyrazolo[1,5-a]pyrimidines lead to the identification of a highly selective casein kinase 2 inhibitor. *Eur. J. Med. Chem.* **2020**, *208*, 112770. [CrossRef]
19. Pierre, F.; Chua, P.C.; O'Brien, S.E.; Siddiqui-Jain, A.; Bourbon, P.; Haddach, M.; Michaux, J.; Nagasawa, J.; Schwaebe, M.K.; Stefan, E.; et al. Discovery and SAR of 5-(3-chlorophenylamino)benzo[c][2,6]naphthyridine-8-carboxylic acid (CX-4945), the first clinical stage inhibitor of protein kinase CK2 for the treatment of cancer. *J. Med. Chem.* **2011**, *54*, 635–654. [CrossRef]
20. Battistutta, R.; Cozza, G.; Pierre, F.; Papinutto, E.; Lolli, G.; Sarno, S.; O'Brien, S.E.; Siddiqui-Jain, A.; Haddach, M.; Anderes, K.; et al. Unprecedented selectivity and structural determinants of a new class of protein kinase CK2 inhibitors in clinical trials for the treatment of cancer. *Biochemistry* **2011**, *50*, 8478–8488. [CrossRef]
21. Kufareva, I.; Bestgen, B.; Brear, P.; Prudent, R.; Laudet, B.; Moucadel, V.; Ettaoussi, M.; Sautel, C.F.; Krimm, I.; Engel, M.; et al. Discovery of holoenzyme-disrupting chemicals as substrate-selective CK2 inhibitors. *Sci. Rep.* **2019**, *9*, 15893. [CrossRef] [PubMed]
22. Meggio, F.; Shugar, D.; Pinna, L.A. Ribofuranosyl-benzimidazole derivatives as inhibitors of casein kinase-2 and casein kinase-1. *Eur. J. Biochem.* **1990**, *187*, 89–94. [CrossRef]
23. Laudet, B.; Moucadel, V.; Prudent, R.; Filhol, O.; Wong, Y.S.; Royer, D.; Cochet, C. Identification of chemical inhibitors of protein-kinase CK2 subunit interaction. *Mol. Cell Biochem.* **2008**, *316*, 63–69. [CrossRef] [PubMed]
24. Moucadel, V.; Prudent, R.; Sautel, C.F.; Teillet, F.; Barette, C.; Lafanechere, L.; Receveur-Brechot, V.; Cochet, C. Antitumoral activity of allosteric inhibitors of protein kinase CK2. *Oncotarget* **2011**, *2*, 997–1010. [CrossRef] [PubMed]
25. De Fusco, C.; Brear, P.; Iegre, J.; Georgiou, K.H.; Sore, H.F.; Hyvönen, M.; Spring, D.R. A fragment-based approach leading to the discovery of a novel binding site and the selective CK2 inhibitor CAM4066. *Bioorg. Med. Chem.* **2017**, *25*, 3471–3482. [CrossRef]
26. Lindenblatt, D.; Applegate, V.; Nickelsen, A.; Klußmann, M.; Neundorf, I.; Götz, C.; Jose, J.; Niefind, K. Molecular Plasticity of Crystalline CK2α′ Leads to KN2, a Bivalent Inhibitor of Protein Kinase CK2 with Extraordinary Selectivity. *J. Med. Chem.* **2022**, *65*, 1302–1312. [CrossRef]
27. Brear, P.; De Fusco, C.; Hadje Georgiou, K.; Francis-Newton, N.J.; Stubbs, C.J.; Sore, H.F.; Venkitaraman, A.R.; Abell, C.; Spring, D.R.; Hyvönen, M. Specific inhibition of CK2α from an anchor outside the active site. *Chem. Sci.* **2016**, *7*, 6839–6845. [CrossRef]
28. Bancet, A.; Frem, R.; Jeanneret, F.; Mularoni, A.; Bazelle, P.; Roelants, C.; Delcros, J.-G.; Guichou, J.-F.; Pillet, C.; Coste, I.; et al. AB668, a novel highly selective protein kinase CK2 inhibitor with a distinct anti-tumor mechanism as compared to CX-4945 and SGC-CK2-1. *bioRxiv* **2022**. [CrossRef]
29. Perea, S.E.; Reyes, O.; Puchades, Y.; Mendoza, O.; Vispo, N.S.; Torrens, I.; Santos, A.; Silva, R.; Acevedo, B.; López, E.; et al. Antitumor effect of a novel proapoptotic peptide that impairs the phosphorylation by the protein kinase 2 (casein kinase 2). *Cancer Res.* **2004**, *64*, 7127–7129. [CrossRef]
30. Gottardo, M.F.; Capobianco, C.S.; Sidabra, J.E.; Garona, J.; Perera, Y.; Perea, S.E.; Alonso, D.F.; Farina, H.G. Preclinical efficacy of CIGB-300, an anti-CK2 peptide, on breast cancer metastasic colonization. *Sci. Rep.* **2020**, *10*, 14689. [CrossRef]
31. Enkvist, E.; Viht, K.; Bischoff, N.; Vahter, J.; Saaver, S.; Raidaru, G.; Issinger, O.-G.; Niefind, K.; Uri, A. A subnanomolar fluorescent probe for protein kinase CK2 interaction studies. *Org. Biomol. Chem.* **2012**, *10*, 8645–8653. [CrossRef] [PubMed]
32. Viht, K.; Saaver, S.; Vahter, J.; Enkvist, E.; Lavogina, D.; Sinijärv, H.; Raidaru, G.; Guerra, B.; Issinger, O.G.; Uri, A. Acetoxymethyl Ester of Tetrabromobenzimidazole-Peptoid Conjugate for Inhibition of Protein Kinase CK2 in Living Cells. *Bioconjugate Chem.* **2015**, *26*, 2324–2335. [CrossRef] [PubMed]
33. Tsien, R.Y. A non-disruptive technique for loading calcium buffers and indicators into cells. *Nature* **1981**, *290*, 527–528. [CrossRef]
34. Vahter, J.; Viht, K.; Uri, A.; Enkvist, E. Oligo-aspartic acid conjugates with benzo[c][2,6]naphthyridine-8-carboxylic acid scaffold as picomolar inhibitors of CK2. *Bioorg. Med. Chem.* **2017**, *25*, 2277–2284. [CrossRef]
35. Wells, C.I.; Al-Ali, H.; Andrews, D.M.; Asquith, C.R.M.; Axtman, A.D.; Dikic, I.; Ebner, D.; Ettmayer, P.; Fischer, C.; Frederiksen, M.; et al. The Kinase Chemogenomic Set (KCGS): An Open Science Resource for Kinase Vulnerability Identification. *Int. J. Mol. Sci.* **2021**, *22*, 566. [CrossRef] [PubMed]
36. Wells, C.; Couñago, R.M.; Limas, J.C.; Almeida, T.L.; Cook, J.G.; Drewry, D.H.; Elkins, J.M.; Gileadi, O.; Kapadia, N.R.; Lorente-Macias, A.; et al. SGC-AAK1-1: A Chemical Probe Targeting AAK1 and BMP2K. *ACS Med. Chem. Lett.* **2019**, *11*, 340–345. [CrossRef]
37. Besnard, J.; Ruda, G.F.; Setola, V.; Abecassis, K.; Rodriguiz, R.M.; Huang, X.P.; Norval, S.; Sassano, M.F.; Shin, A.I.; Webster, L.A.; et al. Automated design of ligands to polypharmacological profiles. *Nature* **2012**, *492*, 215–220. [CrossRef]
38. Kroeze, W.K.; Sassano, M.F.; Huang, X.P.; Lansu, K.; McCorvy, J.D.; Giguère, P.M.; Sciaky, N.; Roth, B.L. PRESTO-Tango as an open-source resource for interrogation of the druggable human GPCRome. *Nat. Struct. Mol. Biol.* **2015**, *22*, 362–369. [CrossRef]
39. Huang, X.P.; Mangano, T.; Hufeisen, S.; Setola, V.; Roth, B.L. Identification of human Ether-à-go-go related gene modulators by three screening platforms in an academic drug-discovery setting. *Assay Drug Dev. Technol.* **2010**, *8*, 727–742. [CrossRef]
40. Vasta, J.D.; Corona, C.R.; Wilkinson, J.; Zimprich, C.A.; Hartnett, J.R.; Ingold, M.R.; Zimmerman, K.; Machleidt, T.; Kirkland, T.A.; Huwiler, K.G.; et al. Quantitative, Wide-Spectrum Kinase Profiling in Live Cells for Assessing the Effect of Cellular ATP on Target Engagement. *Cell Chem. Biol.* **2018**, *25*, 206–214. [CrossRef]
41. Arrowsmith, C.H.; Audia, J.E.; Austin, C.; Baell, J.; Bennett, J.; Blagg, J.; Bountra, C.; Brennan, P.E.; Brown, P.J.; Bunnage, M.E.; et al. The promise and peril of chemical probes. *Nat. Chem. Biol.* **2015**, *11*, 536–541. [CrossRef] [PubMed]

42. Chuaqui, C.E.; Dowling, J.E.; Lyne, P.; Pontz, T.; Ye, Q. *Preparation of Cyanoarylaminocycloalkylaminopyrrolopyri Midine Derivatives for Use as Antitumor Agents*; WO 2013144532A1; AstraZeneca AB: Södertälje, Sweden; AstraZeneca UK Limited: Cambridge, UK, 2013.
43. Dowling, J.E.; Alimzhanov, M.; Bao, L.; Block, M.H.; Chuaqui, C.; Cooke, E.L.; Denz, C.R.; Hird, A.; Huang, S.; Larsen, N.A.; et al. Structure and Property Based Design of Pyrazolo[1,5-a]pyrimidine Inhibitors of CK2 Kinase with Activity in Vivo. *ACS Med. Chem. Lett.* **2013**, *4*, 800–805. [CrossRef] [PubMed]
44. Dowling, J.E.; Alimzhanov, M.; Bao, L.; Chuaqui, C.; Denz, C.R.; Jenkins, E.; Larsen, N.A.; Lyne, P.D.; Pontz, T.; Ye, Q.; et al. Potent and Selective CK2 Kinase Inhibitors with Effects on Wnt Pathway Signaling in Vivo. *ACS Med. Chem. Lett.* **2016**, *7*, 300–305. [CrossRef] [PubMed]
45. Dowling, J.E.; Chuaqui, C.; Pontz, T.W.; Lyne, P.D.; Larsen, N.A.; Block, M.H.; Chen, H.; Su, N.; Wu, A.; Russell, D.; et al. Potent and Selective Inhibitors of CK2 Kinase Identified through Structure-Guided Hybridization. *ACS Med. Chem. Lett.* **2012**, *3*, 278–283. [CrossRef] [PubMed]
46. D'Amore, C.; Borgo, C.; Sarno, S.; Salvi, M. Role of CK2 inhibitor CX-4945 in anti-cancer combination therapy—Potential clinical relevance. *Cell. Oncol.* **2020**, *43*, 1003–1016. [CrossRef] [PubMed]
47. Marschke, R.F.; Borad, M.J.; McFarland, R.W.; Alvarez, R.H.; Lim, J.K.; Padgett, C.S.; Hoff, D.D.V.; O'Brien, S.E.; Northfelt, D.W. Findings from the phase I clinical trials of CX-4945, an orally available inhibitor of CK2. *J. Clin. Oncol.* **2011**, *29*, 3087. [CrossRef]
48. Quezada Meza, C.P.; Ruzzene, M. Protein Kinase CK2 and SARS-CoV-2: An Expected Interplay Story. *Kinases Phosphatases* **2023**, *1*, 141–150. [CrossRef]
49. Licciardello, M.P.; Workman, P. A New Chemical Probe Challenges the Broad Cancer Essentiality of CK2. *Trends Pharmacol. Sci.* **2021**, *42*, 313–315. [CrossRef]
50. Mishra, S.; Kinoshita, C.; Axtman, A.D.; Young, J.E. Evaluation of a selective chemical probe validates that CK2 mediates neuroinflammation in an hiPSC-derived microglial model. *Front. Mol. Neurosci.* **2022**, *15*, 824956. [CrossRef]
51. Forlenza, O.V.; Diniz, B.S.; Talib, L.L.; Mendonça, V.A.; Ojopi, E.B.; Gattaz, W.F.; Teixeira, A.L. Increased serum IL-1beta level in Alzheimer's disease and mild cognitive impairment. *Dement. Geriatr. Cogn. Disord.* **2009**, *28*, 507–512. [CrossRef]
52. Huang, Z.-B.; Sheng, G.-Q. Interleukin-1β with learning and memory. *Neurosci. Bull.* **2010**, *26*, 455–468. [CrossRef]
53. Swardfager, W.; Lanctôt, K.; Rothenburg, L.; Wong, A.; Cappell, J.; Herrmann, N. A meta-analysis of cytokines in Alzheimer's disease. *Biol. Psychiatry* **2010**, *68*, 930–941. [CrossRef] [PubMed]
54. Brosseron, F.; Krauthausen, M.; Kummer, M.; Heneka, M.T. Body fluid cytokine levels in mild cognitive impairment and Alzheimer's disease: A comparative overview. *Mol. Neurobiol.* **2014**, *50*, 534–544. [CrossRef] [PubMed]
55. Scarabino, D.; Peconi, M.; Broggio, E.; Gambina, G.; Maggi, E.; Armeli, F.; Mantuano, E.; Morello, M.; Corbo, R.M.; Businaro, R. Relationship between proinflammatory cytokines (Il-1beta, Il-18) and leukocyte telomere length in mild cognitive impairment and Alzheimer's disease. *Exp. Gerontol.* **2020**, *136*, 110945. [CrossRef]
56. Lyra E Silva, N.M.; Gonçalves, R.A.; Pascoal, T.A.; Lima-Filho, R.A.S.; Resende, E.d.P.F.; Vieira, E.L.M.; Teixeira, A.L.; de Souza, L.C.; Peny, J.A.; Fortuna, J.T.S.; et al. Pro-inflammatory interleukin-6 signaling links cognitive impairments and peripheral metabolic alterations in Alzheimer's disease. *Transl. Psychiatry* **2021**, *11*, 251. [CrossRef]
57. Gyenis, L.; Menyhart, D.; Cruise, E.S.; Jurcic, K.; Roffey, S.E.; Chai, D.B.; Trifoi, F.; Fess, S.R.; Desormeaux, P.J.; Núñez de Villavicencio Díaz, T.; et al. Chemical Genetic Validation of CSNK2 Substrates Using an Inhibitor-Resistant Mutant in Combination with Triple SILAC Quantitative Phosphoproteomics. *Front. Mol. Biosci.* **2022**, *9*, 909711. [CrossRef]
58. Pack, M.; Götz, C.; Wrublewsky, S.; Montenarh, M. SGC-CK2-1 Is an Efficient Inducer of Insulin Production and Secretion in Pancreatic β-Cells. *Pharmaceutics* **2022**, *14*, 19. [CrossRef] [PubMed]
59. Boewe, A.S.; Wemmert, S.; Kulas, P.; Schick, B.; Götz, C.; Wrublewsky, S.; Montenarh, M.; Menger, M.D.; Laschke, M.W.; Ampofo, E. Inhibition of CK2 Reduces NG2 Expression in Juvenile Angiofibroma. *Biomedicines* **2022**, *10*, 966. [CrossRef]
60. Al Shoyaib, A.; Archie, S.R.; Karamyan, V.T. Intraperitoneal Route of Drug Administration: Should it Be Used in Experimental Animal Studies? *Pharm. Res.* **2019**, *37*, 12. [CrossRef]
61. Barrow, J.C.; Lindsley, C.W. The Importance of PK–PD. *J. Med. Chem.* **2023**, *66*, 4273–4274. [CrossRef]
62. Molina, D.M.; Jafari, R.; Ignatushchenko, M.; Seki, T.; Larsson, E.A.; Dan, C.; Sreekumar, L.; Cao, Y.; Nordlund, P. Monitoring Drug Target Engagement in Cells and Tissues Using the Cellular Thermal Shift Assay. *Science* **2013**, *341*, 84–87. [CrossRef] [PubMed]
63. Tolvanen, T.A. Current Advances in CETSA. *Front. Mol. Biosci.* **2022**, *9*, 866764. [CrossRef] [PubMed]
64. Yang, X.; Ong, H.W.; Dickmander, R.J.; Smith, J.L.; Brown, J.W.; Tao, W.; Chang, E.; Moorman, N.J.; Axtman, A.D.; Willson, T.M. Optimization of 3-Cyano-7-cyclopropylamino-pyrazolo[1,5-a]pyrimidines Toward the Development of an In Vivo Chemical Probe for CSNK2A. *bioRxiv* **2023**. [CrossRef]
65. Eroglu, Z.; Cowey, C.L.; Soong, J.; McCormick, D.; Fan, P.; Chen, J.; Elgendy, M.; Jang, S.; Chang, A.L.S. A phase I study of CX-4945 administered orally twice daily to patients with advanced basal cell carcinoma. *J. Clin. Oncol.* **2020**, *38*, TPS10080. [CrossRef]
66. Siddiqui-Jain, A.; Chua, P.; Darjania, L.; Lim, J.; O'Brien, S.; Pierre, F.; Streiner, N.; Trent, K.; Whitten, J.; Rice, W. The discovery and characterization of CX-5011, a highly selective, potent inhibitor of Protein Kinase CK2. *Cancer Res.* **2008**, *68*, 4875.
67. Siddiqui-Jain, A.; Drygin, D.; Streiner, N.; Chua, P.; Pierre, F.; O'Brien, S.E.; Bliesath, J.; Omori, M.; Huser, N.; Ho, C.; et al. CX-4945, an orally bioavailable selective inhibitor of protein kinase CK2, inhibits prosurvival and angiogenic signaling and exhibits antitumor efficacy. *Cancer Res.* **2010**, *70*, 10288–10298. [CrossRef] [PubMed]

68. Pierre, F.; Chua, P.C.; O'Brien, S.E.; Siddiqui-Jain, A.; Bourbon, P.; Haddach, M.; Michaux, J.; Nagasawa, J.; Schwaebe, M.K.; Stefan, E.; et al. Pre-clinical characterization of CX-4945, a potent and selective small molecule inhibitor of CK2 for the treatment of cancer. *Mol. Cell. Biochem.* **2011**, *356*, 37–43. [CrossRef]
69. Castello, J.; Ragnauth, A.; Friedman, E.; Rebholz, H. CK2—An Emerging Target for Neurological and Psychiatric Disorders. *Pharmaceuticals* **2017**, *10*, 7. [CrossRef]
70. Iimoto, D.S.; Masliah, E.; DeTeresa, R.; Terry, R.D.; Saitoh, T. Aberrant casein kinase II in Alzheimer's disease. *Brain Res.* **1990**, *507*, 273–280. [CrossRef]
71. Masliah, E.; Iimoto, D.S.; Mallory, M.; Albright, T.; Hansen, L.; Saitoh, T. Casein kinase II alteration precedes tau accumulation in tangle formation. *Am. J. Pathol.* **1992**, *140*, 263–268.
72. Marshall, C.A.; McBride, J.D.; Changolkar, L.; Riddle, D.M.; Trojanowski, J.Q.; Lee, V.M.Y. Inhibition of CK2 mitigates Alzheimer's tau pathology by preventing NR2B synaptic mislocalization. *Acta Neuropathol. Commun.* **2022**, *10*, 30. [CrossRef] [PubMed]
73. Baum, L.; Masliah, E.; Iimoto, D.S.; Hansen, L.A.; Halliday, W.C.; Saitoh, T. Casein kinase II is associated with neurofibrillary tangles but is not an intrinsic component of paired helical filaments. *Brain Res.* **1992**, *573*, 126–132. [CrossRef] [PubMed]
74. Kim, H.; Lee, K.S.; Kim, A.K.; Choi, M.; Choi, K.; Kang, M.; Chi, S.W.; Lee, M.S.; Lee, J.S.; Lee, S.Y.; et al. A chemical with proven clinical safety rescues Down-syndrome-related phenotypes in through DYRK1A inhibition. *Dis. Model. Mech.* **2016**, *9*, 839–848. [PubMed]
75. Perera, Y.; Farina, H.G.; Gil, J.; Rodriguez, A.; Benavent, F.; Castellanos, L.; Gómez, R.E.; Acevedo, B.E.; Alonso, D.F.; Perea, S.E. Anticancer peptide CIGB-300 binds to nucleophosmin/B23, impairs its CK2-mediated phosphorylation, and leads to apoptosis through its nucleolar disassembly activity. *Mol. Cancer Ther.* **2009**, *8*, 1189–1196. [CrossRef]
76. Perera, Y.; Ramos, Y.; Padrón, G.; Caballero, E.; Guirola, O.; Caligiuri, L.G.; Lorenzo, N.; Gottardo, F.; Farina, H.G.; Filhol, O.; et al. CIGB-300 anticancer peptide regulates the protein kinase CK2-dependent phosphoproteome. *Mol. Cell Biochem.* **2020**, *470*, 63–75. [CrossRef]
77. Rosales, M.; Pérez, G.V.; Ramón, A.C.; Cruz, Y.; Rodríguez-Ulloa, A.; Besada, V.; Ramos, Y.; Vázquez-Blomquist, D.; Caballero, E.; Aguilar, D.; et al. Targeting of Protein Kinase CK2 in Acute Myeloid Leukemia Cells Using the Clinical-Grade Synthetic-Peptide CIGB-300. *Biomedicines* **2021**, *9*, 766. [CrossRef]
78. Perera, Y.; Farina, H.G.; Hernández, I.; Mendoza, O.; Serrano, J.M.; Reyes, O.; Gómez, D.E.; Gómez, R.E.; Acevedo, B.E.; Alonso, D.F.; et al. Systemic administration of a peptide that impairs the protein kinase (CK2) phosphorylation reduces solid tumor growth in mice. *Int. J. Cancer* **2008**, *122*, 57–62. [CrossRef]
79. Solares, A.M.; Santana, A.; Baladrón, I.; Valenzuela, C.; González, C.A.; Díaz, A.; Castillo, D.; Ramos, T.; Gómez, R.; Alonso, D.F.; et al. Safety and preliminary efficacy data of a novel Casein Kinase 2 (CK2) peptide inhibitor administered intralesionally at four dose levels in patients with cervical malignancies. *BMC Cancer* **2009**, *9*, 146. [CrossRef]
80. Soriano-García, J.L.; López-Díaz, A.; Solares-Asteasuainzarra, M.; Baladrón-Castrillo, I.; Batista-Albuerne, N.; García-García, I.; González-Méndez, L.; Perera-Negrín, Y.; Valenzuela-Silva, C.M.; Pedro, A.P.; et al. Pharmacological and safety evaluation of CIGB-300, a casein kinase 2 inhibitor peptide, administered intralesionally to patients with cervical cancer stage IB2/II. *J. Cancer Res. Ther.* **2013**, *1*, 163–173. [CrossRef]
81. Sarduy, M.R.; García, I.; Coca, M.A.; Perera, A.; Torres, L.A.; Valenzuela, C.M.; Baladrón, I.; Solares, M.; Reyes, V.; Hernández, I.; et al. Optimizing CIGB-300 intralesional delivery in locally advanced cervical cancer. *Br. J. Cancer* **2015**, *112*, 1636–1643. [CrossRef]
82. Cruz, L.R.; Baladrón, I.; Rittoles, A.; Díaz, P.A.; Valenzuela, C.; Santana, R.; Vázquez, M.M.; García, A.; Chacón, D.; Thompson, D.; et al. Treatment with an Anti-CK2 Synthetic Peptide Improves Clinical Response in COVID-19 Patients with Pneumonia. A Randomized and Controlled Clinical Trial. *ACS Pharmacol. Transl. Sci.* **2021**, *4*, 206–212. [CrossRef] [PubMed]
83. Sterling, J.; Baker, J.R.; McCluskey, A.; Munoz, L. Systematic literature review reveals suboptimal use of chemical probes in cell-based biomedical research. *Nat. Commun.* **2023**, *14*, 3228. [CrossRef] [PubMed]

kinases and phosphatases

MDPI

Article

Discovery and Exploration of Protein Kinase CK2 Binding Sites Using CK2$\alpha'^{Cys336Ser}$ as an Exquisite Crystallographic Tool

Christian Werner [1], Dirk Lindenblatt [1], Kaido Viht [2], Asko Uri [2] and Karsten Niefind [1,*]

[1] Institute of Biochemistry, Department of Chemistry and Biochemistry, University of Cologne, Zülpicher Str. 47, D-50674 Köln, Germany

[2] Institute of Chemistry, University of Tartu, 14A Ravila St., EST-50411 Tartu, Estonia

* Correspondence: karsten.niefind@uni-koeln.de; Tel.: +49-221-4706444

Abstract: The structural knowledge about protein kinase CK2 is dominated by crystal structures of human CK2α, the catalytic subunit of human CK2, and the product of the *CSNK2A1* gene. In contrast, far fewer structures of CK2α′, its paralogous isoform and the product of the *CSNK2A2* gene, have been published. However, according to a PDB survey, CK2α′ is the superior alternative for crystallographic studies because of the inherent potential of the single mutant CK2$\alpha'^{Cys336Ser}$ to provide crystal structures with atomic resolution. In particular, a triclinic crystal form of CK2$\alpha'^{Cys336Ser}$ is a robust tool to determine high-quality enzyme-ligand complex structures via soaking. In this work, further high-resolution CK2$\alpha'^{Cys336Ser}$ structures in complex with selected ligands emphasizing this trend are described. In one of these structures, the "N-terminal segment site", a small-molecule binding region never found in any eukaryotic protein kinase and holding the potential for the development of highly selective substrate-competitive CK2 inhibitors, was discovered. In order to also address the binding site for the non-catalytic subunit CK2β, which is inaccessible in these triclinic CK2$\alpha'^{Cys336Ser}$ crystals for small molecules, a reliable path to a promising monoclinic crystal form of CK2$\alpha'^{Cys336Ser}$ is presented. In summary, the quality of CK2$\alpha'^{Cys336Ser}$ as an exquisite crystallographic tool is solidified.

Keywords: protein kinase CK2; casein kinase 2; isoenzymes human CK2α and human CK2α′; CSNK2A1; CSNK2A2; N-terminal segment site; protein crystallography; atomic resolution

1. Introduction

Towards the middle of 2023, the protein structure database PDB [1,2] contains 315 entries with homologues of CK2α, the catalytic subunit of protein kinase CK2. 41 of them belong to CK2α from *Zea mays* (UNIPROT_ID P28523) [3,4], which provided the first CK2α crystal structure [5] and dominated the early years of CK2 structural biology. With the crystal structure of the CK2 holoenzyme (heterotetrameric complex of CK2α with the regulatory subunit CK2β) from *Homo sapiens* [6], human CK2α (UNIPROT_ID P68400; product of the *CSNK2A1* gene) entered the PDB in 2001; it is now included in 231 entries, the majority of them being released since 2016 (Figure 1a) and belonging to complexes of human CK2α with ATP-competitive inhibitors [7–10].

In comparison, the PDB contains only 25 entries of human CK2α′, the paralogous isoform of human CK2α (UNIPROT_ID P19784; product of the *CSNK2A2* gene), albeit with an increasing trend (Figure 1a). A main reason for this backlog were solubility issues occurring with wild-type CK2α′ after recombinant expression in bacteria [11], but also in insect cells [12]. The chemical background of this problem became apparent after an inspection of the sequences of human CK2α and CK2α′—they are to 82% identical but differ completely in the C-terminal regions—and the construction of the chimeric variant CK2α_α′ containing its final 24 residues from CK2α′ [13]. This chimera has a conspicuous tendency to form intermolecular disulphide bridges, which drew attention to Cys336 as part of the CK2α′-derived tail; replacing this cysteine with serine led to the full-length variant

CK2α′^Cys336Ser^, which was well soluble and applicable for enzymatic, calorimetric, and crystallographic studies [13]. Alternatively, truncating the C-terminal segment, including Cys336, led to CK2α′ constructs that could be successfully crystallized as well [14,15].

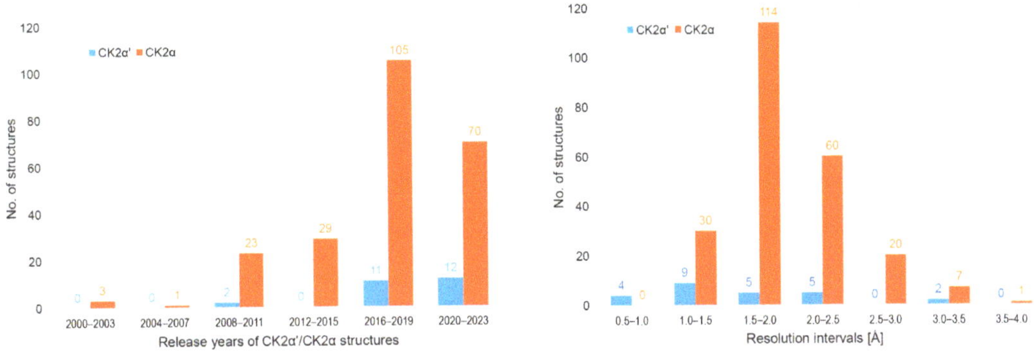

(a) (b)

Figure 1. Distributions of CK2α and CK2α′ crystal structures based on data extracted from the PDB [1,2]. (**a**) Structures clustered into intervals of release years; (**b**) structures clustered into intervals of resolution.

However, CK2α′^Cys336Ser^ was still somewhat problematic for the purpose of crystallization because of its propensity to crystallize as extremely tiny needles under a large variety of conditions. Although these crystal needles grow slightly thicker in the presence of 3-(4,5,6,7-tetrabromo-1*H*-benzotriazol-1-yl)propan-1-ol (MB002; Scheme 1) [13,16] and certain other ATP-competitive inhibitors [17,18], which led to the first crystal structures of CK2α′^Cys336Ser^ [13,17,18], a real breakthrough in growth behaviour only came with a significant increase of the lithium chloride concentration in the crystallization droplets [19]. This—combined with a sophisticated seeding and soaking strategy to replace the originally bound MB002 ligand from the ATP site—resulted in large, compact, and robust CK2α′^Cys336Ser^ crystals. They led to a number of atomic-resolution structures of CK2α′^Cys336Ser^ [19], among them a 1.04-Å complex structure with the benchmark CK2 inhibitor CX-4945 [20–23].

Subsequently, these CK2α′^Cys336Ser^ crystals together with the optimized soaking protocol [19] were systematically exploited:

- For some members of a series of halogenated triazolo pyridines, the exact binding mode at the ATP site could only be clarified via high-resolution complex structures with CK2α′^Cys336Ser^ [24];
- In the case of some 2-aminothiazole compounds supposed to occupy an allosteric binding site [25,26], CK2α′^Cys336Ser^ complex structures revealed that in fact the ATP cavity harboured these inhibitory ligands [27]; with resolutions of 0.833 Å (PDB_ID 6TGU) and 0.922 Å (PDB_ID 6TE2), two of these structures are currently the best resolved among about 4500 X-ray diffraction entries in the PDB [1,2] with protein kinase chains;
- The power of the approach became particularly obvious when the αD pocket, an allosteric site originally discovered with CK2α [28,29], could be occupied via soaking of CK2α′^Cys336Ser^/MB002 crystals, although this required extensive local conformational rearrangements in the crystalline state of the protein [30].

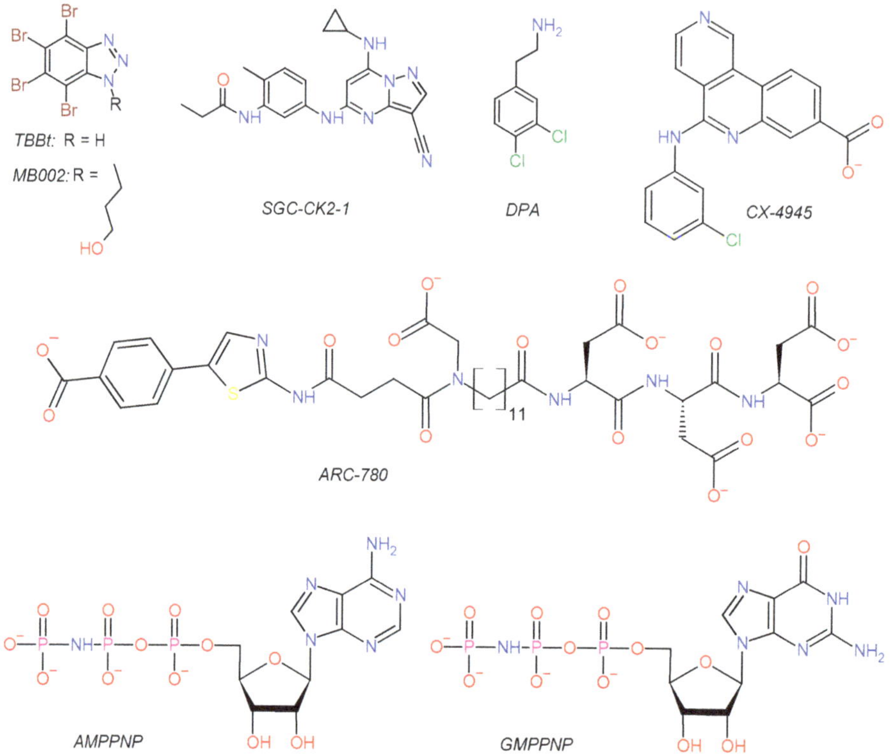

Scheme 1. Structures of CK2 ligands used in this study.

The excellent properties of CK2α′^{Cys336Ser} crystals are responsible for the fact that the resolution distribution of CK2α′ structures is significantly shifted to the high-resolution side compared to CK2α (Figure 1b). In this work, we supplement the collection of CK2α′^{Cys336Ser}/ligand complex structures with further cases. Partially, they were obtained via the crystallization and soaking protocol originally published [19], but we also present selected structural examples resulting from efforts to overcome certain limitations of those crystals and procedures.

2. Results and Discussion

2.1. Complex Structures Determined with Triclinic CK2α′^{Cys336Ser} Crystals

2.1.1. CK2α′^{Cys336Ser} Structure in Complex with the ATP-Site Ligands SGC-CK2-1

The size-optimized CK2α′^{Cys336Ser}/MB002 crystals used by Lindenblatt et al. [19] to determine atomic resolution complex structures belong to the triclinic crystal system (space group P1). In the corresponding crystal packing, the ATP-site is well accessible, so that in particular, high-affinity ligands like CX-4945 can easily displace the crystallization helper compound MB002 [19].

We expected a similar performance for SGC-CK2-1 (Scheme 1), an ATP-competitive CK2 inhibitor with IC_{50} values for CK2α/CK2α′ inhibition in the low nanomolar range and with an extremely high selectivity [31,32]. SGC-CK2-1 has the potential to compete with CX-4945 for the role of benchmark CK2 inhibitor and superior CK2-sensitive tool in cell biology studies, as already demonstrated [33–35]. In fact, soaking of CK2α′^{Cys336Ser}/MB002 crystals in 2.5 mM SGC-CK2-1 led to a high-quality CK2α′^{Cys336Ser}/SGC-CK2-1 complex structure refined to 1.352 Å resolution (Table 1, Figure 2a).

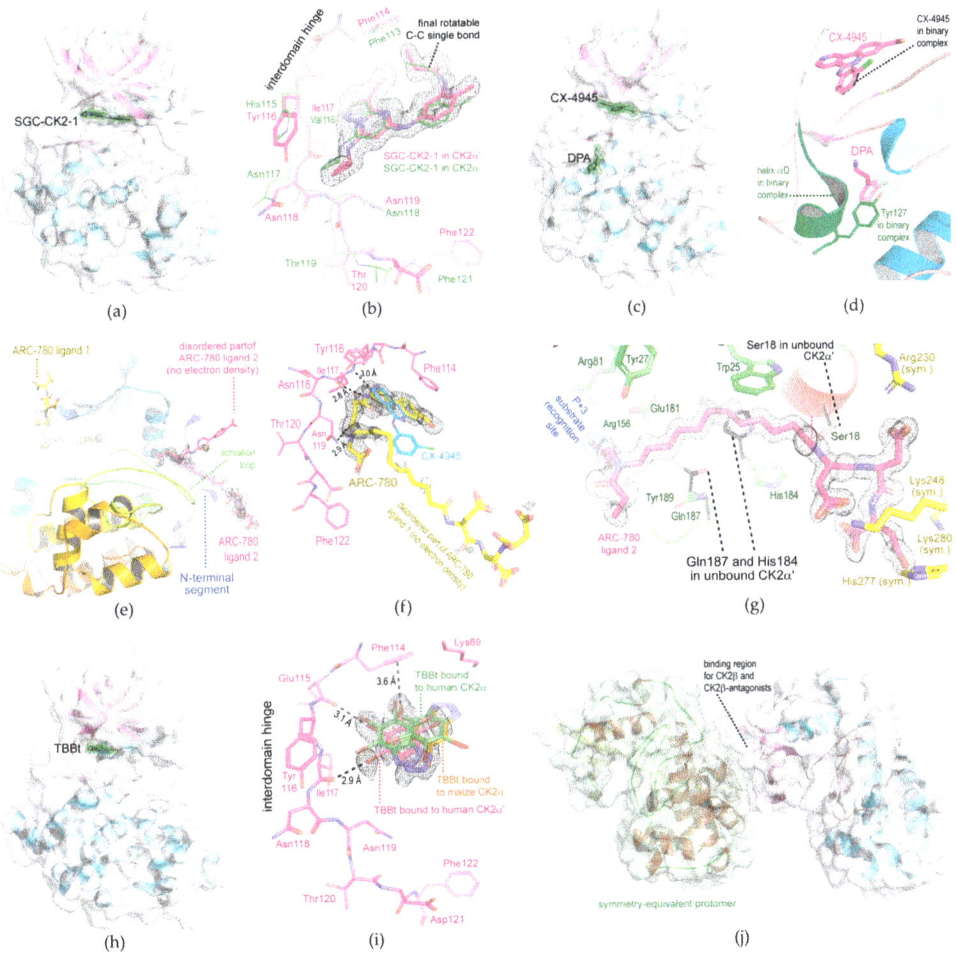

Figure 2. CK2α'^{Cys336Ser} structures in complex with various ligands obtained in triclinic crystal form. The cutoff level for electron density illustration in this figure is generally 1 σ. The structure pictures were produced with PyMol [36]. (**a**) Overview of the CK2α'^{Cys336Ser}/SGC-CK2-1 complex structure. (**b**) SGC-CK2-1 occupying the ATP site in CK2α'^{Cys336Ser} (magenta-coloured C-atoms) and for comparison in CK2α (green C-atoms; PDB_ID 6Z83 [31]). (**c**) Overview of the CK2α'^{Cys336Ser} structure in complex with CX-4945 and DPA. (**d**) Hinge/helix αD region of the ternary CK2α'^{Cys336Ser}/CX-4945/DPA complex (this work) and an overlaid binary CK2α'^{Cys336Ser}/CX-4945 structure (PDB_ID 6HMB [19]). (**e**) Overview of the CK2α'^{Cys336Ser} structure in complex with two molecules of ARC-780. (**f**) ARC-780 ligand 1 occupying the ATP site of CK2α'^{Cys336Ser}; the lengths of three H-bonds between the ligand and the enzyme's hinge region (black dotted lines) are given in Å; for comparison, CX-4945 is drawn from PDB_ID 6HMB [19] after 3D-fit of the protein matrices. (**g**) The ordered part of ARC-780 ligand 2 occupying the novel N-terminal segment site of CK2α'^{Cys336Ser}; side chains of a neighbouring symmetry mate were drawn with yellow C-atoms; Ser18, His184, and Gln187 from unbound (ARC-780-free) CK2α'^{Cys336Ser} were depicted with black C-atoms. (**h**) Overview of the CK2α'^{Cys336Ser}/TBBt complex structure. (**i**) Zoom of TBBt bound to the ATP site of CK2α'^{Cys336Ser} (magenta-coloured C-atoms); for comparison, TBBt was drawn as bound to maize CK2α (orange-coloured C-atoms; PDB_ID 1J91 [37]) or to human CK2α at pH 8.5 (green C-atoms; PDB_ID 7QGE [38]). (**j**) Involvement of the CK2β binding site of CK2α'^{Cys336Ser} in a crystal contact.

Table 1. X-ray diffraction data and refinement statistics for triclinic CK2α′^{Cys336Ser} crystals.

Structure No.	1	2	3	4
CK2α′^{Cys336Ser} ligands	SGC-CK2-1	CX-4945 + DPA	ARC-780	TBBt
PDB code	8Q9S	8QBU	8Q77	8QCD
X-ray diffraction data quality				
Wavelength (Å)	0.9762	0.8856	0.9677	0.8856
Synchrotron (beamline)	P13, EMBL/DESY	P13, EMBL/DESY	MASSIF-3, ESRF	ID23-1, ESRF
Space group	P1	P1	P1	P1
Unit cell: a, b, c (Å) α, β, γ (°)	46.217, 47.682, 50.563 66.827, 89.429, 88.930	46.173, 47.714, 50.586 66.053, 89.722, 88.974	46.603, 47.919, 51.031 66.591, 89.667, 88.163	46.388, 47.701, 50.342 113.481, 90.448, 90.171
Protomers per asymmetric unit	1	1	1	1
Resolution (Å) (highest resolution shell)	32.060–1.352 (1.400–1.352)	46.17–1.095 (1.134–1.095)	46.578–1.255 (1.364–1.255)	23.34–1.033 (1.070–1.033)
R_{sym} (%)	9.7 (148.2) *	10.5 (136.8) *	5.2 (55.9) *	12.8 (55.2) *
CC1/2	0.997 (0.589) *	0.997 (0.608) *	0.998 (0.806) *	0.979 (0.561) *
Signal-to-noise ratio (I/σ_I)	7.8 (1.6) *	6.5 (1.7) *	12.2 (1.6) *	5.7 (1.8) *
No. of unique refl.	56,703 (2835) *	118,499 (5925) *	80,300 (4015) *	149,296 (7465) *
Completeness/spherical (%)	65.3 (11.1) *	72.9 (18.1) *	72.5 (16.4) *	76.9 (21.5) *
Completeness/ellipsoidal (%) §	90.2 (57.4) *	89.7 (53.6) *	82.1 (31.7) *	84.9 (37.0) *
Multiplicity	7.2 (7.1) *	6.5 (6.6) *	3.9 (3.9) *	2.6 (2.6) *
Wilson B-factor (Å^2)	19.46	11.97	10.32	1.45
Structure refinement and quality				
No. of reflections for R_{work}/R_{free}	54,699/1989	116,384/1984	79,069/1214	147,251/2014
R_{work}/R_{free} (%)	13.54/16.88	15.93/17.93	11.99/15.73	14.37/15.62
No. of non-H-atoms	3111	3275	3260	3307
Protein	2822	2898	2793	2876
Ligand/ion	69	176	281	44
Water	253	293	314	406
Average B-factor (Å^2)	26.58	18.80	16.47	7.66
Protein	25.44	17.29	14.16	6.23
Ligand/ion	26.84	24.59	30.78	11.66
water	39.24	32.14	30.06	17.57
RMS deviations				
Bond lengths (Å)	0.008	0.016	0.023	0.009
Bond angles (°)	0.86	1.42	1.67	1.04
Ramachandran plot				
Favoured (%)	96.00	96.93	97.24	97.85
Allowed (%)	4.00	2.76	2.76	2.15
Outliers (%)	0.00	0.31	0.00	0.00

* The values in brackets refer to the highest resolution shell. § After anisotropic analysis with STARANISO [39].

For comparison, a CK2α/SGC-CK2-1 complex structure was published with a resolution of 2.17 Å [31]. An overlay of this structure on the novel CK2α′^{Cys336Ser}/SGC-CK2-1 structure (Figure 2b) reveals that SGC-CK2-1 is bound in a similar way to the two paralogs, albeit with a noteworthy conformational difference in the terminal propionamide moiety: the torsion angle around the final C-C-bond as indicated in Figure 2b is −23.14° in CK2α′^{Cys336Ser}-bound SGC-CK2-1, but 35.24° or 59.65°, respectively, in the two crystallographically independent copies of the CK2α/SGC-CK2-1 structure [31]. This difference is not caused by the direct protein environment around the propionamide moiety since it is identical in the two isoforms. Rather, Figure 2b suggests that the structural background lies in the interdomain hinge where CK2α and CK2α′ have their only sequence difference in the ATP-site region: Tyr116 of CK2α′ is more voluminous than its equivalent His115 of CK2α so that SGC-CK2-1 can approach the hinge less closely in CK2α′. This causes a shift visible at the cyclopropyl group and a constraint at the other side of the molecule, namely at the aforementioned propionamide moiety, which penetrates deeper into the ATP site of CK2α′ than into that of CK2α (Figure 2b). This subtle effect correlates well with the fact that the IC_{50} value of SGC-CK2-1 for CK2α′ inhibition is only half as large as for CK2α inhibition [31], and it could be a first step on the way to the attractive goal of generating isoform-specific CK2 inhibitors [40,41].

2.1.2. Ternary Complex Structure of CK2α′^{Cys336Ser}, CX-4945, and DPA

The αD pocket of CK2α and CK2α′ is a so-called "cryptic site" [42]; this designation was introduced for "hidden" pockets becoming visible and accessible only after conformational changes induced in the presence of a suitable ligand. In the case of the αD pocket, this ligand was 3,4-dichloro phenethylamine (DPA; Scheme 1), which led to the discovery of the αD pocket in 2016 in a fragment-based screen with CK2α crystals [28,29], while in all CK2α structures published before, it was blocked by either a phenylalanine or a tyrosine side chain from the eponymous helix αD. After its discovery, the αD pocket was used to develop the bivalent inhibitor CAM4066 [28,29].

For CK2α′, the existence of an αD pocket was confirmed via soaking DPA into a CK2α′^{Cys336Ser}/MB002 crystal [30]. In the resulting ternary complex structure, the two ligands are 6.9 Å away from each other, a distance that could be chemically bridged and led to the bivalent and highly selective inhibitor KN2 [30]. This success induced the hypothesis that the ATP site and the αD pocket of crystalline CK2α′^{Cys336Ser} can be occupied independently of each other, so that CK2α′^{Cys336Ser} structures in complex with arbitrary pairs of ligands can be obtained via soaking CK2α′^{Cys336Ser}/MB002 crystals.

To test this, we soaked a CK2α′^{Cys336Ser}/MB002 crystal simultaneously with CX-4945 and DPA. In the resulting crystal structure with a resolution below 1.1 Å (Table 1), both ligands were well defined by electron density (Figure 2c), meaning CX-4945 had completely replaced MB002 and DPA had opened and occupied the αD pocket. A 3D-fit of this ternary CK2α′^{Cys336Ser}/CX-4945/DPA complex on the binary CK2α′^{Cys336Ser}/CX-4945 complex structure (Figure 2d) illustrates again the large conformational adaptations occurring in the αD region during soaking. In summary, this experiment confirms that the ATP site and the αD pocket of crystalline CK2α′^{Cys336Ser} cannot only be occupied independently but even simultaneously.

2.1.3. N-Terminal Segment Site: A Novel Ligand Binding Site Discovered in a CK2α′^{Cys336Ser} Structure in Complex with the Bisubstrate Inhibitor ARC-780

ARC-780 (Scheme 1) is a follow-up compound of a series of CK2 bisubstrate inhibitors [43] occupying the ATP site and addressing the recognition region for peptide or protein substrates as well, so that the corresponding K_i values are partly in the picomolar range [43]. ARC-780 contains a long aliphatic linker of 11 methylen groups (Scheme 1), resulting in high hydrophobicity and many rotational degrees of freedom. Therefore, we extended the soaking time of initial CK2α′^{Cys336Ser}/MB002 crystals in ARC-780 containing solutions to eight months. In this time, the concentrations of salts were stepwise decreased from 900 mM LiCl, 500 mM NaCl, and 110 mM Tris/HCl to finally 50 mM LiCl and 10 mM

Tris/HCl, while in parallel, the concentration of DMSO was increased from 0 to 30% (v/v), and the concentration of the precipitant PEG6000 was adopted to saturation.

In spite of these extreme alterations of the surrounding solution, the CK2α'^{Cys336Ser} crystals retained their integrity, and one of them led to a 1.255 Å crystal structure (structure no. 3 in Table 1). Surprisingly, in this structure, two large patches of non-protein electron density were visible. They could be interpreted unambiguously with two separate ARC-780 molecules, and in both cases, large, albeit different, parts of ARC-780 were not covered with significant electron density (Figure 2e).

The first ARC-780 ligand occupies the ATP site (Figure 2f, Video S1): its terminal carboxy phenyl moiety binds next to the Phe114 side chain, and after 3D-fit of the according protein matrices, it overlaps entirely with the corresponding sub-structure of CX-4945. Using its triazole ring and the two subsequent amide bonds, the first ARC-780 ligand forms three close hydrogen bonds with the enzyme's hinge region, while the aliphatic linker and the final peptidic part are completely disordered (Figure 2f).

The second ARC-780 ligand—or at least a considerable part of it—is bound to a region (Figure 2g, Video S1) that, to our knowledge, has never been described before as a small-molecule binding site in CK2α, CK2α', or any other member of the superfamily of eukaryotic protein kinases (EPKs). We call it the "N-terminal segment site" here because it is located close to an N-terminal extension of the EPK-typical N-lobe domain that attaches the likewise EPK-typical activation loop and folds back to the C-lobe domain (Figure 2e). This intramolecular interaction between the N-terminal segment and the activation loop is a distinguishing feature of CK2α/CK2α' among the EPK superfamily and the main structural basis of CK2's constitutive activity since it mimics the intermolecular coordination of the activation loop of cyclin-dependent kinases by activatory cyclin proteins [5].

Just like the αD site, the N-terminal segment site is a cryptic site [42]. Its access for a ligand requires large conformational changes in the side chains of Ser18, His184, and Gln187, which are indicated in Figure 2g and visualized in Video S1. The four carboxy groups in the peptidic part of ARC-780 form ionic interactions with some positively charged side chains of a crystalline CK2α'^{Cys336Ser} neighbour (Figure 2g). Thus, the fact that this peptidic part is well defined by electron density in strong contrast to what has been observed in CK2α complex structures with precursor bisubstrate inhibitors [43] is most likely an artifact of the crystal packing. Insofar, it must remain open in the moment how far the peptidic part of ARC-780 contributes to the compound's affinity to the N-terminal segment site of the enzyme at all.

In contrast to that, the N-linked carboxy methyl group of ARC-780 (Scheme 1) is likely to be an important binding determinant because it interacts ionically with Arg156 (Figure 2g, time point 12 s in Video S1). Together with Arg81, Arg156 forms the P + 3 recognition site for CK2 substrates, which means that this carboxy methyl group would interfere with substrate binding. In the future, this fact could pave the way to developing highly selective, substrate-competitive CK2 inhibitors from the sub-structure of ARC-780 (Figure 2g) that binds to the novel N-terminal segment site with its unique molecular environment.

2.1.4. CK2α'^{Cys336Ser} Structure in Complex with TBBt

MB002 [16] (Scheme 1) is an efficient additive for the crystallization of CK2α'^{Cys336Ser} [13,19], but it has the disadvantage of not being commercially available. We found its head group 4,5,6,7-tetrabromobenzotriazole (TBBt; Scheme 1) to be a suitable and inexpensive substitute: co-crystallization of CK2α'^{Cys336Ser} with TBBt followed by micro- and macro-seeding led to CK2α'^{Cys336Ser}/TBBt crystals, which are isomorphous to the triclinic CK2α'^{Cys336Ser}/MB002 crystals used before, and resulted in a CK2α'^{Cys336Ser}/TBBt complex structure of 1.033 Å resolution (structure no. 4 in Table 1; Figure 2h). For comparison, previously published complex structures with TBBt have resolutions of 2.22 Å (with maize CK2α [37]), 1.88 Å (with human CK2α at pH 7.5 [44]), and 2.27 Å (with human CK2α at pH 8.5 [38]).

For TBBt, a pK_A value of 4.78 was reported [45], so that it is monoanionic at pH 7 and above. Therefore, a "competition between electrostatic interactions and halogen bonding" [38] exists for the interaction of TBBt with the ATP site of CK2α. In fact, in a human CK2α/TBBt complex structure obtained at pH 8.5, two alternative binding modes of TBBt were observed [38] (Figure 2i). In one of them, which had been found before in a maize CK2α/TBBt complex structure as well [37] (Figure 2i), electrostatic forces dominate and direct TBBt via its anionic triazole moiety into the proximity of the highly conserved side chain of Lys68 (which is equivalent to Lys69 of CK2α′ drawn in Figure 2i) [46]. In the other binding mode, however, halogen bonds force TBBt close to the interdomain hinge of human CK2α. It is this second binding mode that we observed exclusively in the $CK2\alpha'^{Cys336Ser}$/TBBt complex (Figure 2i). Apparently, there, the three halogen bonds from the bromo substituents of TBBt to the carbonyl oxygen atoms of Glu115 and Ile117, as well as to the phenyl ring of Phe114, dominate clearly over the electrostatic term.

Noteworthy, the salt concentration during crystallization of the $CK2\alpha'^{Cys336Ser}$/TBBt complex was much higher than that reported for crystallization of the CK2α/TBBt complex [38]. Therefore, follow-up experiments are required to clarify if the difference in TBBt binding between human CK2α and CK2α′ is a crystallization artifact or if it reflects subtle differences between the isoenzymes themselves. In any case, atomic-resolution complex structures of $CK2\alpha'^{Cys336Ser}$ with halogenated inhibitors can help to refine the sophisticated knowledge about halogen bonding in the ATP site of CK2α subunits [38,44,47].

2.2. Complex Structures Determined with Monoclinic $CK2\alpha'^{Cys336Ser}$ Crystals

In order to test if the excellent diffraction of triclinic $CK2\alpha'^{Cys336Ser}$ crystals is restricted to this particular crystal packing, an alternative crystal packing of $CK2\alpha'^{Cys336Ser}$ had to be found. A further motivation to pursue this goal came from the observation that the outer surface of the enzyme's N-lobal anti-parallel CK2β-sheet, which serves as an interface for the binding of the non-catalytic subunit CK2β [6], is involved in a crystal contact in the triclinic $CK2\alpha'^{Cys336Ser}$ crystals (Figure 2j): it is thus inaccessible for small CK2β-antagonistic molecules in soaking approaches and also for co-crystallization because the crystal packing is incompatible with any occupation of the CK2β binding site.

Small peptidic or non-peptidic molecules that compete with CK2β for its binding site and disturb the assembly of the CK2 holoenzyme have been repeatedly described [43,48–54] and, in several cases, structurally characterized in recent years, but exclusively for CK2α. Structures of CK2α′ in complex with such ligands do not exist at present; in order to create the prerequisite for them, a reliable pathway to an alternative crystal form of $CK2\alpha'^{Cys336Ser}$ is desirable.

Since it was demonstrated with lithium sulfate [15] or lithium chloride [19] that the crystallization behavior of CK2α′ constructs is very sensitive to the content of lithium ions, we systematically varied the lithium chloride concentration in $CK2\alpha'^{Cys336Ser}$ crystallization experiments between 500 mM and 900 mM with otherwise unchanged conditions. Already 810 mM LiCl—i.e., a slight reduction of the LiCl concentration compared to the 900 mM in crystallization solutions of the triclinic $CK2\alpha'^{Cys336Ser}$ crystals (Table 1)—led to $CK2\alpha'^{Cys336Ser}$ crystals with monoclinic symmetry (Table 2). In this new crystal form, two $CK2\alpha'^{Cys336Ser}$ protomers per asymmetric unit are present. In one of them, the CK2β binding site is used to form the contact interface to a neighbouring symmetry mate (Figure 3a) in a similar way as it was observed for the triclinic crystals (Figure 2j). In the second protomer, however, the CK2β binding site, although also surrounded by two crystalline neighbours, is basically accessible to ligands of small and medium size (Figure 3b).

Table 2. X-ray diffraction data and refinement statistics for monoclinic CK2α'^{Cys336Ser} crystals.

Structure No.	**5**	**6**
Ligands of CK2α'^{Cys336Ser}	AMPPNP	GMPPNP
PDB code	8QCG	8QF1
	X-ray diffraction data quality	
Wavelength (Å)	0.8856	0.8856
Synchrotron (beamline)	ID23-1, ESRF	ID23-1, ESRF
Space group	$P2_1$	$P2_1$
Unit cell: a, b, c (Å) α, β, γ (°)	46.599, 71.852, 101.984 90.000, 92.423, 90.000	46.628, 71.590, 102.101 90.000, 92.094, 90.000
Protomers per asymmetric unit	2	2
Resolution (Å) (highest resolution shell)	101.893–1.045 (1.157–1.045) *	102.033–1.318 (1.493–1.318) *
R_{sym} (%)	8.5 (97.6)	14.4 (47.2) *
CC1/2	0.997 (0.732) *	0.973 (0.367) *
Signal-to-noise ratio (I/σ_I)	9.5 (2.0) *	4.1 (1.7) *
No. of unique refl.	229,873 (11494) *	91,444 (4572) *
Completeness/spherical (%)	72.6 (13.8) *	57.8 (9.3) *
Completeness/ellipsoidal (%) §	94.1 (62.1) *	90.9 (62.8) *
Multiplicity	6.6 (5.9) *	3.5 (2.8) *
Wilson B-factor (Å^2)	11.47	12.80
	Structure refinement and quality	
No. of reflections for R_{work}/R_{free}	227,816/2005	89,975/1370
R_{work}/R_{free} (%)	15.06/17.03	21.40/23.22
No. of non-H-atoms	6447	6251
Protein	5630	5597
Ligand/ion	91	48
Water	752	619
Average B-factor (Å^2)	20.41	23.67
Protein	18.48	22.39
Ligand/ion	25.21	24.86
Water	34.48	35.26
RMS deviations		
Bond lengths (Å)	0.007	0.004
Bond angles (°)	0.82	0.66
Ramachandran plot		
Favoured (%)	96.91	95.82
Allowed (%)	2.94	4.02
Outliers (%)	0.15	0.15

* The values in brackets refer to the highest resolution shell. § After anisotropic analysis with STARANISO [39].

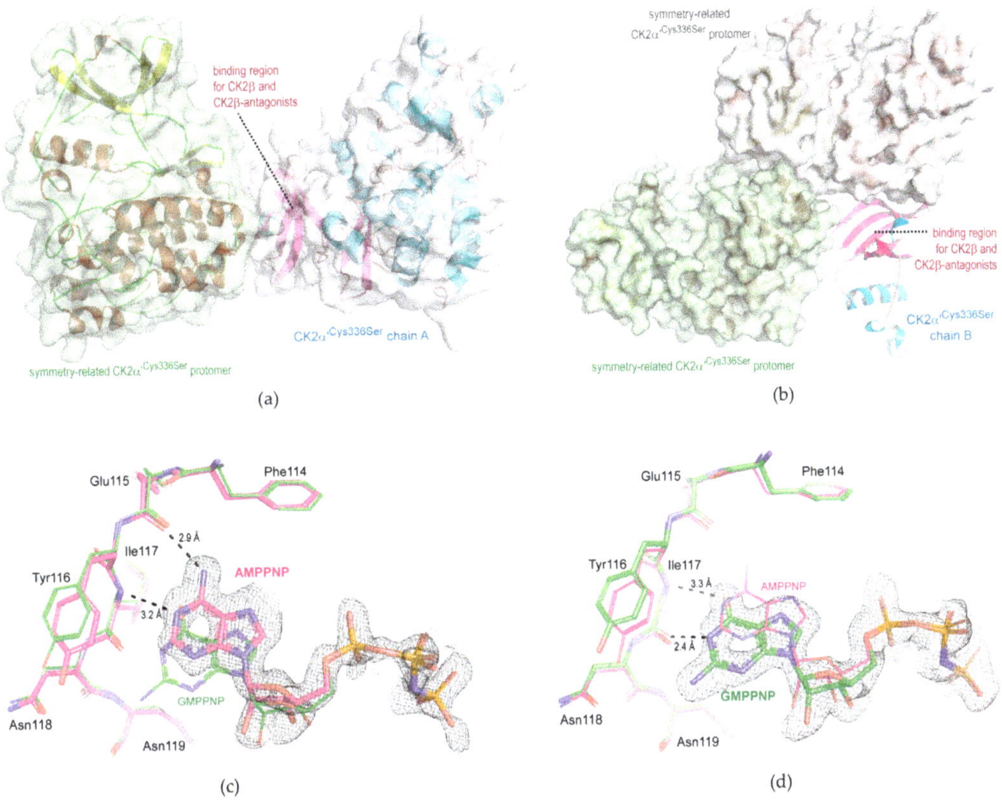

Figure 3. CK2α′^{Cys336Ser} structures obtained with monoclinic crystals. The asymmetric unit contains two CK2α′^{Cys336Ser} chains. (**a**) Crystal contact of the N-terminal domain of CK2α′^{Cys336Ser} chain A with a symmetry-related CK2α′^{Cys336Ser} protomer. (**b**) Crystal packing environment of the N-terminal domain of CK2α′^{Cys336Ser} chain B. (**c**) Cosubstrate binding site of the CK2α′^{Cys336Ser}/AMPPNP complex structure (magenta-coloured C-atoms); for comparison, the CK2α′^{Cys336Ser}/GMPPNP complex structure was drawn with green C-atoms. (**d**) Cosubstrate binding site of the CK2α′^{Cys336Ser}/GMPPNP complex structure (green C-atoms); for comparison, the CK2α′^{Cys336Ser}/AMPPNP complex structure was drawn with magenta-coloured C-atoms. The cutoff level for electron density illustration in this figure is generally 1 σ. The structure pictures were produced with PyMol [36].

The X-ray diffraction capacity of the monoclinic CK2α′^{Cys336Ser} crystals (Table 2) is similar to that of the triclinic crystals (Table 1), i.e., structures with atomic resolution can be achieved and expected. We demonstrate this here with two CK2α′^{Cys336Ser} complex structures with the co-substrate analogues AMPPNP or GMPPNP (Scheme 1), both of which are well visible in electron density at the ATP site (Figure 3c,d), at least in one of the two protomers, respectively.

The ability of CK2 to use GTP as well as ATP as cosubstrate for the kinase reaction has been known since the early 1960s [55]. The first evidence that this dual-cosubstrate specificity is a special property of CK2 compared to other protein kinases emerged in the 1970s [56], but how exceptional this feature of CK2α and CK2α′ really is among EPKs has only been demonstrated in recent years by affinity profiling [57]. Its structural background was clarified with maize CK2α structures in complex of AMPPNP or GMPPNP [58], which revealed essentially what is visible in Figure 3c,d again: the triphospho moieties of the two ligands overlap exactly, but in the region of the purine bases, the different hydrogen-bonding potentials of adenine and guanine enforce a shift of GMPPNP compared to AMPPNP so that finally the pattern of hydrogen bonds between the purine base and the hinge region is shifted by one peptide bond toward the C-terminus.

3. Materials and Methods

3.1. Protein Expression and Purification

For any crystallization experiment shown in this work, we used the point mutant $CK2\alpha^{\prime Cys336Ser}$ with an N-terminal His-tag [13]. The corresponding construct in a pETDuet-1 vector (Merck) was transformed into either chemically competent *E. coli* Gen-X^{TM} (DE3) or chemically competent BL21 Star (DE3) cells. A single clone, respectively, was selected for a preculture. For this, the cells were grown overnight at 30 °C in 100 mL LB medium (10 g/L yeast extract, 20 g/L tryptone, and 20 g/L NaCl) supplemented with 100 µg/mL ampicilin under constant agitation at 180 rpm. An amount of 10 mL of the preculture was used to inocculate 600 mL LB medium.

The subsequent main cultures were grown to an OD_{600} of 0.6 at 37 °C under constant agitation at 180 rpm. Upon reaching an OD600 of 0.6, the temperature was lowered to 18 °C, and isopropyl-β-thiogalactosid (IPTG) was added to a final concentration of 0.5 mM. Expression was subsequently carried out for 18 h. Afterwards, the cells were harvested via centrifugation at 4 °C and 6200× *g* for 30 min. The pellet was washed with a 0.9% (*w*/*v*) sodium chloride solution and afterwards stored at −80 °C. For lysis, the pellet was thawed and then incubated with lysis buffer composed of 500 mM NaCl, 25 mM TRIS-HCl, pH 8.5, 10 µg/mL DNase1, and 1 mg/mL lysozyme for 1 h on ice. Sonification (40% amplitude, 2 s on/4 s off, 4 °C, 3 min total sonification) followed. The lysate was cleared by ultracentrifugation (186,000× *g*, 4 °C, 30 min). The supernatant was filtered and then filled into a superloop for application onto a 5 mL HisTrap FF column (Cytiva) mounted on an ÄKTA Explorer System. Application and washing (15 CV) were carried out using buffer A (40 mM imidazole, 500 mM NaCl, and 25 mM TRIS-HCl. pH 8.5). Afterwards, the protein was eluted using a linear gradient from 0 to 100% buffer B (250 mM imidazole, 500 mM NaCl, 25 mM TRIS-HCl, pH 8.5) over 15 CV. The flowrate was 0.8 mL/min. Elution was monitored via absorption at 280 nm. All fractions within a peak occurring during elution were tested using SDS-PAGE. Fractions containing pure $CK2\alpha^{\prime Cys336Ser}$ were pooled, rebuffered into a standard assay buffer (500 mM NaCl, 25 mM TRIS-HCl, pH 8.5), and concentrated to 5 mg/mL by ultrafiltration using AMICON® tubes with a cut-off of 30 kDa.

3.2. Preparation of ARC-780

While all other CK2 ligands used in this work were either commercially available or (in the case of MB002) were provided by Prof. Maria Bretner, Warsaw, Poland, the substance ARC-780, which had been planned to be a bisubstrate inhibitor, had to be synthesized. For this, $(L\text{-Asp})_3$ peptide with tert-butyl-protected side chains was synthesized on 2-chlorotrityl chloride (2CTC) polystyrene resin (Iris Biotech GmbH) according to common Fmoc-peptide synthesis protocols. Succinic acid and the precursors of residues of 12-[(carboxymethyl)amino]dodecanoic acid and 4-(2-amino-1,3-thiazol-5-yl)benzoic acid were synthesized and attached to the peptide as it was described previously [59]. The compound was cleaved from the resin with a 3 h treatment with TFA:TIPS:H_2O (95:2.5:2.5, *v*:*v*:*v*); subsequent RP-HPLC purification [Shimadzu Prominence LC Solution HPLC system with SPD M20A PDA detector; Phenomenex Gemini C18 RP column, 250 × 4.6 mm, particle size 5 µm, eluted with MeCN/H_2O gradient (0.1% TFA) at flow rate of 1 mL/min; gradient of 20–62% MeCN/14 min, R_t of the title compound: 10.7 min, λ_{max} = 322 nm; Figure S1] yielded ARC-780 with a purity of more than 96.5% (Peak Table insert in Figure S1). The structure was verified using high-resolution mass spectrometry (HRMS) with combined Varian 910-FT-ICR and Varian J-320 3Q spectrometers used in ESI positive ion mode (Figure S2; found: 921.31740 Da [M + H^+]; m/z calcd. $C_{40}H_{52}N_6O_{17}S$ [M + H^+]: 921.31824 Da).

3.3. *Protein Crystallization*

3.3.1. General Procedure

All crystals were grown by applying the sitting drop variant of the vapor diffusion method. For this, 24-well plates (Cryschem) were used. The volume of the reservoir solution was initially 700 µL. All plates were sealed with transparent adhesive film and kept at 20 °C. All microseeding steps were carried out by destroying one crystal from a previous experiment and streaking a loop first through the resulting suspension of crystal seeds and afterwards through the drop that should be inocculated.

3.3.2. Preparation of CK2α′Cys336Ser/SGC-CK2-1 Binary Complex Crystals and of CK2α$'^{Cys336Ser}$/CX-4945/DPA Ternary Complex Crystals

Co-crystals of CK2α$'^{Cys336Ser}$ and MB002 (Scheme 1; provided by Maria Bretner, Warsaw, Poland) were grown according to the previously published protocol [19]. For this, a 5 mg/mL stock solution of CK2α$'^{Cys336Ser}$ was mixed in a 1:10 ratio with a 10 mM stock solution of MB002 in DMSO. After incubation on ice for 30 min and centrifugation (16,100× *g* for 2 min, room temperature), 6 µL of the supernatant were mixed with 3 µL of the reservoir solution (900 mM LiCl, 28% (*w*/*v*) PEG 6000, 100 mM TRIS-HCl, pH 8.5). After equilibration, crystal growth was induced by microseeding. Crystals were then optimized via macroseeding. The resulting co-crystals of CK2α$'^{Cys336Ser}$ and MB002 were purged with reservoir solution (900 mM LiCl, 28% (*w*/*v*) PEG 6000, 100 mM TRIS-HCl, pH 8.5).

SGC-CK2-1 (Sigma-Aldrich) was solved in DMSO at a concentration of 10 mM. This solution was added to CK2α$'^{Cys336Ser}$/MB002 complex crystals to a concentration of 2.5 mM for extensive soaking.

DPA (Sigma-Aldrich, St. Louis, MO, USA) was solved in DMSO at a concentration of 50 mM and CX-4945 (TargetMol, Wellesley Hills, MA, USA) to a concentration of 10 mM likewise in DMSO. 1 µL of each of these solutions, respectively, was added to a CK2α$'^{Cys336Ser}$/MB002 complex crystals for extensive soaking.

3.3.3. Preparation of CK2α$'^{Cys336Ser}$/ARC-780 Complex Crystals

Co-crystals of CK2α$'^{Cys336Ser}$ and MB002 were grown, optimized by micro- and macroseeding, and purged as described above. Then, ARC-780 was added to an initial concentration of 1 mM by adding 1 µL of a 10 mM ARC-780 solution in DMSO in a 1:10 ratio to the droplet. After extensive initial soaking, the salt concentration was successively lowered over a period of 8 months, while in parallel, the concentrations of DMSO and PEG6000 were increased. This was conducted by gradually replacing the reservoir and the droplet solution until any NaCl (which came from the storage solution of the protein) was removed, the LiCl concentration was reduced to 50 mM, the PEG 6000 concentration was increased to saturation, and a DMSO content of 30% was reached. Meanwhile, the ARC-780 ligand was included in any desalting step reaching saturation after the final dilution step.

3.3.4. Co-Crystallization of CK2α$'^{Cys336Ser}$ and TBBt

For this crystallization attempt, the initial co-crystallization with MB002 was avoided. Rather, a 5 mg/mL stock solution of CK2α$'^{Cys336Ser}$ was mixed in a 1:10 ratio with a 20 mM solution of TBBt (Sigma-Aldrich) in DMSO. After incubation on ice for 30 min and centrifugation (16,100× *g* for 2 min, room temperature), 10 µL of the supernatant were mixed with 5 µL of the reservoir solution (900 mM LiCl, 28% (*w*/*v*) PEG 6000, 100 mM TRIS-HCl, pH 8.5). After equilibration, microseeding was carried out to induce crystal growth. Small crystals appeared after one week. One of them was used as a macroseed by transferring it to a second drop prepared in the same manner as the first one.

3.3.5. Growth of CK2α$'^{Cys336Ser}$ Crystals in Complex with AMPPNP or GMPPNP

Monoclinic crystals of CK2α$'^{Cys336Ser}$ were grown in a slightly altered manner compared to the triclinic CK2α$'^{Cys336Ser}$ crystals. 5 mg/mL CK2α$'^{Cys336Ser}$ in storage buffer composed of 500 mM NaCl and 25 mM TRIS-HCl, pH 8.5, were centrifuged immediately after thawing and without mixing it with any inhibitor. 10 µL of the supernatant were mixed with 5 µL of a reservoir solution containing a slightly lowered LiCl concentration of 810 mM, 28% (*w*/*v*) PEG 6000, 100 mM TRIS-HCl, pH 8.5. After equilibration, crystallization was initiated by microseeding, and then crystals were optimized via macroseeding. The ATP-analogue AMPPNP or the GTP-analogue GMPPNP were combined with these crystals by socking. In both cases, a 20 mM solution in 60 mM $MgCl_2$ was prepared. For soaking, 3 µL of the crystal mother liquor were removed and replaced with 3 µL of either 20 mM AMPPNP, 60 mM $MgCl_2$ or 20 mM GMPPNP, 60 mM $MgCl_2$.

3.4. X-ray Diffraction Data Collection and Processing followed by Structure Determination

To prepare X-ray diffraction data collection, any CK2α'^{Cys336Ser}/ligand crystal except for the CK2α'^{Cys336Ser}/ARC-780 co-crystals was cryo-protected before vitrification. For this, 1.4 µL of the reservoir solution and 0.6 µL ethylene glycol were mixed, and the crystals were incubated in this solution for a few seconds. Next, the crystals were flash frozen in liquid nitrogen. Data collections were carried out at beamlines ID 23-1 and MASSIF-3 of the European Synchrotron Radiation Facility (ESRF) in Grenoble (France) or at beamline P13 of the European Molecular Biology Laboratory (EMBL) outstation at DESY in Hamburg (Germany). The temperature during diffraction data collection was 100 K.

The raw diffraction data were processed with the autoPROC toolbox [60] using default settings. The autoPROC pipeline comprises XDS [61] for indexing and integration, POINTLESS [62] and AIMLESS [63] from the CCP4 suite [64] for symmetry determination and scaling, and finally STARANISO [39] for anisotropy analysis. In all cases, the ellipsoidal output data set of STARANISO [39] was used for the further procedure.

All structures were solved by molecular replacement using the CK2α'^{Cys336Ser}/MB002 structure [19] (PDB_ID 6HMQ) as a starting model. The search calculations were performed with PHASER [65] from Phenix [66]. For the subsequent structure refinement, we used the phenix.refine module [67] of Phenix [66] in alternation with Coot [68] for manual model building. Small-molecule ligands were parametrized with eLBOW [69] within the Phenix [66] platform.

4. Conclusions

In this work, six crystal structures of CK2α'^{Cys336Ser} in complex with various ligands and obtained with two different crystal forms are described. In all cases, the high-resolution limit of the underlying X-ray diffraction data is in the range from 1.03 to 1.35 Å. This demonstrates the qualification of CK2α'^{Cys336Ser} as an exquisite tool for CK2 crystallography and emphasizes a tendency to atomic-resolution structures, as indicated already in a survey of the PDB (Figure 1b). In particular, the remarkable robustness of the longer-known triclinic CK2α'^{Cys336Ser} crystals is demonstrated here with an eight-month soaking experiment with ARC-780, a 920 Da molecule designed as a bisubstrate inhibitor, in which the crystals were acclimated to low-salt, DMSO-rich conditions by repeated replacement. In the end, this led to the discovery of the N-terminal segment site, a ligand binding site never observed before in the EPK superfamily that offers the potential to develop highly selective substrate-competitive CK2 inhibitors.

Supplementary Materials: The following supporting information can be downloaded at https://www.mdpi.com/article/10.3390/kinasesphosphatases1040018/s1, Figure S1: RP-HPLC purification of ARC-780; Figure S2: HRMS spectrum of ARC-780; Video S1: binding of ARC-780 to the ATP site and to the novel N-terminal segment site of CK2α'^{Cys336Ser}.

Author Contributions: Conceptualization, C.W., D.L., K.V., A.U. and K.N.; methodology and investigation, C.W., D.L. and K.V.; validation, C.W. and K.N.; data curation, C.W. and K.N.; visualization, D.L. and K.N.; writing—original draft preparation, C.W., K.V. and K.N.; writing—review and editing, C.W., D.L., K.V., A.U. and K.N.; project administration, K.N.; funding acquisition, K.N., K.V. and A.U. All authors have read and agreed to the published version of the manuscript.

Funding: This research was funded by the Deutsche Forschungsgemeinschaft (DFG), grants nos. NI 643/4-1 and NI 643/11-1 to K.N., and by the Estonian Research Council, grant PRG454 to K.V. and A.U.

Institutional Review Board Statement: Not applicable.

Informed Consent Statement: Not applicable.

Data Availability Statement: The atomic coordinates and the structure factors of the six CK2$\alpha'^{Cys336Ser}$ crystal structures documented in Tables 1 and 2 are available from the PDB [2] under the following accession codes: 8Q9S, CK2$\alpha'^{Cys336Ser}$/SGC-CG2-1 complex structure; 8QBU, CK2$\alpha'^{Cys336Ser}$/CX-4945/DPA complex structure; 8Q77, CK2$\alpha'^{Cys336Ser}$/ARC-780 complex structure; 8QCD, CK2$\alpha'^{Cys336Ser}$/TBBt complex structure; 8QCG, CK2$\alpha'^{Cys336Ser}$/AMPPNP complex structure; and 8QF1, CK2$\alpha'^{Cys336Ser}$/GMPPNP complex structure. The digital object identifier (DOI) for the raw X-ray diffraction data underlying the CK2$\alpha'^{Cys336Ser}$/TBBt structure is 10.15151/ESRF-ES-705660733.

Acknowledgments: We thank Professor Ulrich Baumann (University of Cologne) for access to the protein crystallography infrastructure at the Cologne Crystallization facility (C2*f*) and Professor Maria Bretner (Warsaw Technical University) for MB002 (Scheme 1). We are grateful to the staff of the European Synchrotron Radiation Facility (ESRF) in Grenoble (France) and of the European Molecular Biology Laboratory at DESY in Hamburg (Germany) for their assistance with the collection of diffraction data.

Conflicts of Interest: The authors declare no conflict of interest.

References

1. Berman, H.M.; Westbrook, J.; Feng, Z.; Gilliland, G.; Bhat, T.N.; Weissig, H.; Shindyalov, I.N.; Bourne, P.E. The Protein Data Bank. *Nucleic Acids Res.* **2000**, *28*, 235–242. [CrossRef]
2. wwPDB consortium. Protein Data Bank: The single global archive for 3D macromolecular structure data. *Nucleic Acids Res.* **2019**, *47*, D520–D528. [CrossRef] [PubMed]
3. Dobrowolska, G.; Boldyreff, B.; Issinger, O.G. Cloning and sequencing of the casein kinase 2 α subunit from *Zea mays*. *Biochim. Biophys. Acta* **1991**, *1129*, 139–140. [CrossRef] [PubMed]
4. Boldyreff, B.; Meggio, F.; Dobrowolska, G.; Pinna, L.A.; Issinger, O.G. Expression and characterization of a recombinant maize CK-2 α subunit. *Biochim. Biophys. Acta* **1993**, *1173*, 32–38. [CrossRef] [PubMed]
5. Niefind, K.; Guerra, B.; Pinna, L.A.; Issinger, O.G.; Schomburg, D. Crystal structure of the catalytic subunit of protein kinase CK2 from *Zea mays* at 2.1 Å resolution. *EMBO J.* **1998**, *17*, 2451–2462. [CrossRef] [PubMed]
6. Niefind, K.; Guerra, B.; Ermakowa, I.; Issinger, O. Crystal structure of human protein kinase CK2: Insights into basic properties of the CK2 holoenzyme. *EMBO J.* **2001**, *20*, 5320–5331. [CrossRef]
7. Battistutta, R. Protein kinase CK2 in health and disease: Structural bases of protein kinase CK2 inhibition. *Cell. Mol. Life Sci.* **2009**, *66*, 1868–1889. [CrossRef]
8. Cozza, G.; Pinna, L.A.; Moro, S. Protein kinase CK2 inhibitors: A patent review. *Expert Opin. Ther. Pat.* **2012**, *22*, 1081–1097. [CrossRef]
9. Atkinson, E.L.; Iegre, J.; Brear, P.D.; Zhabina, E.A.; Hyvönen, M.; Spring, D.R. Downfalls of Chemical Probes Acting at the Kinase ATP-Site: CK2 as a Case Study. *Molecules* **2021**, *26*, 1977. [CrossRef]
10. Chen, Y.; Wang, Y.; Wang, J.; Zhou, Z.; Cao, S.; Zhang, J. Strategies of Targeting CK2 in Drug Discovery: Challenges, Opportunities, and Emerging Prospects. *J. Med. Chem.* **2023**, *66*, 2257–2281. [CrossRef]
11. Olsen, B.; Boldyreff, B.; Niefind, K.; Issinger, O. Purification and characterization of the CK2α'-based holoenzyme, an isozyme of CK2α: A comparative analysis. *Protein Expr. Purif.* **2006**, *47*, 651–661. [CrossRef] [PubMed]
12. Olsen, B.; Rasmussen, T.; Niefind, K.; Issinger, O. Biochemical characterization of CK2 α and α' paralogues and their derived holoenzymes: Evidence for the existence of a heterotrimeric CK2 α'-holoenzyme forming trimeric complexes. *Mol. Cell. Biochem.* **2008**, *316*, 37–47. [CrossRef]
13. Bischoff, N.; Olsen, B.; Raaf, J.; Bretner, M.; Issinger, O.G.; Niefind, K. Structure of the human protein kinase CK2 catalytic subunit CK2α' and interaction thermodynamics with the regulatory subunit CK2β. *J. Mol. Biol.* **2011**, *407*, 1–12. [CrossRef] [PubMed]
14. Nakaniwa, T.; Kinoshita, T.; Sekiguchi, Y.; Tada, T.; Nakanishi, I.; Kitaura, K.; Suzuki, Y.; Ohno, H.; Hirasawa, A.; Tsujimoto, G. Structure of human protein kinase CK2α2 with a potent indazole-derivative inhibitor. *Acta Crystallogr. F Struct. Biol. Commun.* **2009**, *65*, 75–79. [CrossRef]
15. Tsuyuguchi, M.; Nakaniwa, T.; Kinoshita, T. Crystal structures of human CK2α2 in new crystal forms arising from a subtle difference in salt concentration. *Acta Crystallogr. F Struct. Biol. Commun.* **2018**, *74*, 288–293. [CrossRef] [PubMed]
16. Bretner, M.; Najda-Bernatowicz, A.; Łebska, M.; Muszyńska, G.; Kilanowicz, A.; Sapota, A. New inhibitors of protein kinase CK2, analogues of benzimidazole and benzotriazole. *Mol. Cell. Biochem.* **2008**, *316*, 87–89. [CrossRef] [PubMed]

17. Hochscherf, J.; Lindenblatt, D.; Witulski, B.; Birus, R.; Aichele, D.; Marminon, C.; Bouaziz, Z.; Le Borgne, M.; Jose, J.; Niefind, K. Unexpected Binding Mode of a Potent Indeno[1,2-*b*]indole-Type Inhibitor of Protein Kinase CK2 Revealed by Complex Structures with the Catalytic Subunit CK2α and Its Paralog CK2α′. *Pharmaceuticals* **2017**, *10*, 98. [CrossRef] [PubMed]
18. Niefind, K.; Bischoff, N.; Golub, A.G.; Bdzhola, V.G.; Balanda, A.O.; Prykhod'ko, A.O.; Yarmoluk, S.M. Structural Hypervariability of the Two Human Protein Kinase CK2 Catalytic Subunit Paralogs Revealed by Complex Structures with a Flavonol- and a Thieno[2,3-d]pyrimidine-Based Inhibitor. *Pharmaceuticals* **2017**, *10*, 9. [CrossRef]
19. Lindenblatt, D.; Nickelsen, A.; Applegate, V.M.; Hochscherf, J.; Witulski, B.; Bouaziz, Z.; Marminon, C.; Bretner, M.; Le Borgne, M.; Jose, J.; et al. Diacritic binding of an indenoindole inhibitor by CK2α paralogs explored by a reliable path to atomic resolution CK2α′ structures. *ACS Omega* **2019**, *4*, 5471–5478. [CrossRef] [PubMed]
20. Siddiqui-Jain, A.; Drygin, D.; Streiner, N.; Chua, P.; Pierre, F.; O'Brien, S.E.; Bliesath, J.; Omori, M.; Huser, N.; Ho, C.; et al. CX-4945, an orally bioavailable selective inhibitor of protein kinase CK2, inhibits prosurvival and angiogenic signaling and exhibits antitumor efficacy. *Cancer Res.* **2010**, *70*, 10288–10298. [CrossRef] [PubMed]
21. Battistutta, R.; Cozza, G.; Pierre, F.; Papinutto, E.; Lolli, G.; Sarno, S.; O'Brien, S.E.; Siddiqui-Jain, A.; Haddach, M.; Anderes, K.; et al. Unprecedented selectivity and structural determinants of a new class of protein kinase CK2 inhibitors in clinical trials for the treatment of cancer. *Biochemistry* **2011**, *50*, 8478–8488. [CrossRef]
22. Pierre, F.; Chua, P.C.; O'Brien, S.E.; Siddiqui-Jain, A.; Bourbon, P.; Haddach, M.; Michaux, J.; Nagasawa, J.; Schwaebe, M.K.; Stefan, E.; et al. Pre-clinical characterization of CX-4945, a potent and selective small molecule inhibitor of CK2 for the treatment of cancer. *Mol. Cell. Biochem.* **2011**, *356*, 37–43. [CrossRef] [PubMed]
23. Pierre, F.; Chua, P.C.; O'Brien, S.E.; Siddiqui-Jain, A.; Bourbon, P.; Haddach, M.; Michaux, J.; Nagasawa, J.; Schwaebe, M.K.; Stefan, E.; et al. Discovery and SAR of 5-(3-chlorophenylamino)benzo[*c*][2,6]naphthyridine-8-carboxylic Acid (CX-4945), the First Clinical Stage Inhibitor of Protein Kinase CK2 for the Treatment of Cancer. *J. Med. Chem.* **2011**, *54*, 635–654. [CrossRef] [PubMed]
24. Chojnacki, K.; Lindenblatt, D.; Wińska, P.; Wielechowska, M.; Toelzer, C.; Niefind, K.; Bretner, M. Synthesis, biological properties and structural study of new halogenated azolo[4,5-*b*]pyridines as inhibitors of CK2 kinase. *Bioorganic Chem.* **2021**, *106*, 104502. [CrossRef]
25. Bestgen, B.; Krimm, I.; Kufareva, I.; Kamal, A.A.M.; Seetoh, W.G.; Abell, C.; Hartmann, R.W.; Abagyan, R.; Cochet, C.; Le Borgne, M.; et al. 2-Aminothiazole Derivatives as Selective Allosteric Modulators of the Protein Kinase CK2. 1. Identification of an Allosteric Binding Site. *J. Med. Chem.* **2019**, *62*, 1803–1816. [CrossRef] [PubMed]
26. Bestgen, B.; Kufareva, I.; Seetoh, W.; Abell, C.; Hartmann, R.W.; Abagyan, R.; Le Borgne, M.; Filhol, O.; Cochet, C.; Lomberget, T.; et al. 2-Aminothiazole Derivatives as Selective Allosteric Modulators of the Protein Kinase CK2. 2. Structure-Based Optimization and Investigation of Effects Specific to the Allosteric Mode of Action. *J. Med. Chem.* **2019**, *62*, 1817–1836. [CrossRef]
27. Lindenblatt, D.; Nickelsen, A.; Applegate, V.M.; Jose, J.; Niefind, K. Structural and Mechanistic Basis of the Inhibitory Potency of Selected 2-Aminothiazole Compounds on Protein Kinase CK2. *J. Med. Chem.* **2020**, *63*, 7766–7772. [CrossRef]
28. Brear, P.; De Fusco, C.; Georgiou, K.H.; Francis-Newton, N.J.; Stubbs, C.J.; Sore, H.F.; Venkitaraman, A.R.; Abell, C.; Spring, D.R.; Hyvönen, M. Specific inhibition of CK2α from an anchor outside the active site. *Chem. Sci.* **2016**, *7*, 6839–6845. [CrossRef] [PubMed]
29. De Fusco, C.; Brear, P.; Iegre, J.; Georgiou, K.H.; Sore, H.F.; Hyvönen, M.; Spring, D.R. A fragment-based approach leading to the discovery of a novel binding site and the selective CK2 inhibitor CAM4066. *Bioorganic Med. Chem.* **2017**, *25*, 3471–3482. [CrossRef]
30. Lindenblatt, D.; Applegate, V.; Nickelsen, A.; Klußmann, M.; Neundorf, I.; Götz, C.; Jose, J.; Niefind, K. Molecular Plasticity of Crystalline CK2α′ Leads to KN2, a Bivalent Inhibitor of Protein Kinase CK2 with Extraordinary Selectivity. *J. Med. Chem.* **2022**, *65*, 1302–1312. [CrossRef]
31. Wells, C.I.; Drewry, D.H.; Pickett, J.E.; Tjaden, A.; Krämer, A.; Müller, S.; Gyenis, L.; Menyhart, D.; Litchfield, D.W.; Knapp, S.; et al. Development of a potent and selective chemical probe for the pleiotropic kinase CK2. *Cell Chem. Biol.* **2021**, *28*, 546–558.e10. [CrossRef] [PubMed]
32. Davis-Gilbert, Z.W.; Krämer, A.; Dunford, J.E.; Howell, S.; Senbabaoglu, F.; Wells, C.I.; Bashore, F.M.; Havener, T.M.; Smith, J.L.; Hossain, M.A.; et al. Discovery of a Potent and Selective Naphthyridine-Based Chemical Probe for Casein Kinase 2. *ACS Med. Chem. Lett.* **2023**, *14*, 432–441. [CrossRef] [PubMed]
33. Pack, M.; Götz, C.; Wrublewsky, S.; Montenarh, M. SGC-CK2-1 Is an Efficient Inducer of Insulin Production and Secretion in Pancreatic β-Cells. *Pharmaceutics* **2021**, *14*, 19. [CrossRef] [PubMed]
34. Mishra, S.; Kinoshita, C.; Axtman, A.D.; Young, J.E. Evaluation of a Selective Chemical Probe Validates That CK2 Mediates Neuroinflammation in a Human Induced Pluripotent Stem Cell-Derived Mircroglial Model. *Front. Mol. Neurosci.* **2022**, *15*, 824956. [CrossRef] [PubMed]
35. Boewe, A.S.; Wemmert, S.; Kulas, P.; Schick, B.; Götz, C.; Wrublewsky, S.; Montenarh, M.; Menger, M.D.; Laschke, M.W.; Ampofo, E. Inhibition of CK2 Reduces NG2 Expression in Juvenile Angiofibroma. *Biomedicines* **2022**, *10*, 966. [CrossRef] [PubMed]
36. PyMOL. *The PyMOL Molecular Graphics System, version 1.7*; Schrödinger, LLC: New York, NY, USA, 2013.
37. Battistutta, R.; De Moliner, E.; Sarno, S.; Zanotti, G.; Pinna, L.A. Structural features underlying selective inhibition of protein kinase CK2 by ATP site-directed tetrabromo-2-benzotriazole. *Protein Sci.* **2001**, *10*, 2200–2206. [CrossRef]
38. Winiewska-Szajewska, M.; Czapinska, H.; Kaus-Drobek, M.; Fricke, A.; Mieczkowska, K.; Dadlez, M.; Bochtler, M.; Poznański, J. Competition between electrostatic interactions and halogen bonding in the protein-ligand system: Structural and thermodynamic studies of 5,6-dibromobenzotriazole-hCK2α complexes. *Sci. Rep.* **2022**, *12*, 18964. [CrossRef]

39. Tickle, I.J.; Flensburg, C.; Keller, P.; Paciorek, W.; Sharff, A.; Vonrhein, C.; Bricogne, G. *STARANISO*; Global Phasing Ltd.: Cambridge, UK, 2018.
40. Janeczko, M.; Orzeszko, A.; Kazimierczuk, Z.; Szyszka, R.; Baier, A. CK2α and CK2α′ subunits differ in their sensitivity to 4,5,6,7-tetrabromo- and 4,5,6,7-tetraiodo-*1H*-benzimidazole derivatives. *Eur. J. Med. Chem.* **2012**, *47*, 345–350. [CrossRef] [PubMed]
41. Ikeda, A.; Tsuyuguchi, M.; Kitagawa, D.; Sawa, M.; Nakamura, S.; Nakanishi, I.; Kinoshita, T. Bivalent binding mode of an amino-pyrazole inhibitor indicates the potentials for CK2α1-selective inhibitors. *Biochem. Biophys. Res. Commun.* **2022**, *630*, 30–35. [CrossRef] [PubMed]
42. Cimermancic, P.; Weinkam, P.; Rettenmaier, T.J.; Bichmann, L.; Keedy, D.A.; Woldeyes, R.A.; Schneidman-Duhovny, D.; Demerdash, O.N.; Mitchell, J.C.; Wells, J.A.; et al. CryptoSite: Expanding the Druggable Proteome by Characterization and Prediction of Cryptic Binding Sites. *J. Mol. Biol.* **2016**, *428*, 709–719. [CrossRef]
43. Pietsch, M.; Viht, K.; Schnitzler, A.; Ekambaram, R.; Steinkrüger, M.; Enkvist, E.; Nienberg, C.; Nickelsen, A.; Lauwers, M.; Jose, J.; et al. Unexpected CK2β-antagonistic functionality of bisubstrate inhibitors targeting protein kinase CK2. *Bioorganic Chem.* **2020**, *96*, 103608. [CrossRef] [PubMed]
44. Czapinska, H.; Winiewska-Szajewska, M.; Szymaniec-Rutkowska, A.; Piasecka, A.; Bochtler, M.; Poznański, J. Halogen Atoms in the Protein-Ligand System. Structural and Thermodynamic Studies of the Binding of Bromobenzotriazoles by the Catalytic Subunit of Human Protein Kinase CK2. *J. Phys. Chem. B* **2021**, *125*, 2491–2503. [CrossRef] [PubMed]
45. Wąsik, R.; Wińska, P.; Poznański, J.; Shugar, D. Synthesis and physico-chemical properties in aqueous medium of all possible isomeric bromo analogues of benzo-1H-triazole, potential inhibitors of protein kinases. *J. Phys. Chem. B* **2012**, *116*, 7259–7268. [CrossRef] [PubMed]
46. Battistutta, R.; Mazzorana, M.; Cendron, L.; Bortolato, A.; Sarno, S.; Kazimierczuk, Z.; Zanotti, G.; Moro, S.; Pinna, L.A. The ATP-binding site of protein kinase CK2 holds a positive electrostatic area and conserved water molecules. *Chembiochem* **2007**, *8*, 1804–1809. [CrossRef]
47. Winiewska-Szajewska, M.; Maciejewska, A.M.; Speina, E.; Poznański, J.; Paprocki, D. Synthesis of Novel Halogenated Heterocycles Based on *o*-Phenylenediamine and Their Interactions with the Catalytic Subunit of Protein Kinase CK2. *Molecules* **2021**, *26*, 3163. [CrossRef]
48. Laudet, B.; Barette, C.; Dulery, V.; Renaudet, O.; Dumy, P.; Metz, A.; Prudent, R.; Deshiere, A.; Dideberg, O.; Filhol, O.; et al. Structure-based design of small peptide inhibitors of protein kinase CK2 subunit interaction. *Biochem. J.* **2007**, *408*, 363–373. [CrossRef]
49. Laudet, B.; Moucadel, V.; Prudent, R.; Filhol, O.; Wong, Y.S.; Royer, D.; Cochet, C. Identification of chemical inhibitors of protein-kinase CK2 subunit interaction. *Mol. Cell. Biochem.* **2008**, *316*, 63–69. [CrossRef]
50. Brear, P.; North, A.; Iegre, J.; Hadje Georgiou, K.; Lubin, A.; Carro, L.; Green, W.; Sore, H.F.; Hyvönen, M.; Spring, D.R. Novel non-ATP competitive small molecules targeting the CK2 α/β interface. *Bioorganic Med. Chem.* **2018**, *26*, 3016–3020. [CrossRef]
51. Kufareva, I.; Bestgen, B.; Brear, P.; Prudent, R.; Laudet, B.; Moucadel, V.; Ettaoussi, M.; Sautel, C.F.; Krimm, I.; Engel, M.; et al. Discovery of holoenzyme-disrupting chemicals as substrate-selective CK2 inhibitors. *Sci. Rep.* **2019**, *9*, 15893. [CrossRef]
52. Lindenblatt, D.; Horn, M.; Götz, C.; Niefind, K.; Neundorf, I.; Pietsch, M. Design of CK2β-Mimicking Peptides as Tools To Study the CK2α/CK2β Interaction in Cancer Cells. *ChemMedChem* **2019**, *14*, 833–841. [CrossRef]
53. Tang, S.; Zhang, N.; Zhou, Y.; Cortopassi, W.A.; Jacobson, M.P.; Zhao, L.J.; Zhong, R.G. Structure-based Discovery of Novel CK2α-Binding Cyclic Peptides with Anti-cancer Activity. *Mol. Infor.* **2019**, *38*, e1800089. [CrossRef] [PubMed]
54. Atkinson, E.L.; Iegre, J.; D'Amore, C.; Brear, P.; Salvi, M.; Hyvönen, M.; Spring, D.R. Development of small cyclic peptides targeting the CK2α/β interface. *Chem. Commun.* **2022**, *58*, 4791–4794. [CrossRef] [PubMed]
55. Rodnight, R.; Lavin, B.E. Phosvitin kinase from brain: Activation by ions and subcellular distribution. *Biochem. J.* **1964**, *93*, 84–91. [CrossRef] [PubMed]
56. Hathaway, G.M.; Traugh, J.A. Cyclic nucleotide-independent protein kinases from rabbit reticulocytes. Purification of casein kinases. *J. Biol. Chem.* **1979**, *254*, 762–768. [CrossRef] [PubMed]
57. Becher, I.; Savitski, M.M.; Savitski, M.F.; Hopf, C.; Bantscheff, M.; Drewes, G. Affinity profiling of the cellular kinome for the nucleotide cofactors ATP, ADP, and GTP. *ACS Chem. Biol.* **2013**, *8*, 599–607. [CrossRef] [PubMed]
58. Niefind, K.; Pütter, M.; Guerra, B.; Issinger, O.G.; Schomburg, D. GTP plus water mimic ATP in the active site of protein kinase CK2. *Nat. Struct. Biol.* **1999**, *6*, 1100–1103. [CrossRef] [PubMed]
59. Rahnel, H.; Viht, K.; Lavogina, D.; Mazina, O.; Haljasorg, T.; Enkvist, E.; Uri, A. A Selective Biligand Inhibitor of CK2 Increases Caspase-3 Activity in Cancer Cells and Inhibits Platelet Aggregation. *ChemMedChem* **2017**, *12*, 1723–1736. [CrossRef]
60. Vonrhein, C.; Flensburg, C.; Keller, P.; Sharff, A.; Smart, O.; Paciorek, W.; Womack, T.; Bricogne, G. Data processing and analysis with the autoPROC toolbox. *Acta Crystallogr. D Struct. Biol.* **2011**, *67*, 293–302. [CrossRef]
61. Kabsch, W. XDS. *Acta Crystallogr. D Struct. Biol.* **2010**, *66*, 125–132. [CrossRef]
62. Evans, P. Scaling and assessment of data quality. *Acta Crystallogr. D Struct. Biol.* **2006**, *62*, 72–82. [CrossRef]
63. Evans, P.R.; Murshudov, G.N. How good are my data and what is the resolution? *Acta Crystallogr. D Struct. Biol.* **2013**, *69*, 1204–1214. [CrossRef]
64. Winn, M.D.; Ballard, C.C.; Cowtan, K.D.; Dodson, E.J.; Emsley, P.; Evans, P.R.; Keegan, R.M.; Krissinel, E.B.; Leslie, A.G.; McCoy, A.; et al. Overview of the CCP4 suite and current developments. *Acta Crystallogr. D Struct. Biol.* **2011**, *67*, 235–242. [CrossRef]

65. McCoy, A.J.; Grosse-Kunstleve, R.W.; Adams, P.D.; Winn, M.D.; Storoni, L.C.; Read, R.J. Phaser crystallographic software. *J. Appl. Crystallogr.* **2007**, *40*, 658–674. [CrossRef] [PubMed]
66. Adams, P.D.; Afonine, P.V.; Bunkóczi, G.; Chen, V.B.; Davis, I.W.; Echols, N.; Headd, J.J.; Hung, L.W.; Kapral, G.J.; Grosse-Kunstleve, R.W.; et al. PHENIX: A comprehensive Python-based system for macromolecular structure solution. *Acta Crystallogr. D Struct. Biol.* **2010**, *66*, 213–221. [CrossRef] [PubMed]
67. Afonine, P.V.; Grosse-Kunstleve, R.W.; Echols, N.; Headd, J.J.; Moriarty, N.W.; Mustyakimov, M.; Terwilliger, T.C.; Urzhumtsev, A.; Zwart, P.H.; Adams, P.D. Towards automated crystallographic structure refinement with phenix.refine. *Acta Crystallogr. D Struct. Biol.* **2012**, *68*, 352–367. [CrossRef] [PubMed]
68. Emsley, P.; Lohkamp, B.; Scott, W.G.; Cowtan, K. Features and development of Coot. *Acta Crystallogr. D Struct. Biol.* **2010**, *66*, 486–501. [CrossRef]
69. Moriarty, N.W.; Grosse-Kunstleve, R.W.; Adams, P.D. Electronic Ligand Builder and Optimization Workbench (eLBOW): A tool for ligand coordinate and restraint generation. *Acta Crystallogr. D Struct. Biol.* **2009**, *65*, 1074–1080. [CrossRef]

kinases and phosphatases

MDPI

Brief Report

The CK2/ECE1c Partnership: An Unveiled Pathway to Aggressiveness in Cancer

Karla Villalobos-Nova †, María de los Ángeles Toro †, Pablo Pérez-Moreno, Ignacio Niechi ‡ and Julio C. Tapia *

Laboratorio de Transformación Celular, Programa de Biología Celular y Molecular, Instituto de Ciencias Biomédicas, Facultad de Medicina, Universidad de Chile, Santiago 8380453, Chile; karla.villalobos@ug.uchile.cl (K.V.-N.); maria.dl.angeles.tb@hotmail.com (M.d.l.Á.T.); p.perez@udd.cl (P.P.-M.); ignacio.niechi@uach.cl (I.N.)

* Correspondence: jtapiapineda@uchile.cl

† These authors contributed equally to this work.

‡ Current address: Instituto de Bioquímica y Microbiología, Facultad de Ciencias, Universidad Austral de Chile, Valdivia 5110566, Chile.

Abstract: The endothelin-1 (ET1) peptide has a pathological role in the activation of proliferation, survival and invasiveness pathways in different cancers. ET1's effects rely on its activation by the endothelin-converting enzyme-1 (ECE1), which is expressed as four isoforms, differing only in their cytoplasmic N-terminuses. We already demonstrated in colorectal cancer, glioblastoma, and preliminarily lung cancer, that the isoform ECE1c heightens aggressiveness by promoting cancer stem cell traits. This is achieved through a non-canonical ET1-independent mechanism of enhancement of ECE1c's stability upon CK2-dependent phosphorylation at S18 and S20. Here, a K6 residue is presumably responsible for ECE1c ubiquitination as its mutation to R impairs proteasomal degradation. However, how phosphorylation enhances ECE1c's stability and how this translates into aggressiveness are still open questions. In this brief report, by swapping residues to either phospho-mimetic or phospho-resistant amino acids, we propose that the N-terminus may also be phosphorylated at Y5 and/or T9 by an unknown kinase(s). In addition, N-terminus phosphorylation may lead to a blockage of K6 ubiquitination, increasing ECE1c's stability and presumably activating the Wnt/β-catenin signaling pathway. Thus, a novel CK2/ECE1c partnership may be emerging to promote aggressiveness and thus become a biomarker of poor prognosis and a potential therapeutic target for several cancers.

Keywords: endothelin; CK2; phosphorylation; proteasome; β-catenin; aggressiveness

1. Introduction

Cancer stem cells (CSC) are a marginal cell population responsible for genesis, metastasis, and relapse after chemotherapy in many tumors [1–6]. In recent years, various signaling pathways have garnered attention due to their capacity to provoke CSC development and therefore promote aggressiveness traits. One such signaling pathway, the endothelin-1 (ET1) axis, has been highlighted as playing a pathological role in cancer etiology. In its physiological role, the ET1 axis contributes to the regulation of vascular tone, mainly through binding to its ET_BR receptor. On the other hand, the stimulation of its ET_AR receptor leads to the pathological activation of cancer pathways [7–9]. The ET1 peptide is activated by the cleaving of the endothelin-converting enzyme-1 (ECE1), a membrane-bound protease constituted by three domains: a short N-terminal cytoplasmic domain (which defines four isoforms), followed by a transmembrane domain, and finally a large extracellular C-terminal catalytic domain [9–12].

ECE1 expression has been found to be elevated in patients with various cancers, and increased mRNA and/or protein levels have been detected in several cancer cell lines, with the ECE1c being the most-expressed isoform [13–15]. High levels of ET1 have also been identified in patients with colorectal cancer, suggesting that ECE1 may participate in the disease process [16–18]. Furthermore, an early study reported the increased invasiveness triggered by isoform ECE1c in prostate cancer cells [19]. However, the role of this and of the other ECE1 isoforms in cancer hallmarks beyond invasiveness was an open question for many years.

2. Results and Discussion

2.1. The ECE1c-Dependent Acquisition of a CSC Phenotype

A breakthrough arrived in 2015, when Niechi et al. first reported that isoform ECE1c leads to aggressiveness in colorectal cancer cells [20]. Importantly, these authors demonstrated that the protein kinase CK2 can phosphorylate ECE1c in its N-terminal cytoplasmic domain, greatly enhancing its stability [20]. In fact, the literature shows that CK2 may regulate the stability of many proteins. For example, CK2's phosphorylation of c-myc prevents its proteasomal degradation, enhancing the transcription of genes involved in several cancer hallmarks [21]. Likewise, CK2's phosphorylation of OTUB1 promotes its nuclear deubiquitinating activity and stabilization of chromatin-binding proteins [22]. Indeed, increased CK2 mRNA and protein levels have been found in many types of tumors [23–27]. The findings from Niechi et al. take on special relevance in colorectal cancer, as CK2 regulates many traits related to aggressiveness in this disease, such as survival, resistance to death, metabolic changes, angiogenesis, DNA repair, and tumor growth [28,29]. In consequence, the existence of a non-canonical ET1-independent mechanism underlying cancer cell aggressiveness, occurring through the CK2-dependent phosphorylation of ECE1c, is emerging as an interesting possibility (Figure 1).

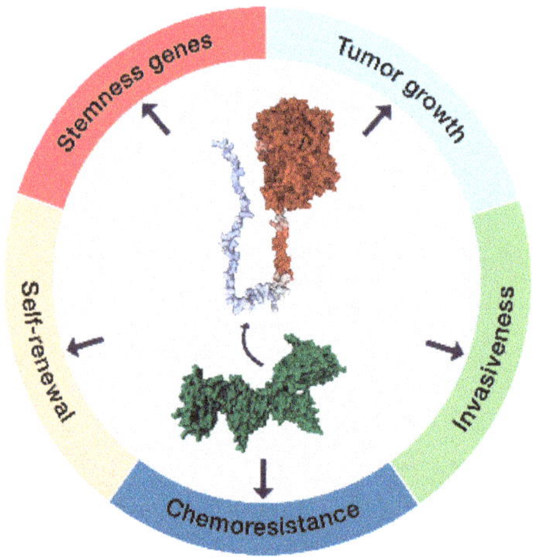

Figure 1. Stable ECE1c leads to CSC traits in various cancer models. Schematic representation of the hallmarks associated with CSCs observed in vitro upon stabilization of ECE1c. Protein stability of ECE1c has been experimentally enhanced by the following mutations at its N-terminus: K6R (ubiquitination site, putative) and S18D/S20D (CK2 phosphorylation sites). As a consequence, traits associated with a CSC phenotype, such as expression of stemness genes, self-renewal, tumor growth, invasiveness and drug resistance, have been found to be significantly augmented in colorectal cancer [30], glioblastoma [31] and lung cancer [32] cells. ECE1 three-dimensional structure (upper) corresponds to a computational prediction (AF-P42892-F1) of isoform B obtained from AlphaFold (https://alphafold.ebi.ac.uk/; accessed on 30 October 2023). The 3D structure is shown in molecular surface representation and is colored by uncertainty/disorder. The 3D structure of human CK2 holoenzyme (lower) corresponds to accession 1JWH obtained from the Protein Data Bank (PDB; https://www.rcsb.org/; accessed on 30 October 2023) and is depicted in molecular surface mode and colored by model index.

2.2. CK2's Phosphorylation of ECE1c and Aggressiveness

The N-terminus of ECE1c is highly conserved in several species, displaying almost a complete identity [15]. It contains three conserved putative phosphorylation sites for CK2: T9, S18, and S20, which are predicted to be excellent substrates by the NetPhos 3.1 software (www.cbs.dtu.dk; accessed 31 July 2023). By designing biphospho-mimetic (i.e., $ECE1c^{S18D/S20D}$) and biphospho-resistant (i.e., $ECE1c^{S18A/S20A}$) mutants at both serines, Pérez-Moreno et al. delved deeper into the mechanism(s) that may enhance the stability of ECE1c. These authors clearly demonstrated that S18 and S20 residues are *bona fide* CK2 phosphorylation sites, which greatly enhance the stability of ECE1c but also lead to an increased invasiveness and other aggressiveness-associated traits in colorectal cancer cells. Surprisingly, while T9 was an excellent putative substrate for CK2, it was not in fact phosphorylated in vitro by this kinase [33]. However, phosphorylation at T9 (or even at Y5, according to NetPhos 3.1) is greatly disfavored when S18/S20 are replaced by alanines, while phosphorylation is significantly enhanced when serines are swapped for phospho-mimetic aspartates (Figure 2a). Moreover, CHO-K1 cells—which express negligible ECE1 levels—were used to show that the triphospho-mimetic $ECE1c^{DDD}$ mutant displays significant resistance to ubiquitination compared to its counterpart, $ECE1c^{AAA}$ (Figure 2b).

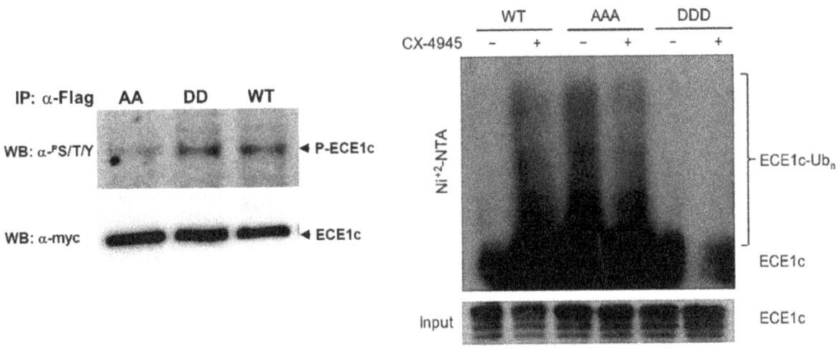

(a) (b)

Figure 2. Phosphorylation of ECE1c blocks its ubiquitination. (**a**) DLD-1 cells expressing either Myc/Flag-tagged ECE1c wild-type (WT) or mutants (AA: S18A/S20A; DD: S18D/S20D) were treated with MG-132. Cell lysates were immunoprecipitated (IP) with an anti-Flag antibody and then ECE1c proteins phosphorylated at any S/T/Y were detected by Western blot (WB) with an anti-pS/pT/pY pan-antibody. Total immunoprecipitated ECE1c was detected by WB with an anti-Myc antibody. (**b**) CHO-K1 cells expressing $ECE1c^{WT}$, $ECE1c^{AAA}$ (i.e., T9A/S18A/S20A), or $ECE1c^{DDD}$ (i.e., T9D/S18D/S20D) were transfected with a plasmid encoding His6-tagged ubiquitin. Cells were treated, or not treated, with the CK2 inhibitor CX-4945 to promote ECE1c degradation. His6-ubiquitinated proteins of each lysate were pulled down with a Ni^{+2}-NTA resin, separated by SDS-PAGE, and detected by WB with an anti-ECE1 pan-antibody (upper). Total ECE1c levels at input are also shown (lower).

The above findings are consistent with a potential hierarchical process in which phospho-serines are a requisite for phosphorylation at Y5 or T9. Alternatively, as reported for some substrates of CK2, the regulatory β subunit may have a docking function in T9 phosphorylation in a given cell context [34–36]. This docking event has been observed, for instance, with the inhibitor of cyclin-dependent kinases, $p27^{KIP1}$, whose phosphorylation via CK2 only occurs in the presence of the β subunit [36]. Finally, it is also plausible that while S18/S20 are CK2 substrates, another kinase(s) actually phosphorylates at Y5 or T9. In this regard, the EGF receptor, although with a low score of 0.389 as predicted by NetPhos 3.1, may phosphorylate ECE1c at Y5. Likewise, PKA with a score of 0.656 may also phosphorylate it at T9.

But beyond phosphorylating Y5/T9, how does ECE1c's phosphorylation translate into enhanced protein stability? The simplest answer is that CK2 phosphorylation induces a conformational change at the N-terminus—a phenomenon already reported for other proteins [36]—that can block protein degradation. On the other hand, many proteins are ubiquitinated in a lysine-dependent fashion to be further degraded by the proteasome [37,38]. In fact, ECE1c contains a conserved K6 residue at its N-terminus [15]. Moreover, the proteasomal inhibitor MG-132 blocks the degradation triggered by the specific CK2 inhibitor silmitasertib in colorectal cancer cells [20]. Thus, CK2 phosphorylation may be linked to greater ECE1c stability by somehow impeding ubiquitination at K6.

To confirm the above hypothesis and correlate increased protein stability with enhanced aggressiveness, Pérez-Moreno et al. mutated K6 to arginine (i.e., ECE1c^{K6R}) to block ubiquitination. As anticipated, protein stability was dramatically increased but, surprisingly and importantly, this mutant protein led to the occurrence of a CSC-like phenotype and a significantly greater aggressiveness of the colorectal cancer cells both in vitro and in vivo [30]. Notably, comparable results have been observed in other cancer models, such as glioblastoma [31] and lung cancer [32].

In terms of the mechanism that could explain the enhanced stability of ECE1c, a conformational change in the phosphorylated N-terminus may prevent K6 ubiquitination. Another potential mechanism is the binding of an adaptor to the phospho-sites. Adaptors that bind to either phospho-Thr or phospho-Ser include proteins containing FHA-, WW-, PoloBox-, or WD40-domains; 14-3-3 proteins; and leucine-rich repeats [39–42]. Nevertheless, whether the underlying mechanism leading to aggressiveness is shared among other types of cancer of different tumor origins remains another interesting but unsolved question.

2.3. The Non-Canonical ET1 Regulation of Signaling Proteins

The effect of the ECE1c^{K6R} mutant has been observed to be independent of its canonical role in activating the ET1 peptide. Levels of this peptide in culture media of ECE1c^{K6R}-expressing cells were indistinguishable from those of ECE1c^{WT}-expressing cells originating from colorectal cancer [30], glioblastoma [31] or lung cancer [32]. Taken together with data obtained using ECE1c inhibitors, ET$_A$R silencers, ET$_A$R antagonists, and ET1 supply (for review [15]), these findings indicate that the promotion of an ECE1c-driven CSC phenotype occurs in parallel to, if not at the expense of, ET1 activation and binding to its ET$_A$R receptor.

Consistent with the above findings, studies using an array of human phosphoproteins from colorectal cancer cells showed that the expression of the highly stable biphospho-mimetic ECE1c^{DD} mutant—functionally similar to ECE1c^{K6R}—promotes significant changes in some signaling proteins (Figure 3a). These proteins include β-catenin, AKT1, SRC, and GSK3β, which are known regulators of the canonical Wnt signaling pathway involved in CSC genesis [1–6]. Upon activation, β-catenin migrates to the nuclei and transactivates the expression of several genes related with stemness, proliferation, differentiation, death, etc. [43–45]. Our data show that the expression of the super-stable ECE1c^{K6R} mutant promotes nuclear localization of β-catenin in colorectal cancer cells (Figure 3b,c), which strongly suggests an activation of the canonical Wnt signaling pathway. In fact, we have already determined a significantly augmented expression of many canonical Wnt target genes as a consequence of the expression of both super-stable ECE1c^{K6R} and biphospho-mimetic ECE1c$^{S18D/S20D}$ enzymes in colorectal cancer cells, such as the stemness genes c-Myc, CD44, Lgr5, Nanog and Snail [30], as well as the proliferation-related genes CCND1 (cyclin-D1) and BIRC5 (survivin) [33], respectively. Notably, whether the same nuclear localization of β-catenin following the expression of the super-stable ECE1c^{K6R} occurs in glioblastoma and lung cancer cells is an interesting but yet unsolved issue, since a group of canonical Wnt target genes, such as c-Myc, CD44, MMP9, Oct-4, Snail, Sox-2 and Twist, have been found to be augmented in these cancer models [31,32].

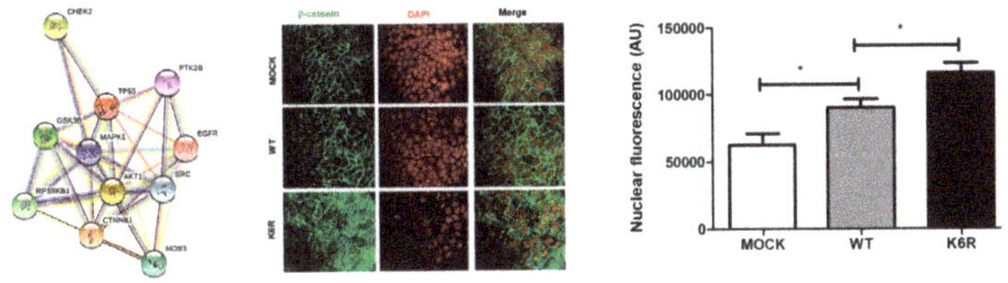

(a) (b) (c)

Figure 3. CSC-linked signaling proteins are regulated by P-ECE1c. (**a**) Lysates from DLD-1 cells expressing ECE1c^{DD}, ECE1c^{AA}, or ECE1c^{WT} were used in a Human Proteome Profiler Array. Phospho-proteins whose levels showed significant variations for ECE1c^{DD} vs. ECE1c^{WT} or ECE1c^{AA} vs. ECE1c^{WT} were: EGF receptor (EGFR), ERK1 (MAPK1), GSK3β, β-catenin (CTNNB1), AKT1, SRC, p53 (TP53), S6K (RPS6KB1), Chk2 (CHEK2), Pyk2 (PTK2B), and eNOS (NOS3). Proteins were analyzed by STRING for protein–protein interactions, including: "known" (cyan: curated databases; pink: experimentally determined), "predicted" (blue: gene co-occurrence), and "other" interactions (green: text mining; black: co-expression; grey: protein homology). (**b**) DLD-1 cells expressing ECE1c^{WT}, ECE1c^{K6R}, or mock were grown under normal conditions for 48 h. β-catenin was detected by confocal IF microscopy with an anti-β-catenin antibody followed of an AF488-conjugated secondary antibody and DAPI for nuclei. (**c**) Nuclear fluorescence (AU: arbitrary units) was quantified in the three clone cells at "b" using the Image J software. Values were plotted as mean ± SE from at least three independent experiments. * $p \leq 0.05$.

Finally, an in silico analysis predicted that all of the proteins detected in the above proteome array may interact with one or more proteins (Figure 3a). However, when ECE1c was incorporated into this analysis, no interactions were predicted with any of the proteins, with the exception of eNOS, which is related to the regulatory role of ECE1 in vascular tone [15]. Moreover, no genetic mutations of Y5, K6, T9, S18, or S20 residues in cancer patients have been reported in the literature [30]. However, it is well known that several signaling proteins are aberrantly elevated in colorectal and other cancers, including CK2 and β-catenin [27,29,45,46]. Thus, whether ECE1c indeed contributes to cancer aggressiveness in a CK2-dependent post-translational manner is an issue that certainly merits continued research.

3. Materials and Methods

Phosphorylation assay. Cells were treated for 3 h with 25 μM MG-132 (Tocris, Bristol, UK). One milligram of cell lysates was immunoprecipitated with 10 μg of rabbit anti-Flag antibody (Cell Signaling Technology, Danvers, MA, USA), and then ECE1c proteins phosphorylated at any S/T/Y were detected by Western blot with a mouse anti-pS/pT/pY pan-antibody (Abcam, Cambridge, UK). Total immunoprecipitated ECE1c was detected by WB with a mouse anti-Myc antibody (Cell Signaling Technology, Danvers, MA, USA).

Ubiquitination assay. Cells were transfected with 5 μg of a plasmid encoding His6-tagged ubiquitin. After 16 h of growing in normal conditions, cells were treated, or not treated, for 24 h with 25 μM of the CK2 inhibitor CX-4945 (ApexBio Technology, Houston, TX, USA) and incubated the last 3 h with 25 μM MG-132 (Cayman, Ann Arbor, MI, USA). His6-ubiquitinated proteins from 1 mg of each lysate were pulled down with a Ni^{+2}-NTA resin (Thermo Fisher Scientific, Waltham, MA, USA), separated by SDS-PAGE, and detected by Western Blot with a rabbit anti-ECE1 pan-antibody (Abcam, Cambridge, UK).

Proteome assay. Cell lysates were used in a Human Proteome Profiler Array (R&D Systems, Minneapolis, MN, USA) following manufacturer's instructions. Phospho-proteins whose levels showed significant variations for ECE1c^{DD} vs. ECE1c^{WT} or ECE1c^{AA} vs. ECE1c^{WT} were analyzed by STRING for protein–protein interactions (https://string-db.org/; accessed on 20 May 2021).

Confocal immunofluorescent microscopy. Cells were grown on glass coverslips under normal conditions for 48 h. After rinsing with PBS, cells were fixed in 4% paraformaldehyde/PBS for 30 min and permeabilized with 0.1% Triton X-100 for 10 min. Cells were incubated with a mouse anti-β-catenin antibody (Becton Dickinson, NJ, USA) followed of an AF488-conjugated secondary antibody (Cell Signaling Technology, Danvers, MA, USA) and DAPI for nuclei. Cells were further mounted onto slides with mowiol (Sigma-Aldrich, St. Louis, MO, USA) and then visualized with an LSM-400 Carl Zeiss confocal microscope Axiovert (Zeiss Group, Jena, Germany) following excitation at 488 nm.

4. Conclusions

A novel CK2/ECE1c functional partnership may be emerging from a hidden non-canonical mechanism that promotes aggressiveness. As tumors progress, the N-terminus of ECE1c is phosphorylated at S18/S20 by CK2 and presumably at Y5/T9 by an unknown kinase(s). This phosphorylation leads to a blockage of ubiquitination at K6, improving the stability of ECE1c, activating CSC-associated signaling pathway(s), and consequently leading to poor prognosis in patients. Therefore, more research is necessary to uncover how this CK2/ECE1c relationship modulates aggressiveness in cancer cells. Undoubtedly, experiments in vitro with cancer cell lines and in vivo with mice will help to define the elusive molecular mechanism(s) governing poor prognosis in cancer patients.

Author Contributions: Conceptualization, J.C.T.; methodology, P.P.-M. and I.N.; investigation, K.V.-N., M.d.l.Á.T., P.P.-M. and I.N.; writing—original draft preparation, J.C.T.; writing—review and editing, P.P.-M. and I.N.; project administration and funding acquisition, J.C.T. All authors have read and agreed to the published version of the manuscript.

Funding: This research was supported by Vicerrectoría de Investigación y Desarrollo de la Universidad de Chile VID ENL10/21; Líneas de apoyo a la investigación financiadas por el ICBM 2021; FONDECYT grant 1220353.

Institutional Review Board Statement: Not applicable.

Data Availability Statement: Data are contained within the article.

Acknowledgments: We thank Ulises Urzua (Universidad de Chile) and Verónica A. Burzio (Universidad Andrés Bello) for their valuable support.

Conflicts of Interest: The authors declare no conflict of interest.

References

1. Ajani, J.A.; Song, S.; Hochster, H.S.; Steinberg, I.B. Cancer Stem Cells: The Promise and the Potential. *Semin. Oncol.* **2015**, *42*, S3–S17. [CrossRef] [PubMed]
2. Barker, N.; Ridgway, R.A.; Van Es, J.H.; Van De Wetering, M.; Begthel, H.; van den Born, M.; Danenberg, E.; Clarke, A.R.; Sansom, O.J.; Clevers, H. Crypt stem cells as the cells-of-origin of intestinal cancer. *Nature* **2009**, *457*, 608–611. [CrossRef] [PubMed]
3. Fanali, C.; Lucchetti, D.; Farina, M.; Corbi, M.; Cufino, V.; Cittadini, A.; Sgambato, A. Cancer stem cells in colorectal cancer from pathogenesis to therapy: Controversies and perspectives. *World J. Gastroenterol.* **2014**, *20*, 923–942. [CrossRef] [PubMed]
4. Jordan, C.T.; Guzman, M.L.; Noble, M. Cancer Stem Cells. *N. Engl. J. Med.* **2006**, *355*, 1253–1261. [CrossRef] [PubMed]
5. Kreso, A.; Dick, J.E. Evolution of the Cancer Stem Cell Model. *Cell Stem Cell* **2014**, *14*, 275–291. [CrossRef]
6. Nguyen, L.V.; Vanner, R.; Dirks, P.; Eaves, C.J. Cancer stem cells: An evolving concept. *Nat. Rev. Cancer* **2012**, *12*, 133–143. [CrossRef] [PubMed]
7. Barton, M.; Yanagisawa, M. Endothelin: 20 Years from Discovery to Therapy. *Can J. Physiol. Pharmacol.* **2008**, *86*, 485–498. [CrossRef]
8. Kawanabe, Y.; Nauli, S.M. Endothelin. *Cell. Mol. Life Sci.* **2011**, *68*, 195–203. [CrossRef]
9. Rosanò, L.; Spinella, F.; Bagnato, A. Endothelin 1 in cancer: Biological implications and therapeutic opportunities. *Nat. Rev. Cancer* **2013**, *13*, 637–651. [CrossRef]
10. Bagnato, A.; Rosanò, L. The endothelin axis in cancer. *Int. J. Biochem. Cell Biol.* **2008**, *40*, 1443–1451. [CrossRef]
11. Khimji, A.-K.; Rockey, D.C. Endothelin—Biology and disease. *Cell. Signal.* **2010**, *22*, 1615–1625. [CrossRef] [PubMed]
12. Jafri, F.; Ergul, A. Nuclear Localization of Endothelin-Converting Enzyme-1: Subisoform Specificity. *Arter. Thromb. Vasc. Biol.* **2003**, *23*, 2192–2196. [CrossRef] [PubMed]

13. Funke-Kaiser, H.; Thomas, A.; Bremer, J.; Kovacevic, S.D.; Scheuch, K.; Bolbrinker, J.; Theis, S.; Lemmer, J.; Zimmermann, A.; Zollmann, F.S.; et al. Regulation of the major isoform of human endothelin-converting enzyme-1 by a strong housekeeping promoter modulated by polymorphic microsatellites. *J. Hypertens.* **2003**, *21*, 2111–2124. [CrossRef] [PubMed]
14. Lindenau, S.; von Langsdorff, C.; Saxena, A.; Paul, M.; Orzechowski, H.-D. Genomic organisation of the mouse gene encoding endothelin-converting enzyme-1 (ECE-1) and mRNA expression of ECE-1 isoforms in murine tissues. *Gene* **2006**, *373*, 109–115. [CrossRef] [PubMed]
15. Tapia, J.C.; Niechi, I. Endothelin-converting enzyme-1 in cancer aggressiveness. *Cancer Lett.* **2019**, *452*, 152–157. [CrossRef]
16. Arun, C.; London, N.; Hemingway, D. Prognostic Significance of Elevated Endothelin-1 Levels in Patients with Colorectal Cancer. *Int. J. Biol. Markers* **2004**, *19*, 32–37. [CrossRef]
17. Simpson, R.A.; Dickinson, T.; Porter, K.E.; London, N.J.M.; Hemingway, D.M. Raised levels of plasma big endothelin 1 in patients with colorectal cancer. *Br. J. Surg.* **2000**, *87*, 1409–1413. [CrossRef]
18. Arun, C.; Swift, B.; Porter, K.; West, K.; London, N.; Hemingway, D. The Role of Big Endothelin-1 in Colorectal Cancer. *Int. J. Biol. Markers* **2002**, *17*, 268–274. [CrossRef]
19. Lambert, L.A.; Whyteside, A.R.; Turner, A.J.; Usmani, B.A. Isoforms of endothelin-converting enzyme-1 (ECE-1) have opposing effects on prostate cancer cell invasion. *Br. J. Cancer* **2008**, *99*, 1114–1120. [CrossRef]
20. Niechi, I.; Silva, E.; Cabello, P.; Huerta, H.; Carrasco, V.; Villar, P.; Cataldo, L.R.; Marcelain, K.; Armisen, R.; Varas-Godoy, M.; et al. Colon cancer cell invasion is promoted by protein kinase CK2 through increase of endothelin-converting enzyme-1c protein stability. *Oncotarget* **2015**, *6*, 42749–42760. [CrossRef]
21. Duncan, J.S.; Litchfield, D.W. Too much of a good thing: The role of protein kinase CK2 in tumorigenesis and prospects for therapeutic inhibition of CK2. *Biochim. Biophys. Acta BBA Proteins Proteom.* **2008**, *1784*, 33–47. [CrossRef] [PubMed]
22. Herhaus, L.; Perez-Oliva, A.B.; Cozza, G.; Gourlay, R.; Weidlich, S.; Campbell, D.G.; Pinna, L.A.; Sapkota, G.P. Casein kinase 2 (CK2) phosphorylates the deubiquitylase OTUB1 at Ser ^{16} to trigger its nuclear localization. *Sci. Signal.* **2015**, *8*, ra35. [CrossRef] [PubMed]
23. St-Denis, N.A.; Litchfield, D.W. From Birth to Death: The Role of Protein Kinase CK2 in the Regulation of Cell Proliferation and Survival. *Cell. Mol. Life Sci.* **2009**, *66*, 1817–1829. [CrossRef] [PubMed]
24. Litchfield, D.W. Protein kinase CK2: Structure, regulation and role in cellular decisions of life and death. *Biochem. J.* **2003**, *369*, 1–15. [CrossRef] [PubMed]
25. Ruzzene, M.; Pinna, L.A. Addiction to protein kinase CK2: A common denominator of diverse cancer cells? *Biochim. Biophys. Acta BBA—Proteins Proteom.* **2010**, *1804*, 499–504. [CrossRef] [PubMed]
26. Liang, L.; Qu, L.; Ding, Y. Protein and mRNA Characterization in Human Colorectal Carcinoma Cell Lines with Different Metastatic Potentials. *Cancer Investig.* **2007**, *25*, 427–434. [CrossRef] [PubMed]
27. Lin, K.-Y.; Tai, C.; Hsu, J.-C.; Li, C.-F.; Fang, C.-L.; Lai, H.-C.; Hseu, Y.-C.; Lin, Y.-F.; Uen, Y.-H. Overexpression of Nuclear Protein Kinase CK2 α Catalytic Subunit (CK2α) as a Poor Prognosticator in Human Colorectal Cancer. *PLoS ONE* **2011**, *6*, e17193. [CrossRef] [PubMed]
28. Borgo, C.; Ruzzene, M. Role of protein kinase CK2 in antitumor drug resistance. *J. Exp. Clin. Cancer Res.* **2019**, *38*, 287. [CrossRef]
29. Borgo, C.; D'amore, C.; Sarno, S.; Salvi, M.; Ruzzene, M. Protein kinase CK2: A potential therapeutic target for diverse human diseases. *Signal Transduct. Target. Ther.* **2021**, *6*, 183. [CrossRef]
30. Pérez-Moreno, P.; Indo, S.; Niechi, I.; Huerta, H.; Cabello, P.; Jara, L.; Aguayo, F.; Varas-Godoy, M.; Burzio, V.A.; Tapia, J.C. Endothelin-converting enzyme-1c promotes stem cell traits and aggressiveness in colorectal cancer cells. *Mol. Oncol.* **2020**, *14*, 347–362. [CrossRef]
31. Niechi, I.; Erices, J.I.; Carrillo-Beltrán, D.; Uribe-Ojeda, A.; Torres, Á.; Rocha, J.D.; Uribe, D.; Toro, M.A.; Villalobos-Nova, K.; Gaete-Ramírez, B.; et al. Cancer Stem Cell and Aggressiveness Traits Are Promoted by Stable Endothelin-Converting Enzyme-1c in Glioblastoma Cells. *Cells* **2023**, *12*, 506. [CrossRef] [PubMed]
32. Almarza, C.; González, M.; Toro, M.; Villalobos-Nova, K.; Niechi, I.; Silva-Pavez, E.; López-Muñoz, R.A.; Varas-Godoy, M.; Burzio, V.A.; Jara, L.; et al. Cisplatin-Resistance and Aggressiveness Are Triggered upon Expression of a Super-Stable Endothelin-Converting Enzyme-1c in Lung Cancer Cells. *Unpublished manuscript*.
33. Pérez-Moreno, P.; Quezada-Meza, C.; Chavez-Almarza, C.; Niechi, I.; Silva-Pavez, E.; Trigo-Hidalgo, C.; Aguayo, F.; Jara, L.; Cáceres-Verschae, A.; Varas-Godoy, M.; et al. Phosphorylation of Endothelin-Converting Enzyme-1c at Serines 18 and 20 by CK2 Promotes Aggressiveness Traits in Colorectal Cancer Cells. *Front. Oncol.* **2020**, *10*, 1004. [CrossRef] [PubMed]
34. Meggio, F.; Pinna, L.A. One-thousand-and-one substrates of protein kinase CK2? *FASEB J.* **2003**, *17*, 349–368. [CrossRef] [PubMed]
35. Marin, O.; Sarno, S.; Boschetti, M.; Pagano, M.A.; Meggio, F.; Ciminale, V.; D'Agostino, D.M.; Pinna, L.A. Unique features of HIV-1 Rev protein phosphorylation by protein kinase CK2 ('casein kinase-2'). *FEBS Lett.* **2000**, *481*, 63–67. [CrossRef] [PubMed]
36. Tapia, J.C.; Bolanos-Garcia, V.M.; Sayed, M.; Allende, C.C.; Allende, J.E. Cell cycle regulatory protein $p27^{KIP1}$ is a substrate and interacts with the protein kinase CK2. *J. Cell. Biochem.* **2004**, *91*, 865–879. [CrossRef]
37. Swatek, K.N.; Komander, D. Ubiquitin modifications. *Cell Res.* **2016**, *26*, 399–422. [CrossRef] [PubMed]
38. Dikic, I. Proteasomal and Autophagic Degradation Systems. *Annu. Rev. Biochem.* **2017**, *86*, 193–224. [CrossRef]
39. Smerdon, S.J.; Yaffe, M.B. Recognition of Phospho-Serine/Threonine Phosphorylated Proteins by Phos-pho-Serine/Threonine-Binding Domains. In *Handbook of Cell Signaling*, 2nd ed.; Academic Press: Cambridge, MA, USA, 2010; Volume 2, pp. 539–550. [CrossRef]

40. Yaffe, M.B.; Smerdon, S.J. PhosphoSerine/Threonine Binding Domains: You Can't pSERious? *Structure* **2001**, *9*, R33–R38. [CrossRef]
41. Almawi, A.W.; Matthews, L.A.; Guarné, A. FHA domains: Phosphopeptide binding and beyond. *Prog. Biophys. Mol. Biol.* **2017**, *127*, 105–110. [CrossRef]
42. Fu, H.; Subramanian, R.R.; Masters, S.C. 14-3-3 Proteins: Structure, Function, and Regulation. *Annu. Rev. Pharmacol. Toxicol.* **2000**, *40*, 617–647. [CrossRef]
43. Wang, B.; Li, X.; Liu, L.; Wang, M. β-Catenin: Oncogenic role and therapeutic target in cervical cancer. *Biol. Res.* **2020**, *53*, 33. [CrossRef] [PubMed]
44. Tominaga, J.; Fukunaga, Y.; Abelardo, E.; Nagafuchi, A. Defining the function of β-catenin tyrosine phosphorylation in cadherin-mediated cell–cell adhesion. *Genes Cells* **2008**, *13*, 67–77. [CrossRef] [PubMed]
45. Nusse, R.; Clevers, H. Wnt/β-Catenin Signaling, Disease, and Emerging Therapeutic Modalities. *Cell* **2017**, *169*, 985–999. [CrossRef] [PubMed]
46. Lian, H.; Su, M.; Zhu, Y.; Zhou, Y.; Soomro, S.H.; Fu, H. Protein Kinase CK2, a Potential Therapeutic Target in Carcinoma Management. *Asian Pac. J. Cancer Prev.* **2019**, *20*, 23–32. [CrossRef]

kinases and phosphatases

MDPI

Review

Scoping Pleiotropy of CK2 in Musculoskeletal Disorders for a Novel Targeting Approach

Venu Pandit, Kailey DeGeorge and Anja Nohe *

Department of Biological Sciences, University of Delaware, Newark, DE 19716, USA; vpandit@udel.edu (V.P.)
* Correspondence: anjanohe@udel.edu

Abstract: Protein kinase CK2 (CK2) influences one-fifth of the cellular phosphoproteome. It regulates almost all cellular pathways and is thus a critical switch between biological processes within a cell. Inhibition of CK2 reverses oncogene addiction of tumor and alters tumor microenvironment. The success of this strategy and its clinical translation opens new opportunities. Targeting CK2 in musculoskeletal disorders is promising. Clinical manifestations of these disorders include dysfunctional inflammation, dysregulated cell differentiation, and senescence. Processes regulated by CK2 include all of these. Its emerging role in senescence also indicates its function's centrality in cellular metabolism. This review summarizes considerations for targeting CK2 in musculoskeletal disorders. We have discussed the implications of CK2-regulated processes in musculoskeletal disorders.

Keywords: casein kinase II; musculoskeletal; osteoarthritis; osteoporosis; CX-4945; CIBG-300; cell signaling; drug development; targeted therapy

1. Introduction

Musculoskeletal disorders affect skeletal muscle, bone, cartilage, and connective tissue. Disorders such as osteoporosis (OP), osteoarthritis (OA), and rheumatoid arthritis (RA) can cause chronic pain, hamper mobility, and reduce quality of life. They are also among the costliest co-morbidities [1]. Traditionally, musculoskeletal disorders were identified as structural dysfunctions of respective physiologies. However, recently, metabolic dysregulation has come up as a significant risk factor in these diseases. Metabolic dysregulation is caused by the defective regulation of biochemical pathways required for homeostasis [2,3]. Emerging studies are investigating the underlying mechanism by which metabolic disorders increase the severity of musculoskeletal disorders. Rheumatoid arthritis (RA) is an autoimmune disorder affecting joints. Researchers are exploring the link between autoimmunity and altered metabolism [4,5]. Likewise, osteoarthritis (OA) is characterized by the progressive degeneration of joints. The pathogenesis of OA is affected by metabolic disorders [6,7]. Small molecular metabolites are assessed for OA-associated biomarker identification [8]. Altered lipid metabolism and immune response during obesity increase the severity of OA symptoms [9]. Osteoporosis (OP) is a disorder associated with low bone mineral density. Several studies investigate the complex relationship between bone homeostasis and metabolic disorders, especially in the case of OP [10–15]. Patients diagnosed with OP are at a higher risk of fractures. An impaired immune system affects the natural process of fracture healing [16]. Defects in fracture healing in obese and insulin-resistant individuals are attributed to the dysregulated innate immunity during the healing-associated inflammatory response [17].

Protein kinase CK2 (formerly called "Casein Kinase 2") is a ubiquitous serine/threonine kinase. The kinase has no extracellular activator [18]. It is not regulated hierarchically by other kinases of vertical signaling cascades. Thus, the regulatory role of CK2 is not limited to the activation of molecular signaling from the plasma membrane to the nucleus. Instead, it crosswise associates and integrates multiple pathways [19,20]. Hence, it is a

'Lateral player' in many biochemical pathways [21,22]. Expression and activity of CK2 are dysregulated in musculoskeletal disorders [23]. Deviation in metabolic processes affects tissue homeostasis and response to endocrine regulation [24]. The role of the inflammatory system and senescence in these diseases is also linked with metabolic dysregulation [25,26]. Moreover, the role of CK2 in modulating immune response, adipogenesis, and mitochondrial function has long been studied [27–29]. The kinase can identify and phosphorylate a vast range of substrates, estimated to be more than 400 today [30,31]. It is predicted to account for almost 20% of the phosphoproteome of cells [32]. Since CK2 is a lateral player, the effects of its dysregulation are manifold.

CK2 is ubiquitously present and expressed in almost all types of cells. The mechanism of pathway regulation by CK2 is different from that of other kinases. The following factors summarize the complexity of CK2's function. First, while most kinases are activated in response to particular stimuli, CK2 is constitutively active [33] and requires no specific stimulus [18,34,35]. Second, the localization and form of CK2 change based on cell type and metabolic status [36]. CK2 has two catalytic subunits, CK2α and CK2α', and a regulatory CK2β subunit. In vivo, it exists as a heterotetramer [37]. The tetramer form of CK2 is also termed CK2 holoenzyme. Holoenzyme comprises catalytic subunits α and α' and two regulatory β subunits. The kinetics of holoenzyme formation and cellular distribution of these subunits change under different stimuli [38]. Third, the β subunit is not strictly a regulatory subunit. It is required to recognize substrates and structural stability of catalytic subunits. However, few substrates are phosphorylated without the β subunit, which makes its role elusive. Fourth, the catalytic subunits CK2α and CK2α' are almost the same in structure, but their involvement in catalytic activity is different [39]. One is preferred over the other in some processes. Finally, the expression of subunits is regulated by various growth factors, and a single subunit's expression level affects the expression and activity of other subunits.

The only clinically approved small molecular inhibitor of CK2, Silmitasertib (CX-4945), is a first-in-class small molecule of its kind [40]. It is an ATP-competitive inhibitor with the highest level of selectivity for CK2. Its use in cancer therapies is under investigation. However, like most currently available CK2 inhibitors, it inhibits CK2 catalytic activity completely. Controlling the inhibition of CK2 activity during specific cellular processes while sparing other activity is not possible. Furthermore, complete inhibition of the catalytic activity of CK2 causes cytotoxicity. This is due to the cells' dependence on the basal phosphorylation level of CK2 substrates for survival [35]. Cytotoxicity is not always desirable, especially in treating musculoskeletal disorders. The technology of modulating the phosphorylation of CK2 substrates taking part in disease pathogenesis rather than inhibiting overall kinase activity is emerging. Focusing on specific CK2–substrate interaction will help bring a pathology-tailored approach for musculoskeletal disorders [41].

One such peptide inhibitor of CK2 named CIGB300 inhibits phosphorylation of specific CK2 substrates. This synthetic peptide binds to the phosphoacceptor domain of CK2 [42]. It was first discovered as an effective peptide in treating cervical cancer. It is also effective in treating Large Cell Lung Carcinoma (LCLC), Non-Small Cell Lung Cancer (NSCLC), advanced cervical cancer, and acute myeloid leukemia [43–46]. Due to its substrate-specific inhibition, it is highly effective and has mild side effects. This drug is under investigation in Phase 2 clinical trials, and studies about its effectiveness will soon be available [29]. The substrate-specific rather than global inhibitory effect of CIGB300 is thus emerging in cancer treatment.

Disease-modifying drugs help reverse the symptoms of disorders; they do so because they are designed to target molecular interactions critical for pathogenesis [47]. This approach re-directs metabolic pathways towards homeostasis. Few disease-modifying drugs, like Sprifermin (recombinant human FGF18, rhFGF18) for OA and methotrexate for RA, are available to treat musculoskeletal diseases [48,49]. Interventions that can restore dysregulated metabolism in these diseases are necessary [47]. CK2 is a lateral player, restoring its activity will effectively re-direct the metabolism to a healthy state. However,

Targeting CK2 is challenging due to the complexity of its function [21,22,50]. Efforts to reveal the complexities of CK2 function in musculoskeletal disorders will help design disease-modifying therapeutics.

For the development of new drugs, the success rate of candidate molecules to move from bench to bedside is only 10%, despite the robustness of preclinical studies and perfect administration of clinical trials. Moreover, an excellent pre-clinical performer may be withdrawn due to the long processing time between drug discovery and commercial production. Substantial costs are involved with this process, and more importantly, the high failure rate delays the advances in better treatment for affected individuals. Lack of biomarker identification, off-target activity, and excess toxicity are a few of the challenges identified that can be addressed while designing new candidates. This process can utilize advanced knowledge of the molecular interactions between the drug and target [51]. In the case of CK2, many small molecular inhibitors have been discovered, most of which are investigated for the treatment of cancers. Yet, very few are approved for clinical use, partly due to their high cytotoxicity. Re-purposing the knowledge about these CK2 inhibitory molecules for treating musculoskeletal disorders is possible. Understanding the critical interactions of CK2 with its substrates in musculoskeletal diseases becomes essential.

In this review, first, we discuss the implications of CK2 in musculoskeletal disorders. Next, we discuss mechanisms of target identification by CK2 and the distinct functions of its subunits. Then, we describe currently available inhibitors of CK2 and their mechanism of action. Finally, we discuss a novel disease-modifying approach for targeting CK2–substrate interactions. This approach achieves CK2 activity modulation using biomimetic peptides targeting specific interactions of CK2 within the signal transduction cascade.

2. Implication of CK2 in Musculoskeletal Disorders

2.1. Rheumatoid Arthritis

Rheumatoid arthritis (RA) is an autoimmune disorder affecting the joints. The exact mechanisms through which RA develops have yet to be fully understood [52,53]. One leading hypothesis is that the interactions between epigenetic modifications and environmental influences facilitate self-antigens production and induce autoimmunity. Self-antigens are then modified by citrullination [5]. As the body cannot recognize citrullinated antigens, the modified self-antigens are then recognized by antigen-presenting cells, which transport them to the lymph nodes. In the lymph nodes, helper T cells and B cells are activated through co-stimulation. The B cells differentiate into plasma cells that produce antibodies against the self-antigens [54]. In this manner, the body produces antibodies against self-antigens and induces tissue inflammation [55]. Synovial hyperplasia and similar disorders may also release cytokines contributing to joint inflammation and autoimmunity. Specifically, the synovial fluid and joint capsule become inflamed during RA, contributing to bone and cartilage erosion [56]. During RA, the balance between the Type I T Helper (Th1) and Type 2 T Helper (Th2) cells is disrupted in favor of the Th1 cells, causing inflammation. Type 17 T Helper (Th17) cells induce the proliferation of fibroblast-like synoviocytes (FLS) [57]. FLSs contribute to the progression of RA. FLSs are found in the synovial intimal lining of healthy tissue; they secrete products that contribute to the synovial fluid and articular cartilage. In RA, they secrete cytokines that promote inflammation and proteases that degrade cartilage [58].

Protein kinase CK2 plays a role in RA through CK2α's control of the Interleukin-12 (IL-12) receptor, which regulates the IL-STAT4 signaling pathway through which Th1 cell differentiation is promoted. The IL-STAT4 pathway is regulated primarily by the expression of IL-12R in CD4+ T cells, though it is also regulated, to a lesser extent, by interferon-α (IFN-α) and interleukin 23 (IL-23). The phosphorylation of the STAT4 pathway induces downstream signaling that ultimately facilitates Th1 cell differentiation [59]. CK2α, CK2α', and CK2β promote Th17 cell differentiation. CK2α also regulates Th1 cell differentiation and suppresses the activity of Th2 cells [59,60].

2.2. Osteoarthritis

Osteoarthritis (OA) is a degenerative disease of the articular cartilage, which is increasingly common with advanced age, especially in women. OA is associated with loss in the number and activity of chondrocytes through increased apoptosis. Reduced activity of chondrocytes reduces the repair of the collagen matrix and diminishes the structural integrity of the cartilage. Oxidative stress is another hallmark of OA. Metabolic disorders affect the severity of OA. Increased serum glucose levels due to type 2 diabetes and metabolic syndrome increase advanced glycation products (AGESs) levels. The AGES are associated with the collagen matrix of cartilage and cause structural damage. They also interact with receptors of AGES called RAGE and cause oxidative stress in chondrocytes [61]. Excess reactive oxygen species (ROS) production leads to oxidative stress response, increasing chondrocyte senescence [62].

CK2 is an inhibitor of apoptosis, and its expression is reduced in chondrocytes of patients diagnosed with OA. Inhibition of CK2, sensitized chondrocytes to Tumor Necrosis Factor-alpha (TNFα)-mediated cell death [63]. Parathyroid hormone-related protein (PTHrP) is a parathyroid hormone homolog. It protects chondrocytes from undergoing excessive apoptosis [64]. PTHrP exerts its protective activity against mitochondria-dependent apoptotic pathway via upregulation of CK2 activity [65,66]. PTHrP is localized to nuclei due to its mid-region bipartite nuclear targeting sequence (NTS) [67]. In one study, treatment with synthetic peptide PTHrP-NTS (the NTS region of PTHrP) protected HEK293 cells from TNFα-activated apoptosis. Exogenous NTS increased nuclear accumulation of CK2. Nuclear retention and activity of CK2 were enhanced. Similar results were obtained in cells treated with intact PTHrP [68]. CK2 is also involved in the oxidative stress response. CK2 signaling is essential for activating transcription factor NF-E2-related factor 2 (Nrf2). Nrf 2 signaling is crucial for redox balancing within cells [69]. It reduces cellular ROS levels and suppresses nuclear factor-κB (NF-κB) localization in the nucleus. Nrf2 upregulates expression of Heme oxygenase-1 (HO-1). Enzyme HO-1 is vital in heme degradation and countering oxidative stress response [70]. This enzyme becomes activated in chondrocytes in response to peroxynitrite-induced oxidative stress [71]. In another study, inhibition of the catalytic activity of CK2 with 4,5,6,7-terabromo-2-azabenzimidazole (TBB) and 5,6-dichlorobenzimidazole 1-β-D-ribofuranoside (DRB) induced senescence and apoptosis in chondrocytes. Overexpression of HO-1 reduced the TBB-induced senescence. Chondrocytes overexpressing HO-1 had reduced sensitivity towards TBB-induced senescence. The knockdown of CK2 reduced type II collagen and increased β catenin expression [72]. The small heat shock protein αB-crystallin is a mediator for the expression of chondrogenic Bone Morphogenetic Protein-2 and collagen type II. Its expression is downregulated in OA [73]. Chondrocytes treated with CK2 inhibitors and αB-crystallin siRNA were sensitized to apoptosis. However, αB-crystallin had a protective effect. Its expression was modulated, and cellular localization was changed after CK2 inhibition [74]. The role of αB-crystallin in aiding CK2 to prevent chondrocyte apoptosis should be explored further. Thus, evidence suggests that CK2 protects chondrocytes from oxidative stress and apoptosis.

2.3. Bone Fracture

Healthy bone is excellent at self-healing in the event of injury. The process occurs roughly through the following phases. The first is the inflammatory phase and hematoma formation. Physical rupture of the bone causes infiltration of immunoregulatory cells, such as Macrophages, at the site. These cells secrete inflammatory cytokines IL-1, IL-6, and TNFα during the early phases of healing [75]. These factors recruit mesenchymal stem cells (MSC) to the fracture site. MSCs undergo chondrogenic and osteogenic differentiation through secreted growth factors. Next, angiogenesis and soft callus formation begin, at which point the central region of the fracture undergoes endochondral ossification during this phase [76]. The MSCs undergo differentiation into osteo-chondroprogenitor cells [77]. Thus, formed chondrocytes form the cartilaginous matrix. Angiogenesis and calcification of the cartilaginous matrix by hypertrophic chondrocytes marks the start of the next phase of hard bone formation. In this phase, the cartilage is replaced by bone via hard calcification. Here, the activity of osteoblasts increases. Finally, in the last phase, bone remodeling occurs. Here, the coordinated function between bone matrix-secreting osteoblasts and bone-resorbing osteoclasts takes place [64]. Bone remodeling is essential in maintaining bone shape. During aging, macrophages, chondrocytes, and osteocytes secrete senescence-associated factors [78]. Their secretion prolongs the inflammatory phase and hampers the bone healing process [79,80].

The bone morphogenic protein (BMP) pathway is essential for fracture healing [81,82]. BMP ligands are critical growth factors for bone, cartilage, joint development, and homeostasis. They drive MSC differentiation. BMP-2 stimulation of senescent bone marrow mesenchymal stem cells (BMSCs) activated adipogenic and cell death pathways like NF-kB or p38-mitogen activated protein kinase (MAPK). In non-senescent bone marrow mesenchymal stem cells (BMSCs), BMP-2 activated bone-forming pathways such as SMAD, BMP, and TGFβ [83]. CK2 negatively regulates BMP-2-activated signaling [84].

Casein kinase 2 interacting protein-1 (CKIP-1) is a negative regulator of BMP signaling [85]. CKIP-1 interacts with the CK2α subunit and regulates signaling between CK2α and effector molecules of BMP signaling [86,87]. CKIP-1 is known to inhibit BMP signaling by promoting Smad1 ubiquitination. The suppression of BMP signaling leads to suppressed osteogenic differentiation [23]. The CKIP-1 knockout mice had abnormally high levels of bone mass. The effects of CKIP-1 on bone growth and repair were age-dependent, with CKIP-1 having a more substantial impact on the bone mass of 18-month-old mice and comparatively little effect on 2-month-old mice. CKIP-1 is a negative regulator of osteogenic differentiation, and age-related inflammation causes an upregulation of CKIP-1, although the exact mechanisms of this upregulation remain unclear [88,89]. Inhibition of interaction between CK2α and CKIP-1 is a possible therapeutic strategy for bone fractures.

2.4. Osteoporosis

Osteoporosis (OP) is a degenerative disease that, as of 2023, affects more than 200 million people. The incidence rate of OP is 1.7% of men and 26% of women over age 50 worldwide [65]. OP is associated with a loss of bone mass and mineral density. This weakens the bones and predisposes them to fractures. It is a musculoskeletal disorder that is very closely related to metabolic dysregulation. OP is characterized by a disruption in the balance between osteoblasts and osteoclasts, cells that generate bone and cells that degrade bone, respectively. One common type of OP is glucocorticoid-induced osteoporosis (GIO). GIO is diagnosed in patients undergoing treatment with glucocorticoids for inflammatory or auto-immune diseases. Glucocorticoids inhibit osteoblast function and decrease the vascularity of the bone [66]. In one study, primary cells from human patients and mice with GIO had elevated levels of CKIP-1 and reduced levels of Smad1/5 compared to controls. CKIP-1 is a non-enzymatic protein that regulates the CK2α subunit of protein kinase CK2. It can be utilized in the localization of protein kinase CK2 in cell [67]. In vitro, elevated expression and activity of CKIP-1 in osteoblasts inhibited Smad-dependent BMP signaling [23]. CKIP-1 regulates BMP signaling and can recruit CK2α to the plasma membrane. Hence, its overexpression can affect the activation of BMP signaling in osteoblasts and osteoclasts. CKIP-1's suppression of BMP signaling inhibits and affects the differentiation of MSC into osteoblasts. These alterations contribute to the reduction in bone mineralization observed in GIO patients. Suppressing the interaction between CKIP-1 and interaction with CK2 could be a novel therapeutic strategy for treating GIO. Upregulation of BMP signaling can increase bone formation and repair [16]. Blocking of the interaction between CK2 and CKIP-1 may induce BMP signaling [68]. A challenge in creating osteoporosis therapeutics is maintaining the optimal balance between osteoblasts and osteoclasts, cells that generate and degrade bone, respectively. Ideally, a therapeutic for OP would increase osteoblast activity while decreasing osteoclast activity, inducing bone formation and repair.

3. Inhibition of CK2

3.1. Molecular Function of CK2

3.1.1. Structure of CK2 and Substrate Recognition

CK2 was discovered as a mitochondrial kinase in 1954; since then, its function has been studied in various biological processes [90]. Recent research has identified its new substrates and allowed us to expand our knowledge about its regulation of biological processes.

The catalytic subunits of CK2 are acidophilic. Its substrates often have acidic amino acids near the phosphorylation site. The consensus sequence on the phosphorylation target ([pS/pT]-(P)-x-[E/D] or [pS/pT]-(P)-x-pS is identified as the minimum identification sequence required for target identification [30,91]. However, due to the short length of this sequence and flexibility for amino acids in the second and third positions, the frequency of occurrence of this sequence across all proteins is high. Using the consensus prediction software Prosite (http://prosite.expasy.org, accessed on 29 January 2024), the total number of sequences containing CK2 phosphorylation motifs comes out as 8640. However, the predicted number of targets of CK2 was much higher than the actual number of targets [92]. Also, CK2 phosphorylates a few substrates that do not have the consensus sequence. Thus, target validation is essential in determining the bona-fide substrates of CK2. It also helps target interactions where alternate kinases cannot nullify the drug's effect. Approaches like phospho-proteomics have helped determine the number of targets this kinase affects.

Chonjowski et al. developed a method for validating genuine targets of CK2, specifically by taking advantage of the co-substrate specificity of CK2. The co-substrate specificity of CK2 means that the kinase can use either adenosine triphosphate (ATP) or guanosine triphosphate (GTP) to phosphorylate its substrates. Briefly, an analog of GTP–guanosine 5′-[γ-thio]triphosphate (GTPγS) is incorporated into the cell suspension. Other endogenous kinases do not use this substrate. Thus, substrates phosphorylated with CK2 are identified by the presence of 'PγS' using Mass Spectrometry. Furthermore, validation of CK2 targets with co-immunoprecipitation is possible with substrate-specific antibodies and pull-down assays. This method allows the use of versatile biological samples and helps capture phosphorylation reactions while the cells are still alive [31,93].

Inhibition of CK2 kinase activity by ATP competitive inhibitors does not alter the phosphorylation of all its targets. Changes in phosphorylation levels of CK2 targets by two CK2 inhibitors, Silmitasertib and GO289, were different. Both inhibitors have very low off-target activity and have an almost overlapping set of affected CK2 phosphorylation targets. However, the extent of reduction in phosphorylation of its targets is very different between these two. Both inhibitors bind the same site on CK2α and cause very different effects. This difference could be attributed to the ability of CK2 to identify its targets under various conditions [18,94].

To identify substrates exclusively phosphorylated by CK2, inhibitor-resistant mutants of CK2 were created. The kinase is known to phosphorylate only 20% of the substrates containing the minimal recognition motif. With the mutants and subsequent use of inhibitors, the expanse of substrates was estimated in C2C12 cell lines. Studies using lysates do not consider the temporal and spatial factors for CK2–substrate interactions. Instead, these studies used the stable isotope labeling using amino acids in cell culture (SILAC) approach. This allowed the study of interaction when the cells performed their normal function. The disparity was observed within popular CK2 inhibitors, with only a proportion of inhibitors showing dose-dependent inhibition of CK2 activity [95].

3.1.2. Function of Subunits

CK2 has catalytic subunits, CK2α and CK2α′, as well as regulatory CK2β subunits. The enzyme functions as a holoenzyme, and each subunit can also work in isolation [37]. Individual subunits of CK2 seem to play diverse roles exclusive to the holoenzyme form. There are many instances where individual subunits of CK2 perform distinct functions [96]. Inhibition of a particular subunit or its depletion in cellular compartments affects the expression and activity of other subunits. Additionally, by performing subunit knockout, the extent of the contribution of individual subunits was determined. This approach is helpful in the creation of subunit-specific drugs. In most cases, the abrogation of catalytic subunits impacts the expression and function of other subunits. These are explained using the following examples.

A coordinated regulation mechanism between the three holoenzyme subunits was observed during skeletal muscle differentiation. The mechanism involved regulating early myogenic regulator genes such as myoblast determination protein 1 (MyoD) and myogenin, followed by the expression of muscle-specific genes such as caveolin-3, troponin, and myomixer. The holoenzyme's individual subunits and catalytic activity also coordinated plasma membrane fusion and the shutting of embedded proteins. In individual knockouts of subunits in C2C12 cells with CRISPR/Cas9, the deletion of one subunit affected the expression of other subunits, demonstrating their interdependence. Deletion of the CK2α subunit downregulated CK2β expression, whereas deletion of the CK2β subunit upregulated CK2α expression. However, deletion of CK2α′ did not alter the levels of the other two units. In knockouts of CK2α and CK2β, MyoD expression was reduced and abrogated, respectively, whereas the deletion of CK2α′ did not have an effect. The reduction in MyoD expression in CK2α deletion was due to the downregulation of CK2β in these mutants. In CK2β null mutants, the expression of this early myogenic regulatory factor (MRF) was not activated until the re-induction of the subunit in CK2β knockdown C2C12 cells already expressing low levels of MyoD. With increasing expression of CK2β in these cells, the level of MyoD increased, which was also reflected as an increase in its mRNA at the transcription level. This indicates that the CK2β with other epigenetic modifiers activate the expression of MyoD. The level of MyoD expression was not affected by varying the catalytic activity of CK2 by pharmacological inhibition or changes in the expression of CK2α and CK2α′ subunits. During the later stages of myogenic differentiation, the levels of MyoD reduce, whereas the expression of muscle-specific genes increases in WT C2C12 cells. Here, pharmacological inhibition of kinase activity in CK2α′ knockout mutants reduced the expression of these markers. This evidence indicates the role of the other catalytic subunit CK2α in the expression of muscle-specific markers in later stages. The role of CK2α′ during myotube formation was indispensable. With the deletion of this subunit, there was a reduction in the number and size of myotubes compared to WT. Exogenous CK2α′ is sufficient to rescue reduced fusogenic activity of muscle fibers because of CK2 deletion [78].

One of the two catalytic subunits, either CK2α or CK2α′, is more critical in some biological processes. This is the case during skeletal muscle development and homeostasis. Here, the activity of the CK2α subunit is crucial [97]. Skeletal muscle specific CK2α knockout mice were produced by breeding floxed mice with human skeletal actin Cre reporter mice. The grip strength of the CK2α knockout mice was decreased compared to the controls, and the difference was more significant in older mice. CK2β expression levels were significantly reduced in the CK2α knockout mice, but expression of CK2α′decreased slightly. Phospho-Akt1 serine 129 and 473 proteins were upregulated in the knockout mice. There was no difference in gastrocnemius and soleus muscles between the CK2α knockout mice and the controls with Hematoxylin and Eosin staining. The muscle sections from the knockout mice had higher levels of centralized nuclei than the controls, indicating their higher propensity for muscular regeneration. The soleus fibers of the knockout mice had lower levels of slow type I muscle fibers but increased levels of fast type II fibers compared to the control. This evidence suggests that CK2α is essential in skeletal muscle regeneration. CK2α knockout mice had elevated expression of several mitophagy markers, including sequestosome-1(SQSTM1), optineurin (OPTN), and microtubule associated protein 1 light chain 3 beta (MAP1LC3B-II). The upregulation of these markers suggests that autophagic processes were increased in the absence of CK2 catalytic activity. These mice also had decreased levels of mitochondrial genomic DNA. Knockout of CK2α also impaired neuromuscular function. The expression of various proteins essential to skeletal muscle function was aberrant [98]. Thus, deleting one catalytic subunit alone was sufficient to hamper the process.

Knockout of CK2 catalytic and regulatory subunits in myogenic C2C12 cells had very different effects. With the knockout of CK2α and CK2α′ subunits, there was a substantial reduction in phosphorylation of predicted CK2 targets (18 out of 24). Expression of the CK2β subunit was reduced with this deletion. One possible explanation could be an increased rate of degradation of CK2β. Phosphorylation was upregulated in some of the non-CK2 phosphorylation targets, which could be explained by changes in the expression and activity of other kinases in the absence of CK2 catalytic subunits. In the knockout of CK2β subunits, there was a proportion of reduction in phosphorylation that was slightly lower than that of the catalytic units (9 out of 15). Here, the catalytic subunit expression was increased compared to the wild type. For some of the CK2 substrates, such as Cdc37 (pS13), the knockout of CK2 did not affect phosphorylation. However, for the substrate, Akt S129, the phosphorylation was drastically reduced to the extent it was almost absent with the knockout of either the catalytic or regulatory subunit. These differential effects on substrates shed light on the function of CK2 subunits as compensatory to each other in some cases or the strict requirements of holoenzymes in others. Changes in the phosphorylation status of predicted CK2 targets and non-targets based on sequence prediction indicated that the consensus sequence alone is not sufficient or essential for target identification and phosphorylation to occur [31].

3.2. Small Molecular Inhibitors of CK2 and Their Mechanism of Action

A critical application of small molecule inhibitors of CK2 is within the treatment of cancer [99,100]. For example, osteosarcoma, a bone malignancy that originates in the osteoblasts, is one such cancer in which these inhibitors are an effective treatment. In osteosarcoma, CK2 is overexpressed. In cloned human osteosarcoma 143B, cell line CK2α and CK2β are upregulated compared to healthy osteoblasts and MSCs. The osteosarcoma cells treated with the CK2 inhibitor Silmitasertib suppressed growth and proliferation and increased apoptosis. Interestingly, the proliferation and differentiation of MSCs were unaffected. The siRNA-induced knockdown of the CK2α and CK2β subunits in vitro suppressed the growth and proliferation of osteosarcoma cells. The 143B osteosarcoma cells were xenografted into mice and treated with Silmitasertib. Similar to in vitro findings, Silmitasertib inhibited the proliferation of the tumor cells and, therefore, constrained the growth of the tumor. These findings support the idea that Silmitasertib is a potential therapeutic for osteosarcoma. It inhibits CK2, which induces the apoptosis of sarcoma cells while having little to no effect on MSCs [74]. The implication of CK2 inhibition in osteosarcoma is explained in Figure 1.

Rhabdomyosarcoma, a cancer initiated in the skeletal muscle. Treatment of rhabdomyosarcoma is another example of the therapeutic implications of CK2 inhibitors. CK2 is upregulated in rhabdomyosarcoma cells. Current research on the pathophysiology of rhabdomyosarcoma uses cloned human tumor cell lines JR1 and Rh30. When these cell lines were treated with the CK2 inhibitor 5,6-dichloro benzimidazole (DRB), the proliferation of pro-apoptotic signals commenced, such as cytochrome c and Smad/DIABLO. This caused widespread cell death. JR1 and Rh30 cells transfected with either short hairpin RNA targeted to CK2α or kinase inactive CK2α/CK2α′, which led to heightened sensitivity to pro-apoptotic signals due to the suppressed CK2 activity. Inhibitors of CK2 have the potential as therapeutics to prevent the growth and metastasis of rhabdomyosarcoma cells [73]. Here, inhibition of kinase activity and knockdown of the α/α′ subunit increased apoptosis.

Additionally, research supports the utility of CK2 inhibition in treating rheumatoid arthritis (RA). In one study, human primary CD4+T lymphocytes isolated from patients diagnosed with RA were treated with the CK2 inhibitor Silmitasertib. Cellular responses in Th1 and Th17 cells were suppressed compared to controls. However, the Th2 cellular activity was enhanced. Th1 cells secrete proinflammatory factors, such as TNF-α and IL-2, while Th2 cells secrete anti-inflammatory factors, such as IL-3, IL-4, and IL-5 [101]. In the same study, for the collagen-induced RA mouse model, the effects of CK2 inhibition were similar [102]. Mice were treated with Silmitasertib via ingestion. The Th1 and Th17 cell responses were inhibited, and their RA symptoms were reduced [57,102].

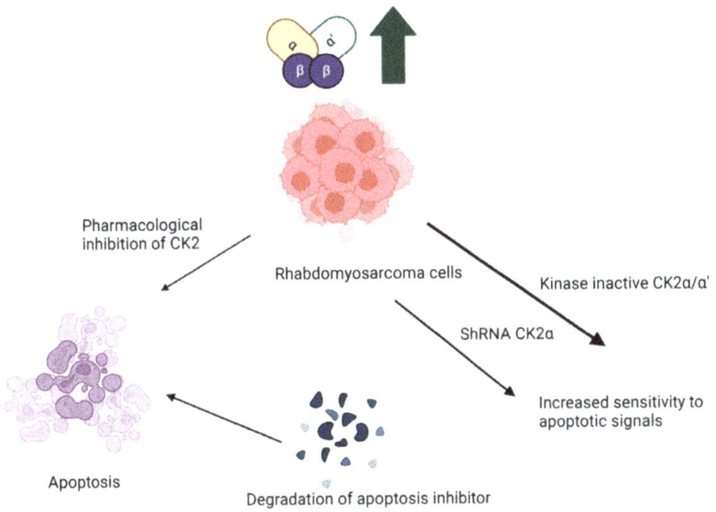

Figure 1. Implication of CK2 in rhabdomyosarcoma and effect of inhibition of CK2 kinase activity. Pharmacological inhibition of CK2 makes the cells more sensitive to apoptotosis due to degradation of apoptosis inhibitor proteins. Abrogation of CK2α by generation of kinase inactive mutants or knockdown with ShRNA make the cells more sensitive apoptotic signals. (Image is created with https://www.biorender.com/ accessed on 9 January 2024).

Another important cellular component in inflammatory pathologies is the primary fibroblast-like synoviocyte (FLS). These are abundant in synovial tissue and function to regulate synovial fluid as well as the extracellular matrix [57]. In one study, primary FLSs from patients diagnosed with RA showed higher levels of CK2 expression and activity than primary FLSs from patients diagnosed with OA, the control. Stimulation of the RA primary FLSs with Silmitasertib suppressed the cell cycle by inhibiting CK2, a key component in regulating the cell cycle. Furthermore, the drug's inhibition of CK2 decreased migration and proliferation of RA-FLSs, ultimately attenuating symptoms of RA, such as inflammation and joint pain [57]. Figure 2 summarizes in vitro and in vivo findings from these two studies.

The two most promising CK2 inhibitors include small molecule Silmitasertib and peptide inhibitor CIBG-300 [29]. Both are under clinical investigation for their use in cancer treatment. The ATP-competitive CK2-specific small molecule inhibitor exploits the differences in this kinase's ATP-binding domain with others. The ATP-binding domain in the CK2α subunit is small compared to other kinases in this family.

Silmitasertib is highly specific for CK2 amongst small molecule inhibitors of CK2, but the drug is not without adverse effects [98]. The inhibitor caused abnormal alternative splicing in CK2 independent manner [103], the CK2α transcript was affected as well [97]. In Cholangiocarcinoma, the drug induced methuosis and caused cell death in a CK2-independent manner. In pancreatic ductal adenocarcinoma (PDAC), the responsiveness to Silmitasertib was tested in different cell lines. Expression of CK2 varied in the cell lines tested, although it was elevated in all of them compared to non-neoplastic cells. Elevated expression of CK2 in tumor cells' responsiveness to Silmitasertib was not correlated to the extent of CK2 upregulation within the cell lines tested [104]. Additionally, inhibition of total CK2 activity within the cell was found to cause uncontrollable events in non-tumor cells [104–106].

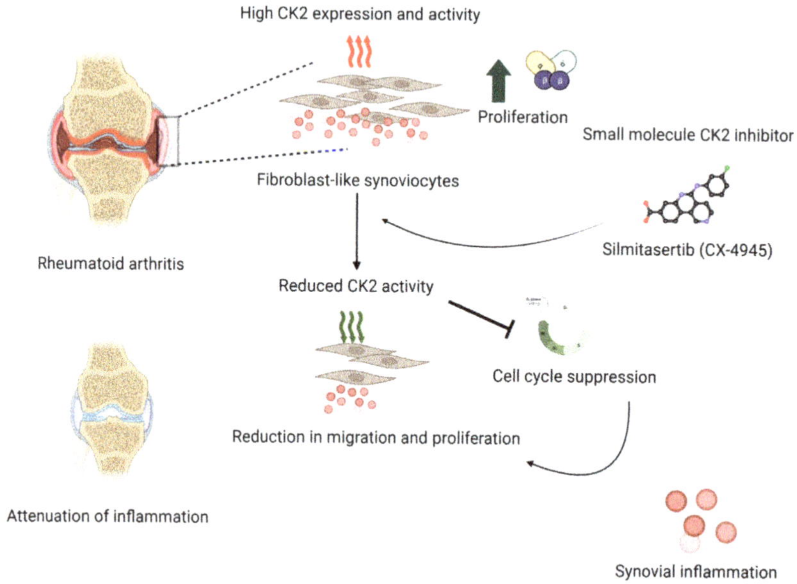

(**a**)

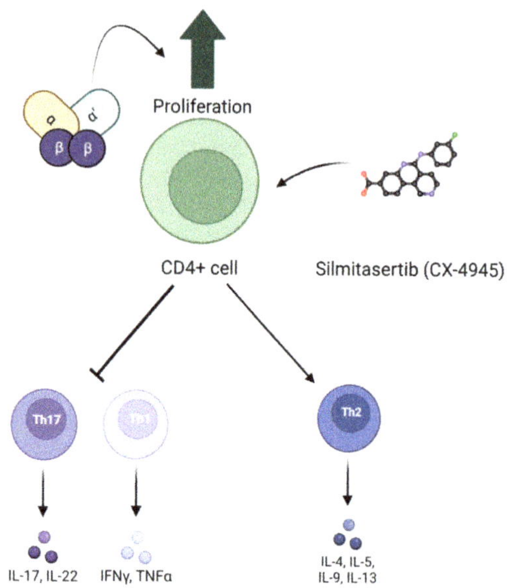

Figure 2. *Cont.*

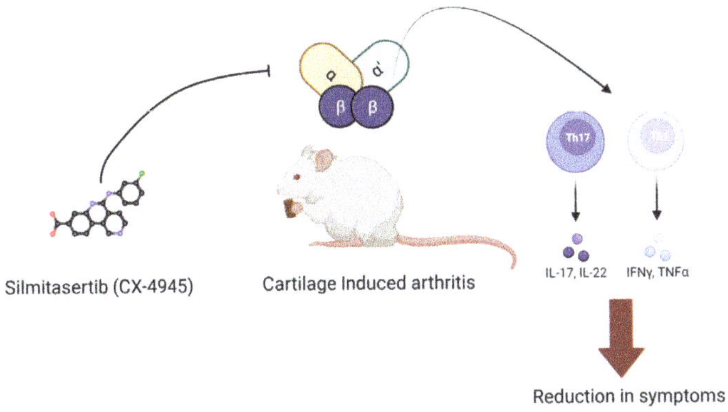

(**b**)

Figure 2. Implication of CK2 in RA and effect of inhibition of CK2 kinase activity. In RA, the expression of CK2 is upregulated. This upregulation increases proliferation and survival of CD4+ cells. Silmitasertib is a small molecule inhibitor of CK2 kinase activity. (**a**) Inhibition of CK2 in fibroblast-like synoviocytes reduced their proliferation and hence reduced the synovial inflammation. (**b**) In RA, CD4+ cells treated with CK2 inhibitors had a reduction in activation of Th1 and Th17 T cell response, and it activated Th2 type cell response. Inhibition of CK2 in CD4+ cells reduced their proliferation, and hence, Th1 and Th17 T cell response was activated. These effects were seen in in vivo conditions as well. (Image created with https://www.biorender.com/ accessed on 9 January 2024).

Silmitasertib also has off target effects. Silmitasertib inhibited dual-specificity tyrosine phosphorylation-regulated kinase 1A (DYRK1A) and glycogen synthase kinase-3β (GSK3β) kinases [107]. Off-target effects are also seen in the case of inhibition of Cdc2-like kinases (Clks). Furthermore, the efficacy of Silmitasertib in cancer is also lower than that of several other inhibitors of CK2, which can be ascribed to its moderate selectivity [99]. The off-target activity of Silmitasertib is reported in the literature [86]. Because Silmitasertib has many off-target effects, a more specific molecule based on the drug's structure is now under development [107].

The utility of CK2 inhibition by Silmitasertib for treating a non-neoplastic disease-osteoporosis was tested. Here, the effect of sub-cytotoxic concentrations of Silmitasertib was tested on osteoblast and osteoclast differentiation. It inhibited differentiation of bone-marrow-derived macrophages (BMM) into osteoclasts through RANKL activation. Inhibition of CK2 reduced phosphorylation of Akt, which caused downregulation in the expression of the transcription factor Nuclear Factor of Activated T Cells 1 (NFATc1), an effector of the Akt signaling cascade. Inhibition of CK2 also reduced RANKL-induced formation of tartrate-resistant acid phosphatase (TRAP), positive multinucleated cell formation, and TRAP activity, which is essential for osteoclast formation. On the other hand, BMP-2-mediated differentiation of myoblastic C2C12 cells into osteoblasts was enhanced with CK2 inhibition. Alkaline Phosphatase (ALP) activity and nuclear smad1/5/8 accumulation increased with increasing Silmitasertib concentration in differentiating cells. There was also an increase in Extracellular receptor Kinase (ERK) 1/2 phosphorylation. Thus, inhibition of CK2 accelerated osteoblast differentiation via the ERK1/2–Smad signaling axis [108].

Allosteric inhibitors bind at a site other than the enzyme's active site. They cause a change in the active conformation of the enzyme, which hampers substrate binding. Thus, they are not competitive for the substrate of the enzyme [109]. Allosteric inhibitors of CK2 are non-ATP competitive [110]. Allosteric inhibitors of CK2 can bind to three different sites [111]. Most effective inhibitors bind at the α and β unit interface [112]. This approach retains the activity of the catalytic subunits and hence only affects the phosphorylation of CK2β-dependent substrates [29]. The regulatory β subunits act as docking sites for a few CK2 substrates and protect the catalytic subunits from degradation. The other two sites where allosteric inhibitors can bind are the αD pocket, the linker region in the ATP binding site [113], and the αC helix region, which is rich in glycine. Detailed descriptions of various CK2 inhibitors and their strategies can be found in the current literature [29]. The structure-activity relation of CK2 inhibitors is reviewed in the literature [29,114–116]. Many of these are either not highly specific or have low cell permeability. Some compounds known to inhibit CK2 do not show cytotoxicity in cancer cell lines. However, their utility in treating musculoskeletal disorders is worth investigating. In these diseases, re-directing pathways involving deregulated CK2 is more critical than causing general cytotoxicity.

Further studies are needed for clinical translation of these inhibitors. Examples of small molecular CK2 inhibitors are included in Table 1. Based on kinase panel assay, their selectivity in inhibiting CK2 is mentioned as CK2 selectivity. The pre-clinical efficacy is described for each one of these.

Table 1. Small molecular inhibitors of CK2.

Name	CK2 Selectivity	Efficacy	Reference
Silmitasertib (CX-4945)	Selective at low concentrations. However, at nanomolar concentrations, it inhibits other kinases, such as DYRK1A.	Currently, it is the most selective CK2 inhibitor in clinical use and has minimal toxicity. Promotes apoptosis while inhibiting the PI3K/Akt signaling pathway and the cell cycle progression. Inhibits angiogenesis.	[108,117–119]
dimethylamino-4,5,6,7-1H-tetrabromobenzimidazole (DMAT)	Selective for CK2 but inhibits DYRK1A	Induces DNA double-strand breaks. Promotes apoptosis. Inhibition of aldosterone, DHEAS, and androstenedione secretion in adenocarcinoma cell line H295R.	[27,120,121]
Emodin	Moderately selective	Natural anthraquinone derivative extracted from rhubarb. Inhibits CK2.	[122–124]
Quinalizarin	Fairly selective	Promotes apoptosis in HEK-293 and Jurkat cells.	[125,126]
IC20	Extremely selective for CK2α	Not cytotoxic in cancer cells	[127–130]
SGC-CK2-1	Selective	Used as a cellular probe to investigate the intracellular function of CK2. Low inhibitory effect on the proliferation of most cancer cells, effective against a small subset of cancer cells.	[131,132]
Tetrabromocinnamic Acid (TBCA)	Selective	Derived from 4,5,6,7-tetrabromobenzotriazole (TBB). It is more potent than TBB. Does not inhibit DYRK1 like TBB. Promotes apoptosis in Jurkat cancer cells. Suppresses platelet aggregation/secretion and the cell cycle progression in prostate cancer cells.	[133,134]
4-(6,8-Dibromo-3-hydroxy-4-oxo-4H-chromo-2-yl)-benzoic acid (FLC26)	Mildly selective	Causes a significant increase in apoptosis in PANC-1 cells	[135,136]
3,8-dibromo-7-hydroxy-4-methylchromen-2-one (DBC)	Poorly selective	Induces apoptosis in Jurkat cells.	[137]
CAM4066	Poorly selective	Acts on the αD region and ATP-binding sites of CK2. The moiety bound to the ATP binding site forms a hydrogen bond with Lys68 and two water molecules. The moiety in the αD site interacts with Pro159 and a conserved water molecule. The linker creates a network of hydrogen bonds. Poor permeability. Methyl ester derivative pro-CAM4066 has better permeability.	[73,113,138]
CAM4712	Highly selective	Anti-proliferative	[109,113]
GO289	High selectivity	Extremely selective, ideal for clinical use. Inhibition of the phosphorylation sites of multiple clock proteins and suppressed the growth/proliferation of cells of a diverse array of cancers. CK2α and CK2α′ are the primary targets of the drug.	[115,119]
HY1-Pt	Highly selective. Derived from Silmitasertib. Overcomes cisplatin-induced resistance.	Reversed cisplatin-induced drug resistance. Suppresses DNA damage repair in cancer cells. It also inhibited the Wnt/beta-catenin signaling pathway while activating the mitochondrial apoptosis pathway. It displayed no toxicity to healthy hepatocytes and could be used as a therapeutic for NSCLC.	[107,139]

It is an effective strategy to target CK2 with other kinases that are either phosphorylated by it or act on the same substrate. Here, Bromodomain-Containing Protein 4 (BRD4) is a kinase that, along with CK2, is highly expressed in several different types of cancer. BRD4 is a transcriptional and epigenetic regulatory factor that belongs to the bromodomain and extraterminal (BET) family of chromatin adapter proteins. Its localization and stability are regulated by its phosphorylation by CK2. The use of inhibitors of BRD4 in cancer treatment is limited due to drug resistance [140]. In lung adenocarcinoma, the mechanism of drug resistance against BRD4 inhibitors was CK2-dependent [141]. A dual inhibitor for CK2 and BRD4 was more effective than targeting CK2 alone. Similarly, proviral integration of Moloney virus-1 (PIM) kinases and CK2 interacts with Myc [142,143]. These two kinases also have functional and structural similarities. In diseases with high expression of PIM and CK2, it was more effective to target both kinases. Both kinases are upregulated in hypoxic conditions in tumors [144]. SR-protein-specific kinase 1 (SRPK1) is involved in angiogenesis and overexpressed in several cancers. SRPIN803 inhibited both SRPK1 and CK2. Its ophthalmic application was also studied. TNIK and DYRK1 help maintain the phosphorylation of key regulators in cancer stem cells. Compound **108600** inhibited TNIK, DYRK1, and CK2. However, there was also an allosteric change in the CK2 α subunit that inhibited holoenzyme formation [109]. Table 2 summarizes the clinical efficacy of dual inhibitors of CK2.

Table 2. Multitarget inhibitors of CK2.

Name	Co-Target(s)	Clinical Efficacy	Reference
Compound **58**	BRD4	Able to overcome drug resistance in cancer treatment.	[114,140]
Compound **60**	BRD4	Highly selective. Reduces tumor growth and lessens cancer symptoms in vivo and in-vitro, with no apparent side effects. It is considered a potential therapeutic in triple-negative breast cancer.	[114,140]
Naphtho[2,1-b:7,6-b′]difuran-2,8-dicarboxylic acid hydrate (CPA), CPB, AMR	PIM	Lack of cell permeability; hence, it cannot be used clinically.	[145]
8-hydroxy-4-methyl-9-nitrobenzol(g)chrome-2-one (NBC)	PIM	Induces apoptosis.	[137,146]
1-β-D-2′-deoxyribofuranosyl-4,5,6,7-tetrabromo-1H-benzimidazole (TDB)	PIM	Extremely high selectivity indicates it has clinical potential.	[147]
Compound **66**	PIM	Cytotoxic against cancer cells but not healthy cells. Inhibits the proliferation of various cancer cell lines. Reduces the viability of cancer cells more effectively than Silmitasertib. It is membrane-permeable.	[146]
6-(4-Hydroxy-3-methoxybenzylidene)-5-imino-2-(trifluoromethyl)-5H-(1,3,4)thiadiazolo[3,2-a]pyrimidin-7(6H)-one (SRPIN803; CK2 inhibitor XIII).	SRPK1	Inhibits aberrant angiogenesis. Significantly inhibits cell viability in Jurkat cell lines. Prevents the formation of intraocular neovascularization in vivo.	[148]
Compound **108600**	TNIK, DYRK1	The inhibitory effect on CK2α' is ten times stronger than on CK2α. Inhibits tumor growth in breast cancer cells and overcomes chemical resistance. In vitro and in vivo studies suggest it is an optimal inhibitor in clinical settings.	[149]

The synthetic peptide CIBG-300 is effective in the treatment of cervical cancer. It is currently in phase 1 and 2 clinical trials [150]. It was also found to be anti-angiogenic [151]. The drug is derived from a cyclic nine-mer peptide. This peptide inhibited phosphorylation of human papillomavirus type-16 E7 (HPV-16 E7) oncoprotein phosphorylation in a phage display assay. Upon conjugating with cell-penetrating peptide Tat (amino acids 48–68) to increase the cell permeability of the peptide, it inhibited phosphorylation of the HPV-16 E7 oncoprotein by CK2 and induced apoptosis in cell cultures [42]. This peptide was then studied in different types of cancer [152]. CIGB-300 interacted more with catalytic subunits and interacted less with the regulatory subunit. Also, it responded with the CK2α' more than the CK2α subunit [43]. The target of this peptide was B23/nucleophosmin, a nucleolar protein that selectively modulates specific genes. It affected protein synthesis, energy metabolism, and biogenesis of ribosomes [140]. These findings have led to a challenge in the defining mechanism of action of CIBG-300. Previously termed as a CK2 inhibitor, its specificity in targeting selected phosphosites rather than generalized inhibition has gained attention.

Inhibitors with a higher specificity can target specific subunits or forms of the CK2 holoenzyme. Some of them, like CIBG-300, are capable of inhibiting selective phosphosites. They are tested for their use in cancer treatment as well as treatment of other diseases. These are listed in Table 3.

Table 3. CK2 inhibitors with pathway or subunit-specific mechanism of action.

Name	Status for Clinical Application	Reference
CIGB-300	Cell-permeable. Inhibits angiogenesis and metastasis. Used in early clinical trials in combination with chemoradiotherapy as a therapeutic against cervical cancer. Administered by injection into the tumor. Targets the phosphoacceptor domain. Releases histamine from the cells, possibly due to higher intracellular calcium levels in the cell.	[42]
4,5,6,7-tetrabromobenzotriazole (TBBt)	Moderately effective as an anti-cancer drug. Induces apoptosis in tumor cells. Inhibits CK2α subunit. They are used in Sepsis-Induced Acute Kidney Injury.	[153,154]
4,5,6,7-tetrabromobenzimidazole (TBBz)	Able to target specific molecular forms of CK2. It is more effective in inducing apoptosis and necrosis in tumor cells than TBBt. Inhibits CK2α subunit activity. It was tested in glioblastoma cell lines.	[153,155]

4. Targeting CK2 Interactions with Its Substrates–Novel Approach

Targeting CK2–substrates interaction critical for pathogenesis for musculoskeletal disorders can be carried out to engineer metabolic pathways to a healthy state. Interfering peptides inspired by the structure of the CK2 substrate can be used for this purpose.

Such biomimetic peptides are designed based on protein-protein interactions (PPIs). PPIs are essential to cellular functioning, and any dysfunction could represent an opportunity for specific targeting [156]. The nature of these interactions is being established using cutting-edge computational methods paired with existing knowledge. These studies aid in the design of drugs targeting very specific PPIs implicated in disease pathology [157]. Peptides and monoclonal antibodies have been widely used to produce new therapeutics to target extracellular PPIs. Still, the development of peptides targeting intracellular PPIs has been far more limited due to the challenges of maintaining the peptide's stability, administration, and bioavailability. Interfering peptides can interfere with PPIs and have been the focus of increasing attention by researchers. The large contact surface associated with PPIs has previously been an obstacle in the development of therapeutics, but interfering peptides have been found to interact more efficiently with large protein surfaces [158]. Peptides offer several advantages when used as therapeutics compared to small molecular drugs. First, they can cover more surface area in the PPI they are inhibiting. Then, their physical properties are easily modifiable based on their application. Moreover, they can be designed to be highly selective and can cover more surface area as inhibitors. Also, they have fewer toxicological effects [159]. Importantly, peptides can be developed to penetrate specific plasma membranes, which aids in targeting them to specific intracellular compartments, a long-standing challenge in therapeutic development [160–163]. Several studies prove that interfering peptides alter cellular processes [155,164–166]. Peptides can be produced in several ways, the simplest being procuring naturally occurring peptides [167]. Another method is to develop large numbers of peptides synthetically and then screen them to evaluate their therapeutic potential. A third method is to use peptides corresponding to fragments at the ends of the PPIs [168].

Disease-Modifying Peptide Drugs-CK2.1 and CK2.3

One of the most integral ways in which CK2 regulates the function of the musculoskeletal system is through the Bone Morphogenetic Protein (BMP) signaling pathway. The BMP signaling pathway regulates chondrogenesis and osteogenesis and maintains connective tissue homeostasis. The BMP-2 ligand interacts with BMPRIa and BMPRII receptors to activate the BMP pathway. CK2 interacts with the BMPRIa receptor in the absence of the BMP-2 ligand. Upon binding the BMP-2 ligand, the BMPRIa receptor undergoes heterodimerization with the BMPRII receptor. Formation of this complex releases of CK2. The release of CK2 initiates the subsequent phosphorylation of downstream signaling, which can cause the differentiation of MSCs into adipocytes, osteoblasts, and chondrocytes, depending on the pathway initiated. However, controlling the cell's fate via the signaling cascade activated by BMP2 is impossible. This led to the design of interfering peptides activating specific branches of the BMP pathway [169]. Three BMPRIa mimetic peptides were synthesized to initiate the BMP signaling pathway without BMP2. These peptides contained one of three CK2 phosphorylation sites on BMPRIa (SLKD, SYED, or SLYD). At the N-terminus, there is the Antennapedia Homeodomain sequence for cellular uptake. Flanking the CK2 phosphorylation motif, there is a BMPRIa homologous sequence. These peptides are named CK2.1, CK2.2, and CK2.3 based on the phosphorylation site they contain [170]. CK2.1 induced chondrogenesis in vitro in mouse MSC line C3H10T1/2 and in vivo in the Destabilized Medial Meniscus (DMM) mouse model. CK2.1 increased proteoglycan synthesis and elevated levels of collagen type II without causing chondrocyte hypertrophy, a frequent occurrence with BMP2-induced signaling [171,172]. Rabbit MSCs were treated with a bilayer peptide-loaded scaffold consisting of CK2.1-coated β-glycerophosphate/chitosan, which resulted in chondrogenesis and osteoblastogenesis. This technique could be beneficial for treating articular osteochondral defects, common in OA patients, involving damage to the cartilage and underlying bone [23]. CK2.2 induced both adipogenesis and osteogenesis, while CK2.3 induced osteogenesis. CK2.3 would be preferred in treating OP and other disorders that reduce bone mass and mineral density because it does not simultaneously induce adipogenesis, as does CK2.2 [171]. CK2.3 activates ERK phosphorylation by preventing CK2 binding to the BMRPIa–BMPRII receptor complex. CK2.3 increases bone area, bone mass, and mineral density [173]. In C2C12 cloned mouse myoblast cells, CK2.3 decreased osteoclastogenesis, increased osteoblastogenesis, and increased mineralization compared to controls. CK2.3 has been tested in an aging mouse model. In vivo, injections of CK2.3 via calvarial injection in mice increased bone area, density, and growth [170]. In 6-to-9-day-old C57BL/6J mice injected with CK2.3 via the calvaria and 8-week-old mice injected via the tail vein, mice showed increased bone formation and increased bone mineral density. At the same time, osteoclast activity appeared to be suppressed, indicating CK2.3 has the potential to alleviate the symptoms of OP by simultaneously enhancing osteoblast activity and inhibiting osteoclast activity, inducing bone growth and repair [174–176]. The principle of design of BMPRIa biomimetic peptides CK2.1 and CK2.3 and their effects are summarized in Figure 3.

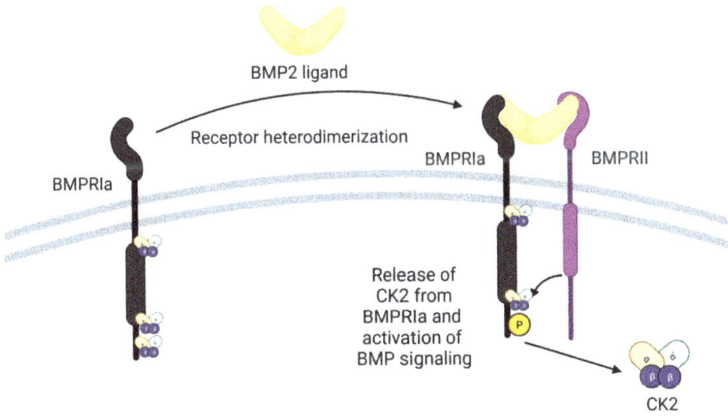

(a)

Figure 3. *Cont.*

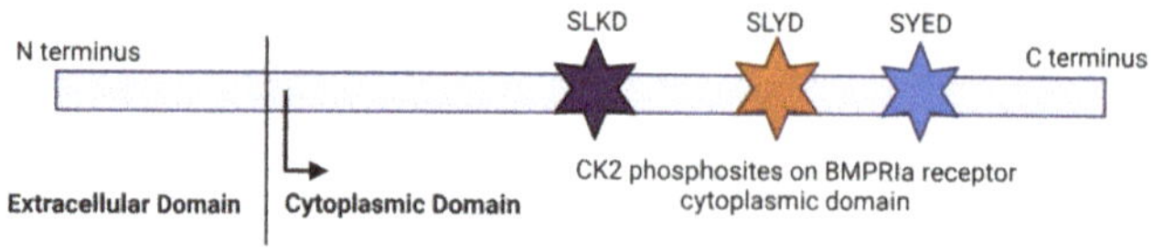

(b)

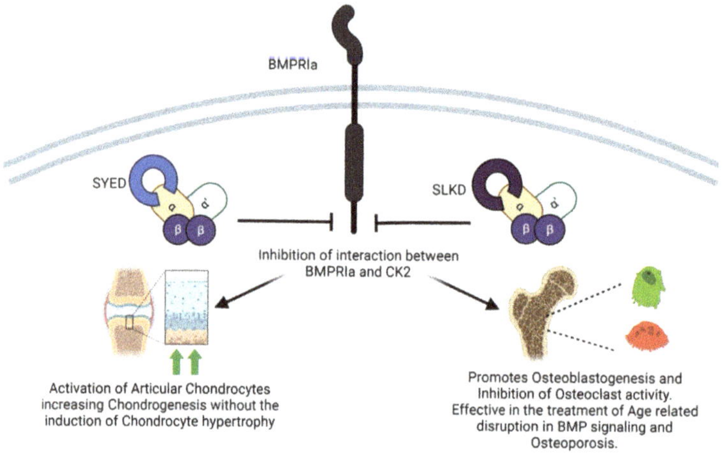

(c)

Figure 3. Inhibition of the interaction between CK2 and BMPRIa is an effective strategy for treating Osteoarthritis and Osteoporosis. (**a**) Stimulation with BMP2 ligand causes heterodimerization of BMPRIa receptor with BMPRII. Release of CK2 from BMPRIa and its phosphorylation by BMPRII activates the BMP signaling pathway. (**b**) BMPRIa receptor has three phosphosites on the cytoplasmic/intracellular domain. These phosphosites were validated using CK2 mutants. (**c**) BMPRIa mimetic peptides containing phosphosite sequences corresponding to 'SYED' activate articular chondrocytes to repair osteoarthritic lesions in knee articular cartilage. The BMPRIa mimetic peptide containing phosphosite sequence corresponding to 'SLKD' corrects the BMP pathway in senile mice. It helps regain balance between Osteoblastogenesis and Osteoclastic activity, which is affected in Osteoporosis. (Image created with https://www.biorender.com/ accessed on 9 January 2024).

5. Discussion

Inhibition of CK2 is proving to be highly successful in treating cancer. In musculoskeletal disorders, the influence of metabolic disorders is a research focus. The kinase CK2 is highly involved in the regulation of cellular metabolism. In rheumatoid arthritis, elevated CK2 activity promotes the inflammatory pathways. In osteoarthritis, a reduction in the activity of CK2 reduces the viability of chondrocytes. In osteoporosis, the imbalance in BMP signaling is due to the dysregulated function of CK2. During fracture healing, aging and senescence cause defective bone formation. CK2 is essential to cell survival and helps the cell counter senescence. Studying the role of CK2 in these diseases will demystify several mechanisms involved.

The pathogenesis of most musculoskeletal disorders has a component of dysregulated cell differentiation, senescence, and inflammation. Causing cytotoxicity is not always the best course of action for these disorders. Instead, correction of underlying biochemical imbalances is an effective treatment. The role of CK2 as the lateral player makes it an ideal protein target for these disorders.

The evolution of small molecular inhibitors of CK2 is mainly focused on their use as cancer therapeutics. Improved specificity and cell permeability are the two main achievements. These inhibitors are commonly used in combination with targeted therapy. However, their use in treating non-neoplastic disorders like musculoskeletal disorders is not common. Also, targeting the kinase activity is only sometimes the most effective method for this group of disorders. The entire phosphoproteome of CK2 is still being experimentally validated. Targeting of redundant interactions and false positive substrates thus stands as a possibility. The peptide drugs target the identified interaction between CK2 and BMPRIa. These are also seen to be highly cell-permeable. Further investigation into their tissue-specific drug delivery and toxicity needs to be undertaken. Evidence of their ability to drive the differentiation of MSCs into different lineages opens many possibilities. Drugs highly specific to kinase substrate interaction can be a molecular engineering tool. It can direct the molecular pathways towards the desired lineage. Targeting the pleiotropic kinase CK2 in this manner is an emerging prospect for designing a new generation of drugs. Figure 4 illustrates the current advances in CK2 inhibitors and the aspects to be addressed by upcoming drugs targeting CK2–substrate interactions.

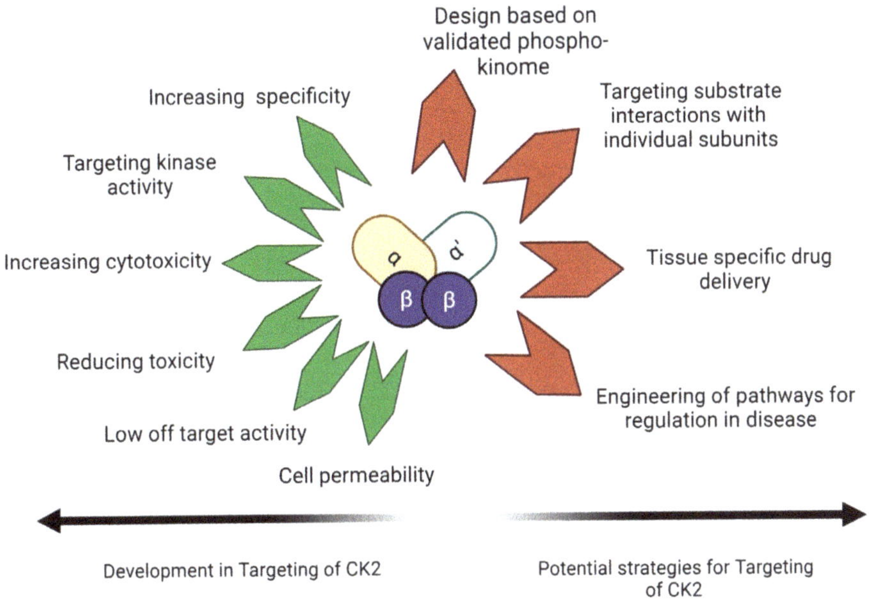

Figure 4. CK2 inhibitors have been designed with increased specificity for CK2, reducing off-target effects and increasing cell permeability. CK2 inhibitors have been found to increase cytotoxicity in anti-cancer drugs. With knowledge of the phosphosites of CK2 and the role of CK2 subunits and molecular forms, future CK2 inhibitors can be designed to target pathology-specific substrate interactions (Image Created with https://www.biorender.com/ accessed on 9 January 2024).

Author Contributions: Conceptualization, V.P. and A.N.; methodology, V.P.; software, V.P.; validation, A.N., V.P. and K.D.; formal analysis, V.P.; investigation, V.P.; resources, A.N.; data curation, V.P. and K.D.; writing—original draft preparation, V.P.; writing—review and editing, A.N., V.P. and K.D.; visualization, V.P. and K.D.; supervision, A.N.; project administration, A.N. All authors have read and agreed to the published version of the manuscript.

Funding: This research received no external funding.

Institutional Review Board Statement: Not applicable.

Informed Consent Statement: Not applicable.

Data Availability Statement: No new data were created or analyzed in this study. Data sharing is not applicable to this article.

Acknowledgments: The authors would like to acknowledge all members of the Nohe Lab, the University of Delaware, and the Delaware Biotechnology Institute for their continued support during this project. The authors thank Daniel Halloran and Kelechi Chukwuocha for their immense help and valuable suggestions in writing this review.

Conflicts of Interest: The authors declare no conflict of interest.

References

1. El Batawi, M.A. Work-related diseases. A new program of the World Health Organization. *Scand. J. Work. Environ. Health* **1984**, *10*, 341–346. [CrossRef]
2. Khan, M.A.; Zubair, H.; Anand, S.; Srivastava, S.K.; Singh, S.; Singh, A.P. Dysregulation of metabolic enzymes in tumor and stromal cells: Role in oncogenesis and therapeutic opportunities. *Cancer Lett.* **2020**, *473*, 176–185. [CrossRef]
3. Egami, R.; Kokaji, T.; Hatano, A.; Yugi, K.; Eto, M.; Morita, K.; Ohno, S.; Fujii, M.; Hironaka, K.-I.; Uematsu, S.; et al. Trans-omic analysis reveals obesity-associated dysregulation of inter-organ metabolic cycles between the liver and skeletal muscle. *iScience* **2021**, *24*, 102217. [CrossRef]
4. Comertpay, B.; Gov, E. Immune cell-specific and common molecular signatures in rheumatoid arthritis through molecular network approaches. *Biosystems* **2023**, *234*, 105063. [CrossRef] [PubMed]
5. Liu, M.; Li, S.; Cao, N.; Wang, Q.; Liu, Y.; Xu, Q.; Zhang, L.; Sun, C.; Xiao, X.; Yao, J. Intestinal flora, intestinal metabolism, and intestinal immunity changes in complete Freud's adjuvant-rheumatoid arthritis C57BL/6 mice. *Int. Immunopharmacol.* **2023**, *125 Pt A*, 111090. [CrossRef]
6. Mobasheri, A.; Rayman, M.P.; Gualillo, O.; Sellam, J.; van der Kraan, P.; Fearon, U. The role of metabolism in the pathogenesis of osteoarthritis. *Nat. Rev. Rheumatol.* **2017**, *13*, 302–311. [CrossRef]
7. Cho, Y.; Jeong, S.; Kim, H.; Kang, D.; Lee, J.; Kang, S.-B.; Kim, J.-H. Disease-modifying therapeutic strategies in osteoarthritis: Current status and future directions. *Exp. Mol. Med.* **2021**, *53*, 1689–1696. [CrossRef]
8. Liao, Z.; Han, X.; Wang, Y.; Shi, J.; Zhang, Y.; Zhao, H.; Zhang, L.; Jiang, M.; Liu, M. Differential Metabolites in Osteoarthritis: A Systematic Review and Meta-Analysis. *Nutrients* **2023**, *15*, 4191. [CrossRef] [PubMed]
9. Su, Z.; Zong, Z.; Deng, J.; Huang, J.; Liu, G.; Wei, B.; Cui, L.; Li, G.; Zhong, H.; Lin, S. Lipid Metabolism in Cartilage Development, Degeneration, and Regeneration. *Nutrients* **2022**, *14*, 3984. [CrossRef] [PubMed]
10. Xi, Y.; Shen, J.; Li, X.; Bao, Y.; Zhao, T.; Li, B.; Qin, D. Regulatory Effects of Quercetin on Bone Homeostasis: Research Updates and Future Perspectives. *Am. J. Chin. Med.* **2023**, *51*, 2077–2094. [CrossRef]
11. Robin, F.; Chappard, D.; Leroyer, P.; Latour, C.; Mabilleau, G.; Monbet, V.; Cavey, T.; Horeau, M.; Derbré, F.; Roth, M.; et al. Differences in bone microarchitecture between genetic and secondary iron-overload mouse models suggest a role for hepcidin deficiency in iron-related osteoporosis. *FASEB J.* **2023**, *37*, e23245. [CrossRef] [PubMed]
12. Alghadir, A.H.; Gabr, S.A.; Iqbal, A. Hand grip strength, vitamin D status, and diets as predictors of bone health in 6–12 years old school children. *BMC Musculoskelet. Disord.* **2023**, *24*, 830. [CrossRef] [PubMed]
13. Ribeiro, M.S.; Venturini, L.G.; Speck-Hernandez, C.A.; Alabarse, P.V.; Xavier, T.; Taira, T.M.; Duffles, L.F.; Cunha, F.Q.; Fukada, S.Y. AMPKα1 negatively regulates osteoclastogenesis and mitigates pathological bone loss. *J. Biol. Chem.* **2023**, *299*, 105379. [CrossRef] [PubMed]
14. Zhu, Z.; Liu, M.; Zhang, Y.; Wu, J.; Gao, M.; Lei, T.; Huang, F.; Chen, H.; Wu, M. Risk factors for the comorbidity of osteoporosis/osteopenia and kidney stones: A cross-sectional study. *Arch. Osteoporos.* **2023**, *18*, 128. [CrossRef] [PubMed]
15. Yoon, H.; Sung, E.; Kang, J.-H.; Kim, C.-H.; Shin, H.; Yoo, E.; Kim, M.; Lee, M.Y.; Shin, S. Association between body fat and bone mineral density in Korean adults: A cohort study. *Sci. Rep.* **2023**, *13*, 17462. [CrossRef] [PubMed]
16. Claes, L.; Recknagel, S.; Ignatius, A. Fracture healing under healthy and inflammatory conditions. *Nat. Rev. Rheumatol.* **2012**, *8*, 133–143. [CrossRef] [PubMed]
17. Khajuria, D.K.; Reider, I.; Kamal, F.; Norbury, C.C.; Elbarbary, R.A. Distinct defects in early innate and late adaptive immune responses typify impaired fracture healing in diet-induced obesity. *Front. Immunol.* **2023**, *14*, 1250309. [CrossRef] [PubMed]
18. Borgo, C.; D'amore, C.; Cesaro, L.; Sarno, S.; Pinna, L.A.; Ruzzene, M.; Salvi, M. How can a traffic light properly work if it is always green? The paradox of CK2 signaling. *Crit. Rev. Biochem. Mol. Biol.* **2021**, *56*, 321–359. [CrossRef]
19. Ruzzene, M.; Pinna, L.A. Addiction to protein kinase CK2: A common denominator of diverse cancer cells? *Biochim. Biophys. Acta* **2010**, *1804*, 499–504. [CrossRef]
20. St-Denis, N.A.; Litchfield, D.W. Protein kinase CK2 in health and disease: From birth to death: The role of protein kinase CK2 in the regulation of cell proliferation and survival. *Cell Mol. Life Sci.* **2009**, *66*, 1817–1829. [CrossRef]
21. Halloran, D.; Pandit, V.; Nohe, A. The Role of Protein Kinase CK2 in Development and Disease Progression: A Critical Review. *J. Dev. Biol.* **2022**, *10*, 31. [CrossRef] [PubMed]

22. Borgo, C.; D'amore, C.; Sarno, S.; Salvi, M.; Ruzzene, M. Protein kinase CK2: A potential therapeutic target for diverse human diseases. *Signal Transduct. Target. Ther.* **2021**, *6*, 183. [CrossRef] [PubMed]
23. Liu, J.; Lu, C.; Wu, X.; Zhang, Z.; Li, J.; Guo, B.; Li, D.; Liang, C.; Dang, L.; Pan, X.; et al. Targeting osteoblastic casein kinase-2 interacting protein-1 to enhance Smad-dependent BMP signaling and reverse bone formation reduction in glucocorticoid-induced osteoporosis. *Sci. Rep.* **2017**, *7*, 41295. [CrossRef] [PubMed]
24. Rea, I.M.; Gibson, D.S.; McGilligan, V.; McNerlan, S.E.; Alexander, H.D.; Ross, O.A. Age and Age-Related Diseases: Role of Inflammation Triggers and Cytokines. *Front. Immunol.* **2018**, *9*, 586. [CrossRef] [PubMed]
25. McGarry, T.; Biniecka, M.; Veale, D.J.; Fearon, U. Hypoxia, oxidative stress and inflammation. *Free Radic. Biol. Med.* **2018**, *125*, 15–24. [CrossRef]
26. Song, J.; Bae, Y.S. CK2 Down-Regulation Increases the Expression of Senescence-Associated Secretory Phenotype Factors through NF-κB Activation. *Int. J. Mol. Sci.* **2021**, *22*, 406. [CrossRef]
27. Pagano, M.A.; Andrzejewska, M.; Ruzzene, M.; Sarno, S.; Cesaro, L.; Bain, J.; Elliott, M.; Meggio, F.; Kazimierczuk, Z.; Pinna, L.A. Optimization of Protein Kinase CK2 Inhibitors Derived from 4,5,6,7-Tetrabromobenzimidazole. *J. Med. Chem.* **2004**, *47*, 6239–6247. [CrossRef]
28. Sarno, S.; Pinna, L.A. Protein kinase CK2 as a druggable target. *Mol. Biosyst.* **2008**, *4*, 889–894. [CrossRef]
29. Borgo, C.; Ruzzene, M. Protein kinase CK2 inhibition as a pharmacological strategy. *Adv. Protein Chem. Struct. Biol.* **2021**, *124*, 23–46. [PubMed]
30. Meggio, F.; Pinna, L.A. One-thousand-and-one substrates of protein kinase CK2? *FASEB J.* **2003**, *17*, 349–368. [CrossRef] [PubMed]
31. Franchin, C.; Borgo, C.; Cesaro, L.; Zaramella, S.; Vilardell, J.; Salvi, M.; Arrigoni, G.; Pinna, L.A. Re-evaluation of protein kinase CK2 pleiotropy: New insights provided by a phosphoproteomics analysis of CK2 knockout cells. *Cell. Mol. Life Sci.* **2018**, *75*, 2011–2026. [CrossRef] [PubMed]
32. Salvi, M.; Cesaro, L.; Pinna, L.A. Variable contribution of protein kinases to the generation of the human phosphoproteome: A global weblogo analysis. *Biomol. Concepts* **2010**, *1*, 185–195. [CrossRef] [PubMed]
33. Olsen, B.B.; Guerra, B.; Niefind, K.; Issinger, O.G. Structural basis of the constitutive activity of protein kinase CK2. *Methods Enzymol.* **2010**, *484*, 515–529. [PubMed]
34. Pinna, L.A. Protein kinase CK2: A challenge to canons. *J. Cell Sci.* **2002**, *115 Pt 20*, 3873–3878. [CrossRef] [PubMed]
35. Pinna, L.A. Protein kinase CK2. *Int. J. Biochem. Cell Biol.* **1997**, *29*, 551–554. [CrossRef]
36. Filhol, O.; Cochet, C. Protein kinase CK2 in health and disease: Cellular functions of protein kinase CK2: A dynamic affair. *Cell Mol. Life Sci.* **2009**, *66*, 1830–1839. [CrossRef] [PubMed]
37. Niefind, K.; Guerra, B.; Ermakowa, I.; Issinger, O. Crystal structure of human protein kinase CK2: Insights into basic properties of the CK2 holoenzyme. *EMBO J.* **2001**, *20*, 5320–5331. [CrossRef]
38. Olsten, M.E.; Litchfield, D.W. Order or chaos? An evaluation of the regulation of protein kinase CK2. *Biochem. Cell Biol.* **2004**, *82*, 681–693. [CrossRef]
39. Montenarh, M.; Götz, C. Protein Kinase CK2α', More than a Backup of CK2α. *Cells* **2023**, *12*, 2834. [CrossRef]
40. Pierre, F.; Chua, P.C.; O'Brien, S.E.; Siddiqui-Jain, A.; Bourbon, P.; Haddach, M.; Michaux, J.; Nagasawa, J.; Schwaebe, M.K.; Stefan, E.; et al. Discovery and SAR of 5-(3-Chlorophenylamino)benzo[c][2,6]naphthyridine-8-carboxylic Acid (CX-4945), the First Clinical Stage Inhibitor of Protein Kinase CK2 for the Treatment of Cancer. *J. Med. Chem.* **2011**, *54*, 635–654. [CrossRef] [PubMed]
41. Zanin, S.; Sandre, M.; Cozza, G.; Ottaviani, D.; Marin, O.; Pinna, L.A.; Ruzzene, M. Chimeric peptides as modulators of CK2-dependent signaling: Mechanism of action and off-target effects. *Biochim. Biophys. Acta* **2015**, *1854 Pt B*, 1694–1707. [CrossRef]
42. Perea, S.E.; Baladrón, I.; Valenzuela, C.; Perera, Y. CIGB-300: A peptide-based drug that impairs the Protein Kinase CK2-mediated phosphorylation. *Semin. Oncol.* **2018**, *45*, 58–67. [CrossRef] [PubMed]
43. Pérez, G.V.; Rosales, M.; Ramón, A.C.; Rodríguez-Ulloa, A.; Besada, V.; González, L.J.; Aguilar, D.; Vázquez-Blomquist, D.; Falcón, V.; Caballero, E.; et al. CIGB-300 Anticancer Peptide Differentially Interacts with CK2 Subunits and Regulates Specific Signaling Mediators in a Highly Sensitive Large Cell Lung Carcinoma Cell Model. *Biomedicines* **2022**, *11*, 43. [CrossRef] [PubMed]
44. Cirigliano, S.M.; Bessone, M.I.D.; Berardi, D.E.; Flumian, C.; Bal de Kier Joffé, E.D.; Perea, S.E.; Farina, H.G.; Todaro, L.B.; Urtreger, A.J. The synthetic peptide CIGB-300 modulates CK2-dependent signaling pathways affecting the survival and chemoresistance of non-small cell lung cancer cell lines. *Cancer Cell Int.* **2017**, *17*, 42. [CrossRef] [PubMed]
45. Sarduy, M.R.; García, I.; Coca, M.A.; Perera, A.; Torres, L.A.; Valenzuela, C.M.; Baladrón, I.; Solares, M.; Reyes, V.; Hernández, I.; et al. Optimizing CIGB-300 intralesional delivery in locally advanced cervical cancer. *Br. J. Cancer* **2015**, *112*, 1636–1643. [CrossRef] [PubMed]
46. Vázquez-Blomquist, D.; Ramón, A.C.; Rosales, M.; Pérez, G.V.; Rosales, A.; Palenzuela, D.; Perera, Y.; Perea, S.E. Gene expression profiling unveils the temporal dynamics of CIGB-300-regulated transcriptome in AML cell lines. *BMC Genom.* **2023**, *24*, 373. [CrossRef] [PubMed]
47. Rodriguez-Merchan, E.C. The Current Role of Disease-modifying Osteoarthritis Drugs. *Arch. Bone Jt. Surg.* **2023**, *11*, 11–22.
48. Song, Z.; Li, Y.; Shang, C.; Shang, G.; Kou, H.; Li, J.; Chen, S.; Liu, H. Sprifermin: Effects on Cartilage Homeostasis and Therapeutic Prospects in Cartilage-Related Diseases. *Front. Cell Dev. Biol.* **2021**, *9*, 786546. [CrossRef]
49. Maksimovic, V.; Pavlovic-Popovic, Z.; Vukmirovic, S.; Cvejic, J.; Mooranian, A.; Al-Salami, H.; Mikov, M.; Golocorbin-Kon, S. Molecular mechanism of action and pharmacokinetic properties of methotrexate. *Mol. Biol. Rep.* **2020**, *47*, 4699–4708. [CrossRef]

50. Chua, M.M.J.; Lee, M.; Dominguez, I. Cancer-type dependent expression of CK2 transcripts. *PLoS ONE* **2017**, *12*, e0188854. [CrossRef]
51. Sun, D.; Gao, W.; Hu, H.; Zhou, S. Why 90% of clinical drug development fails and how to improve it? *Acta Pharm. Sin B* **2022**, *12*, 3049–3062. [CrossRef]
52. Lee, D.M.; Weinblatt, M.E. Rheumatoid arthritis. *Lancet* **2001**, *358*, 903–911. [CrossRef]
53. Gibofsky, A. Epidemiology, pathophysiology, and diagnosis of rheumatoid arthritis: A Synopsis. *Am. J. Manag. Care* **2014**, *20*, S128–S135.
54. Huang, J.; Fu, X.; Chen, X.; Li, Z.; Huang, Y.; Liang, C. Promising Therapeutic Targets for Treatment of Rheumatoid Arthritis. *Front. Immunol.* **2021**, *12*, 686155. [CrossRef]
55. Mcinnes, I.B.; Schett, G. The pathogenesis of rheumatoid arthritis. *N. Engl. J. Med.* **2011**, *365*, 2205–2219. [CrossRef] [PubMed]
56. Radu, A.; Bungao, S.G. Management of Rheumatoid Arthritis: An Overview. *Cells* **2021**, *10*, 2857. [CrossRef] [PubMed]
57. Luo, Y.; Lei, Y.; Guo, X.; Zhu, D.; Zhang, H.; Guo, Z.; Xu, Z.; Zhao, H.; Xi, Y.; Peng, X.; et al. CX-4945 inhibits fibroblast-like synoviocytes functions through the CK2-p53 axis to reduce rheumatoid arthritis disease severity. *Int. Immunopharmacol.* **2023**, *119*, 110163. [CrossRef] [PubMed]
58. Bartok, B.; Firestein, G.S. Fibroblast-like synoviocytes: Key effector cells in rheumatoid arthritis. *Immunol. Rev.* **2009**, *1*, 233–255. [CrossRef] [PubMed]
59. Yang, W.; Gibson, S.A.; Yan, Z. Protein kinase 2 (CK2) controls CD4(+) T cell effector function in the pathogenesis of colitis. *Mucosal Immunol.* **2020**, *13*, 788–798. [CrossRef] [PubMed]
60. Ulges, A.; Klein, M.; Reuters, S. Protein kinase CK2 enables regulatory T cells to suppress excessive TH2 responses in vivo. *Nat. Immunol.* **2015**, *16*, 267–275. [CrossRef] [PubMed]
61. Zheng, L.; Zhang, Z.; Sheng, P.; Mobasheri, A. The role of metabolism in chondrocyte dysfunction and the progression of osteoarthritis. *Ageing Res. Rev.* **2021**, *66*, 101249. [CrossRef] [PubMed]
62. Henrotin, Y.; Kurz, B.; Aigner, T. Oxygen and reactive oxygen species in cartilage degradation: Friends or foes? *Osteoarthr. Cartil.* **2005**, *13*, 643–654. [CrossRef] [PubMed]
63. Lee, S.W.; Song, Y.S.; Lee, S.Y.; Yoon, Y.G.; Lee, S.H.; Park, B.S.; Yun, I.; Choi, H.; Kim, K.; Chung, W.T.; et al. Downregulation of protein kinase CK2 activity facilitates tumor necrosis factor-α-mediated chondrocyte death through apoptosis and autophagy. *PLoS ONE* **2011**, *6*, e19163. [CrossRef] [PubMed]
64. Nishimori, S.; Lai, F.; Shiraishi, M.; Kobayashi, T.; Kozhemyakina, E.; Yao, T.-P.; Lassar, A.B.; Kronenberg, H.M. PTHrP targets HDAC4 and HDAC5 to repress chondrocyte hypertrophy. *J. Clin. Investig.* **2019**, *4*, e97903. [CrossRef] [PubMed]
65. Hui, W.; A Young, D.; Rowan, A.D.; Xu, X.; E Cawston, T.; Proctor, C.J. Oxidative changes and signalling pathways are pivotal in initiating age-related changes in articular cartilage. *Ann. Rheum. Dis.* **2016**, *75*, 449–458. [CrossRef] [PubMed]
66. Librizzi, M.; Naselli, F.; Abruscato, G.; Luparello, C.; Caradonna, F. Parathyroid Hormone Related Protein (PTHrP)-Associated Molecular Signatures in Tissue Differentiation and Non-Tumoral Diseases. *Biology* **2023**, *12*, 950. [CrossRef]
67. Aarts, M.M.; Levy, D.; He, B.; Stregger, S.; Chen, T.; Richard, S.; Henderson, J.E. Parathyroid Hormone-related Protein Interacts with RNA. *J. Biol. Chem.* **1999**, *274*, 4832–4838. [CrossRef]
68. Okoumassoun, L.E.; Russo, C.; Denizeau, F.; Averill-Bates, D.; Henderson, J.E. Parathyroid hormone-related protein (PTHrP) inhibits mitochondrial-dependent apoptosis through CK2. *J. Cell. Physiol.* **2007**, *212*, 591–599. [CrossRef]
69. Saha, S.; Buttari, B.; Panieri, E.; Profumo, E.; Saso, L. An Overview of Nrf2 Signaling Pathway and Its Role in Inflammation. *Molecules* **2020**, *25*, 5474. [CrossRef]
70. Soares, M.P.; Seldon, M.P.; Gregoire, I.P.; Vassilevskaia, T.; Berberat, P.O.; Yu, J.; Tsui, T.-Y.; Bach, F.H. Heme Oxygenase-1 Modulates the Expression of Adhesion Molecules Associated with Endothelial Cell Activation. *J. Immunol.* **2004**, *172*, 3553–3563. [CrossRef]
71. Park, Y.C.; Kim, K.M.; Song, J.D.; Chung, H.T. Protein kinase CK2 mediates peroxynitrite-induced heme oxygenase-1 expression in articular chondrocytes. *Int. J. Mol. Med.* **2012**, *29*, 1039–1044. [CrossRef]
72. Kim, K.M.; Sohn, D.H.; Kim, K.; Park, Y.C. Inhibition of protein kinase CK2 facilitates cellular senescence by inhibiting the expression of HO-1 in articular chondrocytes. *Int. J. Mol. Med.* **2019**, *43*, 1033–1040. [CrossRef]
73. Lindenblatt, D.; Applegate, V.; Nickelsen, A.; Klußmann, M.; Neundorf, I.; Götz, C.; Jose, J.; Niefind, K. Molecular Plasticity of Crystalline CK2α′ Leads to KN2, a Bivalent Inhibitor of Protein Kinase CK2 with Extraordinary Selectivity. *J. Med. Chem.* **2022**, *65*, 1302–1312. [CrossRef]
74. Lee, S.W.; Rho, J.H.; Lee, S.Y.; Yoo, S.H.; Kim, H.Y.; Chung, W.T.; Yoo, Y.H. Alpha B-Crystallin Protects Rat Articular Chondrocytes against Casein Kinase II Inhibition-Induced Apoptosis. *PLoS ONE* **2016**, *11*, e0166450. [CrossRef]
75. Muire, P.J.; Mangum, L.H.; Wenke, J.C. Time Course of Immune Response and Immunomodulation During Normal and Delayed Healing of Musculoskeletal Wounds. *Front. Immunol.* **2020**, *11*, 1056. [CrossRef]
76. Prein, C.; Beier, F. ECM signaling in cartilage development and endochondral ossification. *Curr. Top. Dev. Biol.* **2019**, *133*, 25–47. [PubMed]
77. PPajarinen, J.; Lin, T.; Gibon, E.; Kohno, Y.; Maruyama, M.; Nathan, K.; Lu, L.; Yao, Z.; Goodman, S.B. Mesenchymal stem cell-macrophage crosstalk and bone healing. *Biomaterials* **2019**, *196*, 80–89. [CrossRef] [PubMed]

78. Recknagel, S.D.; Bindl, R.; Brochhausen, C.; Göckelmann, M.D.; Wehner, T.; Schoengraf, P.; Huber-Lang, M.; Claes, L.; Ignatius, A.D. Systemic inflammation induced by a thoracic trauma alters the cellular composition of the early fracture callus. *J. Trauma Inj. Infect. Crit. Care* **2013**, *74*, 531–537. [CrossRef] [PubMed]
79. Saul, D.; Khosla, S. Fracture Healing in the Setting of Endocrine Diseases, Aging, and Cellular Senescence. *Endocr. Rev.* **2022**, *43*, 984–1002. [CrossRef] [PubMed]
80. Takayama, H.; La Rochelle, W.J.; Anver, M.; E Bockman, D.; Merlino, G. Scatter factor/hepatocyte growth factor as a regulator of skeletal muscle and neural crest development. *Proc. Natl. Acad. Sci. USA* **1996**, *93*, 5866–5871. [CrossRef]
81. Majidinia, M.; Sadeghpour, A.; Yousefi, B. The roles of signaling pathways in bone repair and regeneration. *J. Cell Physiol.* **2018**, *233*, 2937–2948. [CrossRef] [PubMed]
82. Dumic-Cule, I.; Peric, M.; Kucko, L.; Grgurevic, L.; Pecina, M.; Vukicevic, S. Bone morphogenetic proteins in fracture repair. *Int. Orthop.* **2018**, *42*, 2619–2626. [CrossRef] [PubMed]
83. Cho, J.H.; Lee, J.H.; Lee, K.M.; Lee, C.-K.; Shin, D.-M. BMP-2 Induced Signaling Pathways and Phenotypes: Comparisons Between Senescent and Non-senescent Bone Marrow Mesenchymal Stem Cells. *Calcif. Tissue Int.* **2021**, *110*, 489–503. [CrossRef] [PubMed]
84. Bragdon, B.; Thinakaran, S.; Moseychuk, O.; King, D.; Young, K.; Litchfield, D.W.; Petersen, N.O.; Nohe, A. Casein kinase 2 beta-subunit is a regulator of bone morphogenetic protein 2 signaling. *Biophys. J.* **2010**, *99*, 897–904. [CrossRef] [PubMed]
85. Yu, B.; Huo, L.; Liu, Y.; Deng, P.; Szymanski, J.; Li, J.; Luo, X.; Hong, C.; Lin, J.; Wang, C.Y. PGC-1α Controls Skeletal Stem Cell Fate and Bone-Fat Balance in Osteoporosis and Skeletal Aging by Inducing TAZ. *Cell Stem Cell* **2018**, *23*, 193–209.e5. [CrossRef]
86. Nie, J.; Liu, L.; He, F.; Fu, X.; Han, W.; Zhang, L. CKIP-1: A scaffold protein and potential therapeutic target integrating multiple signaling pathways and physiological functions. *Ageing Res. Rev.* **2013**, *12*, 276–281. [CrossRef]
87. Fu, L.; Zhang, L. Physiological functions of CKIP-1: From molecular mechanisms to therapy implications. *Ageing Res. Rev.* **2019**, *53*, 100908. [CrossRef]
88. Yuan, Y.; Sun, J.; Zhou, H.; Wang, S.; He, C.; Chen, T.; Fang, M.; Li, S.; Kang, S.; Huang, X.; et al. The effect of QiangGuYin on osteoporosis through the AKT/mTOR/autophagy signaling pathway mediated by CKIP-1. *Aging* **2022**, *14*, 892–906. [CrossRef]
89. Peng, X.; Wu, X.; Zhang, J.; Zhang, G.; Li, G.; Pan, X. The role of CKIP-1 in osteoporosis development and treatment. *Bone Jt. Res.* **2018**, *7*, 173–178. [CrossRef]
90. Litchfield, D.W. Protein kinase CK2: Structure, regulation and role in cellular decisions of life and death. *Biochem. J.* **2003**, *369 Pt 1*, 1–15. [CrossRef]
91. Salvi, M.; Sarno, S.; Cesaro, L.; Nakamura, H.; Pinna, L.A. Extraordinary pleiotropy of protein kinase CK2 revealed by weblogo phosphoproteome analysis. *Biochim. Biophys. Acta (BBA)-Mol. Cell Res.* **2009**, *1793*, 847–859. [CrossRef]
92. Franchin, C.; Borgo, C.; Zaramella, S.; Cesaro, L.; Arrigoni, G.; Salvi, M.; Pinna, L.A. Exploring the CK2 Paradox: Restless, Dangerous, Dispensable. *Pharmaceuticals* **2017**, *10*, 11. [CrossRef]
93. Chojnowski, J.E.; Mcmillan, E.A.; Strochlic, T.I. Identification of Novel CK2 Kinase Substrates Using a Versatile Biochemical Approach. *J. Vis. Exp.* **2019**, *21*, e59037.
94. Borgo, C.; Cesaro, L.; Hirota, T.; Kuwata, K.; D'amore, C.; Ruppert, T.; Blatnik, R.; Salvi, M.; Pinna, L.A. Comparing the efficacy and selectivity of Ck2 inhibitors a phosphoproteomics approach. *Eur. J. Med. Chem.* **2021**, *214*, 113217. [CrossRef] [PubMed]
95. Gyenis, L.; Menyhart, D.; Cruise, E.S.; Jurcic, K.; Roffey, S.E.; Chai, D.B.; Trifoi, F.; Fess, S.R.; Desormeaux, P.J.; Díaz, T.N.d.V.; et al. Chemical Genetic Validation of CSNK2 Substrates Using an Inhibitor-Resistant Mutant in Combination with Triple SILAC Quantitative Phosphoproteomics. *Front. Mol. Biosci.* **2022**, *9*, 909711. [CrossRef]
96. Borgo, C.; Cesaro, L.; Hirota, T.; Kuwata, K.; D'Amore, C.; Ruppert, T.; Blatnik, R.; Salvi, M.; Pinna, L.A. Analysis of the phosphoproteome of CK2α((-/-))/$\Delta\alpha'$ C2C12 myoblasts compared to the wild-type cells. *Open Biol.* **2023**, *13*, 220220. [CrossRef] [PubMed]
97. Kim, H.; Choi, K.; Kang, H.; Lee, S.-Y.; Chi, S.-W.; Lee, M.-S.; Song, J.; Im, D.; Choi, Y.; Cho, S. Identification of a Novel Function of CX-4945 as a Splicing Regulator. *PLoS ONE* **2014**, *9*, e94978. [CrossRef] [PubMed]
98. Merholz, M.; Jian, Y.; Wimberg, J.; Gessler, L.; Hashemolhosseini, S. In Skeletal Muscle Fibers, Protein Kinase Subunit CSNK2A1/CK2α Is Required for Proper Muscle Homeostasis and Structure and Function of Neuromuscular Junctions. *Cells* **2022**, *11*, 3962. [CrossRef]
99. Salvi, M.; Borgo, C.; Pinna, L.A.; Ruzzene, M. Targeting CK2 in cancer: A valuable strategy or a waste of time? *Cell Death Discov.* **2021**, *7*, 325. [CrossRef] [PubMed]
100. Trembley, J.H.; Kren, B.T.; Afzal, M.; Scaria, G.A.; Klein, M.A.; Ahmed, K. Protein kinase CK2—Diverse roles in cancer cell biology and therapeutic promise. *Mol. Cell. Biochem.* **2022**, *478*, 899–926. [CrossRef]
101. Jiang, Q.; Yang, G.; Liu, Q.; Wang, S.; Cui, D. Function and Role of Regulatory T Cells in Rheumatoid Arthritis. *Front. Immunol.* **2021**, *12*, 626193. [CrossRef]
102. Ye, H.; Fu, D.; Fang, X.; Xie, Y.; Zheng, X.; Fan, W.; Hu, F.; Li, Z. Casein Kinase II exacerbates rheumatoid arthritis via promoting Th1 and Th17 cell inflammatory responses. *Expert. Opin. Ther. Targets* **2021**, *25*, 1017–1024. [CrossRef] [PubMed]
103. Lee, J.Y.; Yun, J.-S.; Kim, W.-K.; Chun, H.-S.; Jin, H.; Cho, S.; Chang, J.H. Structural Basis for the Selective Inhibition of Cdc2-Like Kinases by CX-4945. *BioMed Res. Int.* **2019**, *2019*, 6125068. [CrossRef]
104. Ma, Y.; Sender, S.; Sekora, A.; Kong, W.; Bauer, P.; Ameziane, N.; Krake, S.; Radefeldt, M.; Al-Ali, R.; Weiss, F.U.; et al. Inhibitory Response to CK II Inhibitor Silmitasertib and CDKs Inhibitor Dinaciclib Is Related to Genetic Differences in Pancreatic Ductal Adenocarcinoma Cell Lines. *Int. J. Mol. Sci.* **2022**, *23*, 4409. [CrossRef]

105. Lertsuwan, J.; Lertsuwan, K.; Sawasdichai, A.; Tasnawijitwong, N.; Lee, K.Y.; Kitchen, P.; Afford, S.; Gaston, K.; Jayaraman, P.S.; Satayavivad, J. CX-4945 Induces Methuosis in Cholangiocarcinoma Cell Lines by a CK2-Independent Mechanism. *Cancers* **2018**, *10*, 283. [CrossRef]
106. Silva-Pavez, E.; Villar, P.; Trigo, C.; Caamaño, E.; Niechi, I.; Pérez, P.; Muñoz, J.P.; Aguayo, F.; Burzio, V.A.; Varas-Godoy, M.; et al. CK2 inhibition with silmitasertib promotes methuosis-like cell death associated to catastrophic massive vacuolization of colorectal cancer cells. *Cell Death Dis.* **2019**, *10*, 73. [CrossRef] [PubMed]
107. Wang, Y.; Wang, X.; Xu, G.; Gou, S. Novel CK2-Specific Pt(II) Compound Reverses Cisplatin-Induced Resistance by Inhibiting Cancer Cell Stemness and Suppressing DNA Damage Repair in Non-small Cell Lung Cancer Treatments. *J. Med. Chem.* **2021**, *64*, 4163–4178. [CrossRef] [PubMed]
108. Son, Y.H.; Moon, S.H.; Kim, J. The Protein Kinase 2 Inhibitor CX-4945 Regulates Osteoclast and Osteoblast Differentiation In Vitro. *Mol. Cells* **2013**, *36*, 417–423. [CrossRef]
109. Chen, X.; Li, C.; Wang, D.; Chen, Y.; Zhang, N. Recent Advances in the Discovery of CK2 Allosteric Inhibitors: From Traditional Screening to Structure-Based Design. *Molecules* **2020**, *25*, 870. [CrossRef]
110. Moucadel, V.; Prudent, R.; Sautel, C.F.; Teillet, F.; Barette, C.; Lafanechere, L.; Receveur-Brechot, V.; Cochet, C. Antitumoral activity of allosteric inhibitors of protein kinase CK2. *Oncotarget* **2011**, *2*, 997–1010. [CrossRef]
111. Li, C.; Zhang, X.; Zhang, N.; Zhou, Y.; Sun, G.; Zhao, L.; Zhong, R. Identification and Biological Evaluation of CK2 Allosteric Fragments through Structure-Based Virtual Screening. *Molecules* **2020**, *25*, 237. [CrossRef]
112. Brear, P.; North, A.; Iegre, J.; Georgiou, K.H.; Lubin, A.; Carro, L.; Green, W.; Sore, H.F.; Hyvönen, M.; Spring, D.R. Novel non-ATP competitive small molecules targeting the CK2 α/β interface. *Bioorg Med. Chem.* **2018**, *26*, 3016–3020. [CrossRef] [PubMed]
113. Iegre, J.; Brear, P.; De Fusco, C.; Yoshida, M.; Mitchell, S.L.; Rossmann, M.; Carro, L.; Sore, H.F.; Hyvönen, M.; Spring, D.R. Second-generation CK2α inhibitors targeting the αD pocket. *Chem. Sci.* **2018**, *9*, 3041–3049. [CrossRef] [PubMed]
114. Chen, Y.-H.; Zhang, X.; Attarian, D.; Kraus, V.B. Synergistic roles of CBX4 chromo and SIM domains in regulating senescence of primary human osteoarthritic chondrocytes. *Arthritis Res. Ther.* **2023**, *25*, 197. [CrossRef] [PubMed]
115. Oshima, T.; Niwa, Y.; Kuwata, K.; Srivastava, A.; Hyoda, T.; Tsuchiya, Y.; Kumagai, M.; Tsuyuguchi, M.; Tamaru, T.; Sugiyama, A.; et al. Cell-based screen identifies a new potent and highly selective CK2 inhibitor for modulation of circadian rhythms and cancer cell growth. *Sci. Adv.* **2019**, *5*, eaau9060. [CrossRef] [PubMed]
116. Chen, Y.; Wang, Y.; Wang, J.; Zhou, Z.; Cao, S.; Zhang, J. Strategies of Targeting CK2 in Drug Discovery: Challenges, Opportunities, and Emerging Prospects. *J. Med. Chem.* **2023**, *66*, 2257–2281. [CrossRef] [PubMed]
117. Ferguson, A.D.; Sheth, P.R.; Basso, A.D.; Paliwal, S.; Gray, K.; Fischmann, T.O.; Le, H.V. Structural basis of CX-4945 binding to human protein kinase CK2. *FEBS Lett.* **2011**, *585*, 104–110. [CrossRef] [PubMed]
118. Siddiqui-Jain, A.; Drygin, D.; Streiner, N.; Chua, P.; Pierre, F.; O'Brien, S.E.; Bliesath, J.; Omori, M.; Huser, N.; Ho, C.; et al. CX-4945, an orally bioavailable selective inhibitor of protein kinase CK2, inhibits prosurvival and angiogenic signaling and exhibits antitumor efficacy. *Cancer Res.* **2010**, *70*, 10288–10298. [CrossRef] [PubMed]
119. Atkinson, E.L.; Iegre, J.; Brear, P.; A Zhabina, E.; Hyvönen, M.; Spring, D. Downfalls of Chemical Probes Acting at the Kinase ATP-Site: CK2 as a Case Study. *Molecules* **2021**, *26*, 1977. [CrossRef]
120. Schneider, C.C.; Hessenauer, A.; Götz, C.; Montenarh, M. DMAT, an inhibitor of protein kinase CK2 induces reactive oxygen species and DNA double strand breaks. *Oncol. Rep.* **2009**, *21*, 1593–1597.
121. Pagano, M.A.; Meggio, F.; Ruzzene, M.; Andrzejewska, M.; Kazimierczuk, Z.; Pinna, L.A. 2-Dimethylamino-4,5,6,7-tetrabromo-1H-benzimidazole: A novel powerful and selective inhibitor of protein kinase CK2. *Biochem. Biophys. Res. Commun.* **2004**, *321*, 1040–1044. [CrossRef] [PubMed]
122. Yim, H.; Lee, Y.H.; Lee, C.H.; Lee, S.K. Emodin, an Anthraquinone Derivative Isolated from the Rhizomes of *Rheum palmatum*, Selectively Inhibits the Activity of Casein Kinase II as a Competitive Inhibitor. *Planta Medica* **1999**, *65*, 9–13. [CrossRef] [PubMed]
123. Feng, Y.; Huang, S.L.; Dou, W.; Zhang, S.; Chen, J.H.; Shen, Y.; Shen, J.H.; Leng, Y. Emodin, a natural product, selectively inhibits 11beta-hydroxysteroid dehydrogenase type 1 and ameliorates metabolic disorder in diet-induced obese mice. *Br. J. Pharmacol.* **2010**, *161*, 113–126. [CrossRef]
124. Sarno, S.; Moro, S.; Meggio, F.; Zagotto, G.; Ben, D.D.; Ghisellini, P.; Battistutta, R.; Zanotti, G.; Pinna, L.A. Toward the rational design of protein kinase casein kinase-2 inhibitors. *Pharmacol. Ther.* **2002**, *93*, 159–168. [CrossRef]
125. Cozza, G.; Mazzorana, M.; Papinutto, E.; Bain, J.; Elliott, M.; di Maira, G.; Gianoncelli, A.; Pagano, M.A.; Sarno, S.; Ruzzene, M.; et al. Quinalizarin as a potent, selective and cell-permeable inhibitor of protein kinase CK2. *Biochem. J.* **2009**, *421*, 387–395. [CrossRef]
126. Franchin, C.; Cesaro, L.; Salvi, M.; Millioni, R.; Iori, E.; Cifani, P.; James, P.; Arrigoni, G.; Pinna, L. Quantitative analysis of a phosphoproteome readily altered by the protein kinase CK2 inhibitor quinalizarin in HEK-293T cells. *Biochim. Biophys. Acta (BBA)—Proteins Proteom.* **2014**, *1854*, 609–623. [CrossRef] [PubMed]
127. Bullock, A.N.; Debreczeni, J.; Fedorov, O.Y.; Nelson, A.; Marsden, B.D.; Knapp, S. Structural Basis of Inhibitor Specificity of the Human Protooncogene Proviral Insertion Site in Moloney Murine Leukemia Virus (PIM-1) Kinase. *J. Med. Chem.* **2005**, *48*, 7604–7614. [CrossRef]
128. Mathison, C.J.N.; Chianelli, D.; Rucker, P.V.; Nelson, J.; Roland, J.; Huang, Z.; Yang, Y.; Jiang, J.; Xie, Y.F.; Epple, R.; et al. Efficacy and Tolerability of Pyrazolo [1,5-a]pyrimidine RET Kinase Inhibitors for the Treatment of Lung Adenocarcinoma. *ACS Med. Chem. Lett.* **2020**, *11*, 558–565. [CrossRef]

129. Sacks, D.; Baxter, B.; Campbell, B.C.; Carpenter, J.S.; Cognard, C.; Dippel, D.; Eesa, M.; Fischer, U.; Hausegger, K.; Hirsch, J.A. Multisociety Consensus Quality Improvement Revised Consensus Statement for Endovascular Therapy of Acute Ischemic Stroke. *Int. J. Stroke* **2018**, *13*, 612–632. [CrossRef]
130. Krämer, A.; Kurz, C.G.; Berger, B. T.; Celik, I.E.; Tjaden, A.; Greco, F.A.; Knapp, S.; Hanke, T. Optimization of pyrazolo[1,5-a]pyrimidines lead to the identification of a highly selective casein kinase 2 inhibitor. *Eur. J. Med. Chem.* **2020**, *208*, 112770. [CrossRef]
131. Licciardello, M.P.; Workman, P. A New Chemical Probe Challenges the Broad Cancer Essentiality of CK2. *Trends Pharmacol. Sci.* **2021**, *42*, 313–315. [CrossRef]
132. Wells, C.I.; Drewry, D.H.; Pickett, J.E.; Tjaden, A.; Krämer, A.; Müller, S.; Gyenis, L.; Menyhart, D.; Litchfield, D.W.; Knapp, S.; et al. Development of a potent and selective chemical probe for the pleiotropic kinase CK2. *Cell Chem. Biol.* **2021**, *28*, 546–558.e10. [CrossRef]
133. Yao, K.; Youn, H.; Gao, X.; Huang, B.; Zhou, F.; Li, B.; Han, H. Casein kinase 2 inhibition attenuates androgen receptor function and cell proliferation in prostate cancer cells. *Prostate* **2012**, *72*, 1423–1430. [CrossRef] [PubMed]
134. Pagano, M.A.; Poletto, G.; Di Maira, G.; Cozza, G.; Ruzzene, M.; Sarno, S.; Bain, J.; Elliott, M.; Moro, S.; Zagotto, G.; et al. Tetrabromocinnamic Acid (TBCA) and Related Compounds Represent a New Class of Specific Protein Kinase CK2 Inhibitors. *ChemBioChem* **2007**, *8*, 129–139. [CrossRef] [PubMed]
135. Golub, A.G.; Bdzhola, V.G.; Kyshenia, Y.V.; Sapelkin, V.M.; Prykhod'ko, A.O.; Kukharenko, O.P.; Ostrynska, O.V.; Yarmoluk, S.M. Structure-based discovery of novel flavonol inhibitors of human protein kinase CK2. *Mol. Cell. Biochem.* **2011**, *356*, 107–115. [CrossRef]
136. Guerra, B.; Issinger, O.-G. Protein Kinase CK2 in Human Diseases. *Curr. Med. Chem.* **2008**, *15*, 1870–1886. [CrossRef] [PubMed]
137. Meggio, F.; Pagano, M.A.; Moro, S.; Zagotto, G.; Ruzzene, M.; Sarno, S.; Cozza, G.; Bain, J.; Elliott, M.; Deana, A.D.; et al. Inhibition of Protein Kinase CK2 by Condensed Polyphenolic Derivatives. An in Vitro and in Vivo Study. *Biochemistry* **2004**, *43*, 12931–12936. [CrossRef] [PubMed]
138. Brear, P.; De Fusco, C.; Georgiou, K.H.; Francis-Newton, N.J.; Stubbs, C.J.; Sore, H.F.; Venkitaraman, A.R.; Abell, C.; Spring, D.R.; Hyvönen, M. Specific inhibition of CK2α from an anchor outside the active site. *Chem. Sci.* **2016**, *7*, 6839–6845. [CrossRef]
139. Wang, X.; Wang, Y.; Gou, S. A platinum(II) complex HY1-Pt overcomes cisplatin-induced resistance and attenuates metastasis of epithelial ovarian cancer by cancer cell stemness inhibition. *Int. J. Biochem. Cell Biol.* **2023**, *157*, 106395. [CrossRef]
140. Zhang, J.; Tang, P.; Zou, L.; Zhang, J.; Chen, J.; Yang, C.; He, G.; Liu, B.; Liu, J.; Chiang, C.M.; et al. Discovery of Novel Dual-Target Inhibitor of Bromodomain-Containing Protein 4/Casein Kinase 2 Inducing Apoptosis and Autophagy-Associated Cell Death for Triple-Negative Breast Cancer Therapy. *J. Med. Chem.* **2021**, *64*, 18025–18053. [CrossRef]
141. Calder, J.; Nagelberg, A.; Luu, J.; Lu, D.; Lockwood, W.W. Resistance to BET inhibitors in lung adenocarcinoma is mediated by casein kinase phosphorylation of BRD4. *Oncogenesis* **2021**, *10*, 27. [CrossRef] [PubMed]
142. Channavajhala, P.; Seldin, D.C. Functional interaction of protein kinase CK2 and c-Myc in lymphomagenesis. *Oncogene* **2002**, *21*, 5280–5288. [CrossRef] [PubMed]
143. Wang, J.; Kim, J.; Roh, M.; O E Franco, O.; Hayward, S.W.; Wills, M.L.; A Abdulkadir, S. Pim1 kinase synergizes with c-MYC to induce advanced prostate carcinoma. *Oncogene* **2010**, *29*, 2477–2487. [CrossRef]
144. Wińska, P.; Wielechowska, M.; Koronkiewicz, M.; Borowiecki, P. Synthesis and Anticancer Activity of Novel Dual Inhibitors of Human Protein Kinases CK2 and PIM-1. *Pharmaceutics* **2023**, *15*, 1991. [CrossRef] [PubMed]
145. Prudent, R.; Moucadel, V.; Sautel, C.F.; Barette, C.; Lafanechère, L.; Mouawad, L.; Grierson, D.; Schmidt, F.; Filippakopoulos, P.; Bullock, A.N.; et al. New potent dual inhibitors of CK2 and Pim kinases: Discovery and structural insights. *FASEB J.* **2010**, *24*, 3171–3185.
146. Sarno, S.; Mazzorana, M.; Traynor, R.; Ruzzene, M.; Cozza, G.; Pagano, M.A.; Meggio, F.; Zagotto, G.; Battistutta, R.; Pinna, L.A. Structural features underlying the selectivity of the kinase inhibitors NBC and dNBC: Role of a nitro group that discriminates between CK2 and DYRK1A. *Cell. Mol. Life Sci.* **2011**, *69*, 449–460. [CrossRef] [PubMed]
147. Łukowska-Chojnacka, E.; Wińska, P.; Wielechowska, M.; Poprzeczko, M.; Bretner, M. Synthesis of novel polybrominated benzimidazole derivatives-potential CK2 inhibitors with anticancer and proapoptotic activity. *Bioorg Med. Chem.* **2016**, *24*, 735–741. [CrossRef]
148. Morooka, S.; Hoshina, M.; Kii, I.; Okabe, T.; Kojima, H.; Inoue, N.; Okuno, Y.; Denawa, M.; Yoshida, S.; Fukuhara, J.; et al. Identification of a Dual Inhibitor of SRPK1 and CK2 That Attenuates Pathological Angiogenesis of Macular Degeneration in Mice. *Mol. Pharmacol.* **2015**, *88*, 316–325. [CrossRef]
149. Sato, K.; Padgaonkar, A.A.; Baker, S.J.; Cosenza, S.C.; Rechkoblit, O.; Subbaiah, D.R.C.V.; Domingo-Domenech, J.; Bartkowski, A.; Port, E.R.; Aggarwal, A.K.; et al. Simultaneous CK2/TNIK/DYRK1 inhibition by 108600 suppresses triple negative breast cancer stem cells and chemotherapy-resistant disease. *Nat. Commun.* **2021**, *12*, 4671. [CrossRef]
150. Perera, Y.; Ramos, Y.; Padrón, G.; Caballero, E.; Guirola, O.; Caligiuri, L.G.; Lorenzo, N.; Gottardo, F.; Farina, H.G.; Filhol, O.; et al. CIGB-300 anticancer peptide regulates the protein kinase CK2-dependent phosphoproteome. *Mol. Cell. Biochem.* **2020**, *470*, 63–75. [CrossRef]
151. Farina, H.G.; Acero, F.B.; Perera, Y.; Rodríguez, A.; Perea, S.E.; Castro, B.A.; Gomez, R.; Alonso, D.F.; Gomez, D.E. CIGB-300, a proapoptotic peptide, inhibits angiogenesis in vitro and in vivo. *Exp. Cell Res.* **2011**, *317*, 1677–1688. [CrossRef]

152. Gottardo, M.F.; Capobianco, C.S.; Sidabra, J.E.; Garona, J.; Perera, Y.; Perea, S.E.; Alonso, D.F.; Farina, H.G. Preclinical efficacy of CIGB-300, an anti-CK2 peptide, on breast cancer metastasic colonization. *Sci. Rep.* **2020**, *10*, 14689. [CrossRef]
153. Zien, P.; Duncan, J.S.; Skierski, J.; Bretner, M.; Litchfield, D.W.; Shugar, D. Tetrabromobenzotriazole (TBBt) and tetrabromobenzimidazole (TBBz) as selective inhibitors of protein kinase CK2: Evaluation of their effects on cells and different molecular forms of human CK2. *Biochim. Biophys. Acta (BBA)—Proteins Proteom.* **2005**, *1754*, 271–280. [CrossRef]
154. Koo, J.-H.; Yu, H.C.; Nam, S.; Kim, D.-C.; Lee, J.H. Casein Kinase 2 Alpha Inhibition Protects against Sepsis-Induced Acute Kidney Injury. *Int. J. Mol. Sci.* **2023**, *24*, 9783. [CrossRef]
155. Nitta, R.T.; Gholamin, S.; Feroze, A.H.; Agarwal, M.; Cheshier, S.H.; Mitra, S.S.; Li, G. Casein kinase 2α regulates glioblastoma brain tumor-initiating cell growth through the β-catenin pathway. *Oncogene* **2014**, *34*, 3688–3699. [CrossRef]
156. Wang, T.; Yang, N.; Liang, C.; Xu, H.; An, Y.; Xiao, S.; Zheng, M.; Liu, L.; Wang, G.; Nie, L. Detecting Protein-Protein Interaction Based on Protein Fragment Complementation Assay. *Curr. Protein Pept. Sci.* **2020**, *21*, 598–610. [CrossRef] [PubMed]
157. Dai, B.; Bailey-Kellogg, C. Protein interaction interface region prediction by geometric deep learning. *Bioinformatics* **2021**, *37*, 2580–2588. [CrossRef] [PubMed]
158. Apostolopoulos, V.; Bojarska, J.; Chai, T.-T.; Elnagdy, S.; Kaczmarek, K.; Matsoukas, J.; New, R.; Parang, K.; Lopez, O.P.; Parhiz, H.; et al. A Global Review on Short Peptides: Frontiers and Perspectives. *Molecules* **2021**, *26*, 430. [CrossRef] [PubMed]
159. Wang, L.; Wang, N.; Zhang, W.; Cheng, X.; Yan, Z.; Shao, G.; Wang, X.; Wang, R.; Fu, C. Therapeutic peptides: Current applications and future directions. *Signal Transduct. Target. Ther.* **2022**, *7*, 48. [CrossRef] [PubMed]
160. Berillo, D.; Yeskendir, A.; Zharkinbekov, Z.; Raziyeva, K.; Saparov, A. Peptide-Based Drug Delivery Systems. *Medicina* **2021**, *57*, 1209. [CrossRef] [PubMed]
161. Hao, M.; Zhang, L.; Chen, P. Membrane Internalization Mechanisms and Design Strategies of Arginine-Rich Cell-Penetrating Peptides. *Int. J. Mol. Sci.* **2022**, *23*, 9038. [CrossRef]
162. De Oliveira, E.C.L.; da Costa, K.S.; Taube, P.S.; Lima, A.H.; Junior, C.D.S.D.S. Biological Membrane-Penetrating Peptides: Computational Prediction and Applications. *Front. Cell Infect. Microbiol.* **2022**, *12*, 838259. [CrossRef]
163. Lai, Y.; Fois, G.; Flores, J.R.; Tuvim, M.J.; Zhou, Q.; Yang, K.; Leitz, J.; Peters, J.; Zhang, Y.; Pfuetzner, R.A.; et al. Inhibition of calcium-triggered secretion by hydrocarbon-stapled peptides. *Nature* **2022**, *603*, 949–956. [CrossRef]
164. Dong, C.Z.; Bruzzoni-Giovanelli, H.; Yu, Y.; Dorgham, K.; Parizot, C.; Zini, J.M.; Brossas, J.Y.; Tuffery, P.; Rebollo, A. Identification of peptides interfering with the LRRK2/PP1 interaction. *PLoS ONE* **2020**, *15*, e0237110. [CrossRef]
165. Dergunova, L.V.; Filippenkov, I.B.; Limborska, S.A.; Myasoedov, N.F. Neuroprotective Peptides and New Strategies for Ischemic Stroke Drug Discoveries. *Genes* **2023**, *14*, 953. [CrossRef]
166. Simón-Gracia, L.; Loisel, S.; Sidorenko, V.; Scodeller, P.; Parizot, C.; Savier, E.; Haute, T.; Teesalu, T.; Rebollo, A. Preclinical Validation of Tumor-Penetrating and Interfering Peptides against Chronic Lymphocytic Leukemia. *Mol. Pharm.* **2022**, *19*, 895–903. [CrossRef]
167. Wang, J.; Wu, Y.; Chen, Z.; Chen, Y.; Lin, Q.; Liang, Y. Exogenous Bioactive Peptides Have a Potential Therapeutic Role in Delaying Aging in Rodent Models. *Int. J. Mol. Sci.* **2022**, *23*, 1421. [CrossRef]
168. Bruzzoni-Giovanelli, H.; Alezra, V.; Wolff, N.; Dong, C.Z.; Tuffery, P.; Rebollo, A. Interfering peptides targeting protein-protein interactions: The next generation of drugs? *Drug Discov. Today* **2018**, *23*, 272–285. [CrossRef] [PubMed]
169. Lisberg, A.; Ellis, R.; Nicholson, K.; Moku, P.; Swarup, A.; Dhurjati, P.; Nohe, A. Mathematical modeling of the effects of CK2.3 on mineralization in osteoporotic bone. *CPT Pharmacomet. Syst. Pharmacol.* **2017**, *6*, 208–215. [CrossRef] [PubMed]
170. Bragdon, B.; Thinakaran, S.; Moseychuk, O.; Gurski, L.; Bonor, J.; Price, C.; Wang, L.; Beamer, W.G.; Nohe, A. Casein kinase 2 regulates in vivo bone formation through its interaction with bone morphogenetic protein receptor type Ia. *Bone* **2011**, *49*, 944–954. [CrossRef] [PubMed]
171. Akkiraju, H.; Bonor, J.; Nohe, A. CK2.1, a novel peptide, induces articular cartilage formation in vivo. *J. Orthop. Res.* **2016**, *35*, 876–885. [CrossRef]
172. Akkiraju, H.; Srinivasan, P.P.; Xu, X.; Jia, X.; Safran, C.B.K.; Nohe, A. CK2.1, a bone morphogenetic protein receptor type Ia mimetic peptide, repairs cartilage in mice with destabilized medial meniscus. *Stem Cell Res. Ther.* **2017**, *8*, 82. [CrossRef]
173. Takahashi, K.; Setoguchi, T.; Tsuru, A.; Saitoh, Y.; Nagano, S.; Ishidou, Y.; Maeda, S.; Furukawa, T.; Komiya, S. Inhibition of casein kinase 2 prevents growth of human osteosarcoma. *Oncol. Rep.* **2016**, *37*, 1141–1147. [CrossRef]
174. Halloran, D.; Pandit, V.; MacMurray, C.; Stone, V.; DeGeorge, K.; Eskander, M.; Root, D.; McTague, S.; Pelkey, H.; Nohe, A. Age-Related Low Bone Mineral Density in C57BL/6 Mice Is Reflective of Aberrant Bone Morphogenetic Protein-2 Signaling Observed in Human Patients Diagnosed with Osteoporosis. *Int. J. Mol. Sci.* **2022**, *23*, 11205. [CrossRef] [PubMed]
175. Vrathasha, V.; Weidner, H.; Nohe, A. Mechanism of CK2.3, a Novel Mimetic Peptide of Bone Morphogenetic Protein Receptor Type IA, Mediated Osteogenesis. *Int. J. Mol. Sci.* **2019**, *10*, 2500. [CrossRef] [PubMed]
176. Weidner, H.; Gao, V.Y.; Dibert, D.; McTague, S.; Eskander, M.; Duncan, R.; Wang, L.; Nohe, A. CK2.3, a Mimetic Peptide of the BMP Type I Receptor, Increases Activity in Osteoblasts over BMP2. *Int. J. Mol. Sci.* **2019**, *20*, 5877. [CrossRef] [PubMed]

kinases and phosphatases

MDPI

Review

CK2 Inhibitors Targeting Inside and Outside the Catalytic Box

Sophie Day-Riley [1], Rebekah M. West [1], Paul D. Brear [2], Marko Hyvönen [2] and David R. Spring [1,*]

[1] Yusuf Hamied Department of Chemistry, University of Cambridge, Lensfield Road, Cambridge CB2 1EW, UK; sed61@cam.ac.uk (S.D.-R.); rw603@cam.ac.uk (R.M.W.)

[2] Department of Biochemistry, Sanger Building, University of Cambridge, 80 Tennis Court Road, Cambridge CB2 1GA, UK

* Correspondence: spring@ch.cam.ac.uk

Abstract: CK2 is a protein kinase that plays an important role in numerous cellular pathways involved in cell growth, differentiation, proliferation, and death. Consequently, upregulation of CK2 is implicated in many disease types, in particular cancer. As such, CK2 has gained significant attention as a potential therapeutic target in cancer, and over 40 chemical probes targeting CK2 have been developed in the past decade. In this review, we highlighted several chemical probes that target sites outside the conventional ATP-binding site. These chemical probes belong to different classes of molecules, from small molecules to peptides, and possess different mechanisms of action. Many of the chemical probes discussed in this review could serve as promising new candidates for drugs selectively targeting CK2.

Keywords: CK2; casein kinase II; CSNK2A1; CSNK2A2; CSNK2B; protein phosphorylation; human diseases; signal transduction; protein kinase inhibitors

1. Introduction

1.1. An Overview of CK2

The human protein kinome, comprising over 500 kinases, regulates almost all fundamental cellular processes responsible for cell growth, proliferation, differentiation, and death [1]. Kinases phosphorylate their substrates by catalyzing the transfer of a terminal phosphate group from adenosine triphosphate (ATP) or guanosine triphosphate (GTP) to its substrate, depending on the type. This ultimately activates or deactivates crucial cell signaling pathways. Therefore, normal cell function depends on precise kinase regulation [2]. Unsurprisingly, gene mutations that cause aberrant kinase function are implicated in the progression of many malignant and benign disorders; the implications of kinase mutations are most documented in cancer progression, and the pursuit of kinase inhibition is prominent in pharmaceutical research. As of today, there are 75 FDA-approved kinase inhibitors, and this number is expected to grow as drug development efforts continue [3].

CK2 is a highly conserved and ubiquitously expressed kinase belonging to the CMGC (cyclin-dependent kinases (CDKs), mitogen-activated protein kinases (MAPKs), glycogen synthase kinases (GSKs), and Cdc2-like kinases (CLKs)) family, which contains 63 family members [4,5]. CK2 was first discovered by Burnett and Kennedy in 1954, named originally as casein kinase 2 after casein that was used in the original work and was considered an in vivo substrate of CK2 [6]. However, further studies elucidated that CK2 can only phosphorylate casein in vitro; therefore, the kinase is no longer referred to as casein kinase 2, and the shorthand name CK2 is used [7]. CK2 is a serine/threonine protein kinase that exists as a heterotetrameric holoenzyme and adopts a butterfly-shaped conformation, as shown in Figure 1. The heterotetrameric holoenzyme is composed of two catalytic subunits (α and/or α') and two non-catalytic regulatory β subunits. The β subunits dimerize through a zinc finger domain and bind the α or α' kinase subunits [8]. The heterotetrameric structure can take the forms $\alpha\alpha\beta\beta$, $\alpha'\alpha\beta\beta$, or $\alpha'\alpha'\beta\beta$, where the α subunit is on occasion replaced by the α' isoform [9,10]. Both the CK2α and CK2α' subunits and the CK2 holoenzyme itself are constitutively active. This is unusual for a eukaryotic kinase and means the enzyme does not rely on an upstream phosphorylation event for its functionality [11]. This unusual feature is thought to contribute to the multifunctionality and pathogenic potential of CK2 [12].

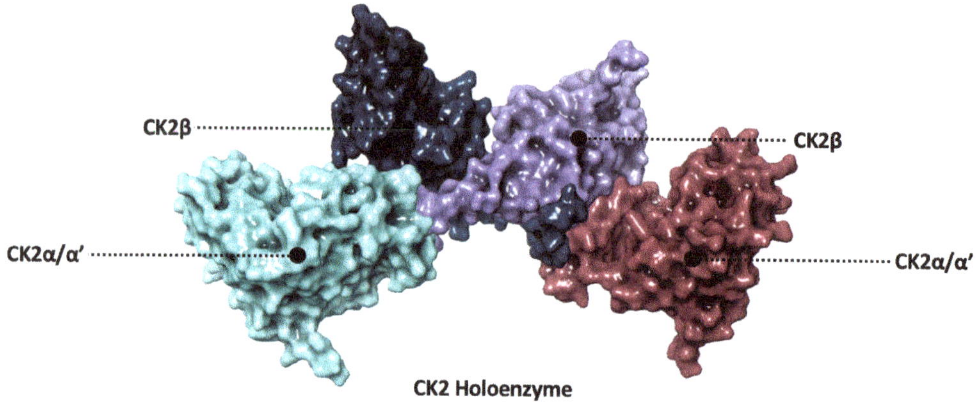

Figure 1. The heterotetrameric structure of protein kinase CK2. The catalytic α/α' subunits are shown in cyan and burgundy; the regulatory β subunits are shown in navy and lilac (PDB: 1JWH).

This highly pleiotropic kinase has over 760 identified substrates in humans, according to the PhosphoSitePlus database, https://www.phosphosite.org/ (accessed on 1 January 2024), generating a large proportion of the human phosphoproteome [13,14]. A large portion of CK2's substrates are involved in various cell signaling pathways related to cancer progression, such as phosphoinositide 3-kinase (PI3K)/Protein kinase B (PKB, also known as Akt); inhibitor of nuclear factor-κB kinase (IKK)/nuclear factor-κB (NFκB); Janus kinase 2 (JAK2)/signal transducer and activator of transcription protein 3 (SAT3); wingless-related integration site (Wnt)/β-catenin; Hedgehog, and neurogenic locus notch homolog protein 1 (Notch 1) [15–21]. A few of these pathways are detailed in Figure 2. Through phosphoproteomic studies, CK2 has also been found to phosphorylate several key constituents in drug efflux, DNA damage, and DNA repair pathways. CK2 expression within healthy eukaryotic cells only increases during mitosis, whilst in cancerous cells CK2 is commonly overexpressed, aiding in proliferation, tumorigenesis, metastasis, drug resistance, and the ability to evade apoptosis [10]. The extent to which CK2 potentiates each cell signaling pathway is proportional to its expression [21]. The survival of a plethora of cancer types, including, but not limited to, glioblastoma, medulloblastoma, cholangiocarcinoma, and breast and renal cell carcinoma, has been shown to be negatively impacted by the downregulation of CK2 [22]. Thus, CK2 is considered an extremely attractive target for cancer therapy.

It is important to note that CK2 is not only found within the cytoplasm but is found in nearly every compartment of eukaryotic cells [23]. The translocation of CK2 from cytoplasm to nucleus is correlated with elevated levels of CK2 and cell proliferation. This indicates that the subcellular localization of CK2 is a dynamic process, adapting to the varying needs of CK2 within different cellular compartments.

The role of CK2 is not only prominent in the pathogenesis of cancer but also in the progression of many other diseases, such as Parkinson's disease, Alzheimer's disease, and amyotrophic lateral scoliosis (ALS) [10,22]. Additionally, siRNA knockdown of CK2 has shown that CK2 is implicated in the regulation of the human papilloma virus (HPV) life cycle [24]. Furthermore, CK2 inhibition has been suggested as a potential antiviral agent against SARS-CoV-2; upregulation and then interaction of CK2 with the nucleocapsid of

SARS-CoV-2 has been found in host cells [25]. Therefore, targeting CK2 may serve as a valid antiviral approach against viruses such as HPV and SARS-CoV-2 in the future.

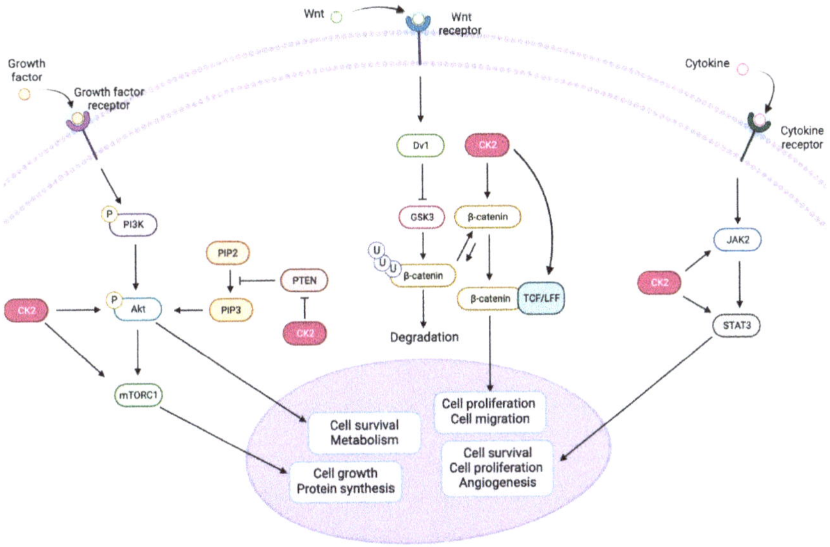

Figure 2. A schematic diagram depicting several biological pathways that CK2 is known to be involved in that are implicated in cancer progression. Pathways shown from right to left are PI3k/Akt, Wnt/β-catenin, and JAK2/STAT3. Created with BioRender.com (Accessed on 23 October 2023).

From small molecule inhibitors to proteolysis targeting chimeras (PROTACs), peptides, peptidomimetics, and polyoxometalates, there are many drug modalities that can be utilized to target CK2. Predominantly, these modalities are class I kinase ligands, which typically occupy the ATP-binding site, hence impeding substrate phosphorylation. Unfortunately, the structure of the ATP-binding site is highly conserved across the human kinome, which can lead to off-target activity and adverse side effects [26]. This poses a serious impediment in the development of new CK2 inhibitors with high selectivity. This drawback is highlighted in the case of CX-4945, commercially known as silmitasertib, a potent CK2α ATP-competitive inhibitor in phase II clinical trials (ClinicalTrials.gov identifier NCT02128282), where strong inhibitory activity has been detected against several isoforms of Cdc2-like kinases (CLKs) [23,27,28]. In fact, CX-4945 exhibited stronger inhibition for CLK2 than for CK2 (IC_{50} = 3.8 nM against CLK2 and IC_{50} = 14.7 nM against CK2) [28]. Therefore, CX-4945 cannot be classified as a selective CK2 inhibitor and could perhaps be considered a CK2/CLK2 dual inhibitor. Alternative approaches have been explored that aim to achieve high CK2 selectivity, such as endogenous substrate displacement, inhibition of holoenzyme formation, and allosteric inhibition of CK2 [29].

This review will provide an overview of the molecular and structural biology of CK2, mechanisms of inhibition, and highlight inhibitors that target the ATP site. Most importantly, we will discuss chemical probes that have been developed to target CK2 outside the catalytic ATP site. Through this review, we hope to inspire further investigation into this promising area of research.

1.2. Structure of CK2

The ATP site comprises a deep hydrophobic binding pocket flanked by the hinge region and a catalytic Lys68 residue, making it an ideal location for aromatic compounds that contain hydrogen bonding substituents [8]. The Lys68 residue is essential for catalytic activity as it aids in the binding of the phosphates of ATP in the active site; this residue is conserved across all human protein kinases [30]. The structure of the ATP site is shown in Figure 3.

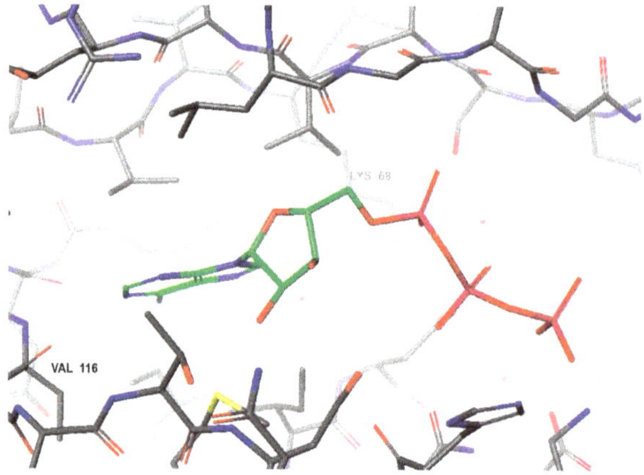

Figure 3. The crystal structure of adenosine triphosphate (ATP) bound to CK2; key interactions are shown in magenta; red points indicate the presence of a water molecule.

The α and α′ subunits are encoded by different genes, CSNK2A1 and CSNK2A2, respectively [31]. CK2α contains 391 amino acid residues and CK2α′ contains 350 amino acid residues; both isoforms share 90% sequence identity [10]. Both catalytic subunits adopt a bilobal structure that contains a lysine-rich N-terminus, and a C-terminus rich in α-helices. The ATP site is situated between the N-terminal and C-terminal domains, linked by the αD region, a region of the protein that has been exploited in the development of selective CK2 inhibitors [32]. The N-terminal segment contains five β-sheets, named β1-5, and one α-helix, named αC. The αC helix establishes substrate contact and, owing to its abundance of lysine residues, confers a tendency to favor acidic substrates. The C-terminal segment comprises seven α-helices and one β-sheet, which collectively form the structural foundation for both the ATP-binding site and activation loop. The activation loop is conformationally fixed by numerous stabilizing interactions between itself and the N-terminal segment. These stable interactions essentially "lock" CK2 in an active conformation, making it constitutively active without the need for an upstream phosphorylation event [8,33].

Many of CK2's substrates do not require the presence of β-subunits for phosphorylation [34,35]. The β-subunits, each containing 215 amino acids, are encoded by the *CSNK2B* gene [36]. Although the presence of CK2β is not fundamental for substrate phosphorylation, the subunit plays a crucial role in enhancing the tetrameric complex's thermostability, thus enhancing catalytic activity. Additionally, it aids in substrate recruitment by establishing both polar and hydrophobic interactions with the substrate, essentially acting as a "docking station" [37]. In this respect, substrates such as p53, nuclear phosphoprotein 140 (Nopp140), Fas-associated Factor 1 (FAS1), and topoisomerase II interact with CK2 via CK2β [28]. CK2β also regulates kinase activity by facilitating the shuttling of the kinase between the intracellular compartments, enabling the holoenzyme to enter the nucleus and gain access to most of CK2's substrates [38,39].

1.3. CK2 in Cancer

The disease type in which the role of CK2 is most well-documented is cancer [40,41]. There is evidence to suggest that CK2 is directly involved in each of Hanahan and Weinberg's six hallmarks of cancer: proliferative signaling, resisting cell death, evading growth suppressors, inducing angiogenesis, enabling replicative immortality, and activating invasion and mortality [42,43]. This involvement is highlighted in Figure 4.

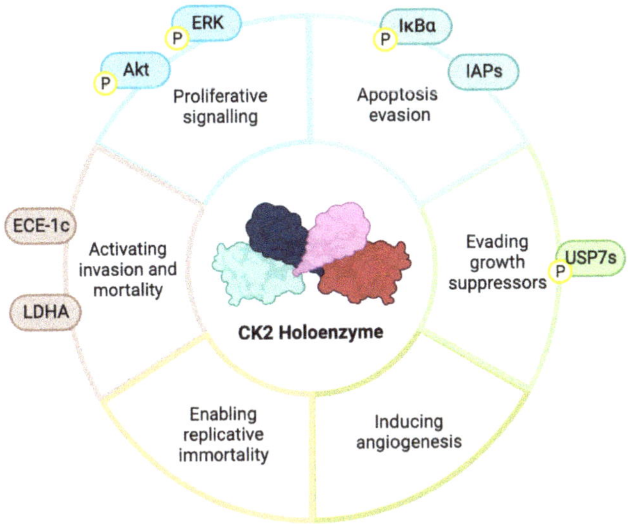

Figure 4. A schematic diagram showing CK2's involvement in the six hallmarks of cancer, and examples of proteins directly regulated by CK2. Substrates marked with a P indicate they are phosphorylated by CK2. CK2 is involved in the stabilization of endothelin converting enzyme 1c (ECE-1c) and inhibitor of apoptosis proteins (IAPs) and increases expression of lactate dehydrogenase A (LDHA). Despite known CK2 involvement in enabling replicative immortality and inducing angiogenesis, the specific pathways that CK2 is involved in are unknown. Created with BioRender.com (Accessed on 23 October 2023).

The upregulation of CK2 has been found within the nucleus of a multitude of different cancer cell types, such as lung, breast, colorectal, and head and neck carcinomas [14,44–46]. Therefore, elevated levels of CK2 serve as a prognostic marker in cancer progression. However, CK2 is not considered an oncogene itself as it is ubiquitously expressed within healthy cells. Cancer cells exhibit a "non-oncogene addiction" to CK2, heavily relying on the kinase for survival [22,47].

Both CK2α and CK2α' subunits are implicated in promoting tumor progression more than CK2β. The question of which isoform contributes most to CK2's oncogenic potential remains the subject of ongoing debate [40]. However, the involvement of CK2α is more commonly reported than CK2α'. A study by Zou et al. showed that CK2α plays an essential role in the progression of colorectal carcinoma [48]. The suppression of CK2α via siRNA in LoVo cells led to G_0/G_1 phase arrest, induced cell senescence, elevated expression of p53/p21, and decreased expression of c-Myc. In 2015, Zhang et al. showed that silencing CK2α in hepatocellular carcinoma (HCC) induced HCC cell apoptosis and inhibited HCC cell migration, proliferation, and angiogenesis both in vitro and in vivo [49]. In line with more of a "tumor suppressor-like" role, CK2β prevents the phosphorylation of substrates vital for apoptosis evasion, such as caspase-3 [50]. Additionally, the role of CK2 in drug resistance has been linked to upregulation of CK2α, not CK2β [51]. However, CK2α' has been shown to reduce migration in the mouse gonadotropin-releasing hormone (GnRH) neuronal cell line GN11, and CK2β promotes migration [36]. Furthermore, Takahashi et al. determined that the expression of CK2α and CK2β is elevated in human osteosarcoma, and siRNA knockdown of either CK2α or CK2β inhibited human osteosarcoma cell proliferation [52].

The pro-oncogenic function of each subunit cannot be objectively determined as this is dependent on cancer type, which CK2 substrates are present, and which isoform is needed to phosphorylate the substrates. However, CK2α/α' and CK2β have differing roles in cancer progression, which is supportive of monomeric CK2 being more related to CK2's oncogenic phenotype than tetrameric CK2.

2. Targeting CK2 within the ATP Site

2.1. ATP-Competitive Inhibition

The ATP site of CK2 is a primary target for inhibition as it is a highly ligandable pocket. As this site is conserved across the human kinome, selectivity issues often arise with ATP site binders.

Small-molecule ATP-competitive inhibitors of CK2 can be divided into four main classes: polyhalogenated benzimidazole and benzotriazole derivatives; anthraquinone derivatives; pyrazolo-triazines and pyrazolo-pyrimidines; and indoloquinazolines such as CX-4945. Some details of these classes of inhibitors are outlined below. However, for further details, the reader is directed towards an up-to-date and comprehensive review on ATP-competitive CK2 inhibitors [53].

2.1.1. Polyhalogenated Benzimidazole and Benzotriazole Derivatives

The nucleoside analogue 5,6-dichloro-1-β-D-ribofuranosylbenzimidazole (DRB) **1**, Figure 5, was initially recognized for its biological activity in 1954 [54]. However, it was not until 1986 when Zandomeni et al. reported inhibition of CK2 by DRB, although its activity against CK2 is only moderate (IC_{50} = 15 μM, K_i = 23 μM)* [55]. DRB has been found to be active against several other kinases (CK1, for example) with similar affinities to CK2. Additionally, it is also capable of binding to the CK2α/β interface. Despite its promiscuity, DRB has served as a foundation for many studies that have led to the development of numerous potent CK2 inhibitors that are in use today.

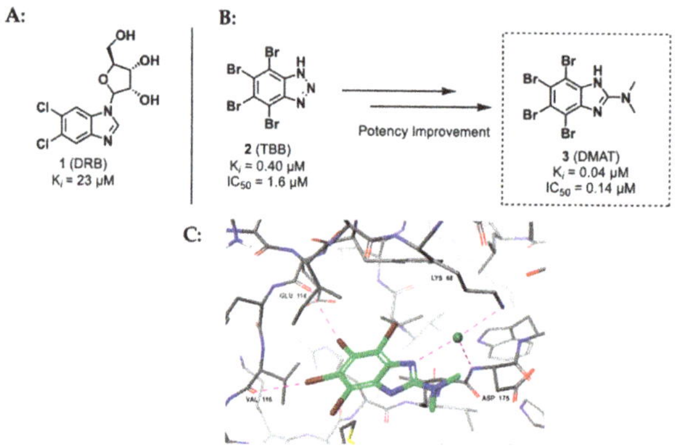

Figure 5. (**A**) Structure of CK2α inhibitor DRB **1**; (**B**) structures of CK2α inhibitors TBB **2** and DMAT **3**; (**C**) crystal structure of DMAT bound to CK2α; the green sphere represents a chloride; bonding interactions are shown in magenta (PDB 1ZOE).

The first significant improvement regarding DRB stemmed from two key modifications: the elimination of the sugar moiety and the substitution of chlorine atoms with bulkier bromines. This resulted in the formation of 4,5,6,7-tetrabromo-1H-benzotriazole TBB **2**, Figure 5, (IC_{50} = 0.14 μM, K_i = 0.40), and exhibited substantially improved cell permeability compared to DRB [56,57]. A screening of 10 μM TBB against 70 kinases unfortunately led to significant inhibition of over 90% of them, again highlighting the promiscuous nature of ATP-competitive kinase inhibitors.

Following the development of 4,5,6,7-tetrabromo-benzotriazole (TBB), subsequent structure–activity relationship studies led to the development of 2-dimethylamino-4,5,6,7-tetrabromo-benzimidazole (DMAT) **3**, Figure 5, which exhibited even greater potency towards CK2 (K_i = 0.04 μM) [58]. However, DMAT was found to be less selective for CK2 compared to TBB; ten kinases were more than 90% inhibited by 10 μM DMAT, and eight kinases were more than 90% inhibited by 10 μM TBB [59]. Both TBB and DMAT have been used extensively and in vivo [60–62].

2.1.2. Anthraquinone Derivatives

Anthraquinones constitute a class of natural products containing phenolic substituents [63]. An important example is emodin **4**, Figure 6, which is found in rhubarb rhizomes and inhibits numerous targets, including CK2 (IC_{50} = 2 μM, K_i = 7.2 μM) [64]. Several studies have been conducted to enhance anthraquinone-based inhibition of CK2, resulting in the development of MNA **5** (IC_{50} = 0.30 μM, K_i = 0.78 μM) and MNX **6** (IC_{50} = 0.40 μM, K_i = 0.80 μM), Figure 6 [65,66]. The presence of a nitro group in these derivatives increases polarization of the para-hydroxyl substituent through the electron-withdrawing effect. On the other hand, an alternative emodin derivative DAA **7**, Figure 6, lacks a nitro group yet exhibits a lower K_i value (K_i = 0.35 μM, IC_{50} = 0.30 μM) than MNA and MNX [67]. This is attributed to the formation of additional hydrogen bonds to Glu114 and Val116.

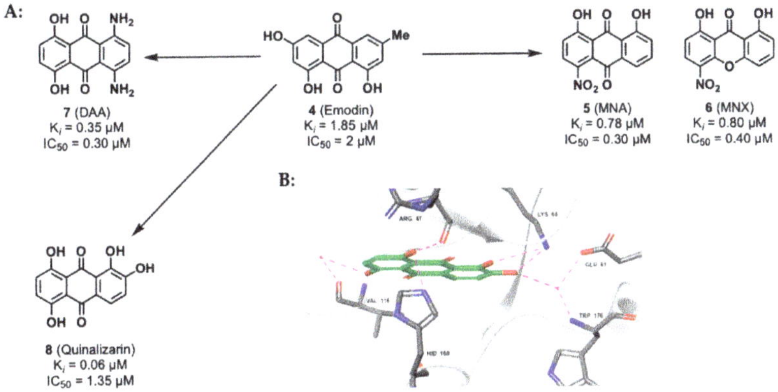

Figure 6. (**A**) Structures of CK2α inhibitors DAA **7**, Emodin **4**, MNA **5**, MNX **6**, and quinalizarin **8**; (**B**) crystal structure of quinalizarin **8** bound to CK2α; bonding interactions are shown in magenta; red points indicate the presence of a water molecule (PDB 3FL5).

Among further emodin derivatives is quinalizarin **8** (1,2,5,8-tetrahydroxyanthraquinone) (K_i = 60 nm), discovered via virtual screening [68]. Although structurally like emodin, quinalizarin is particularly potent and selective for CK2, more so than its predecessor. A selectivity profile of 1 μM quinalizarin was performed on a panel of 140 protein kinases, which found only 8% residual CK2 activity, and none of the other 139 kinases displayed residual activity of less than 50%. Moreover, quinalizarin showed the ability to differentiate between isolated CK2α and the CK2 holoenzyme [69]. Quinalizarin was found to be more active against the CK2 holoenzyme (IC_{50} = 0.15 μM and IC_{50} = 1.35 μM for CK2 holoenzyme and CK2α, respectively) and, therefore, could be used as a tool to quantify the presence of intracellular CK2 holoenzyme and CK2α.

2.1.3. Pyrazolo-Triazines and Pyrazolo-Pyrimidines

A series of pyrazolo-triazines (PT) were designed for CK2 inhibition by Nie et al. in 2007 after a co-crystal structure of CK2 and pyrazolo-triazine **9** was obtained, Figure 7 [70]. The co-crystal structure revealed that the pyrazolo-triazine core occupied the adenine pocket within the ATP site and was anchored in place via two hydrogen bonds in the hinge region.

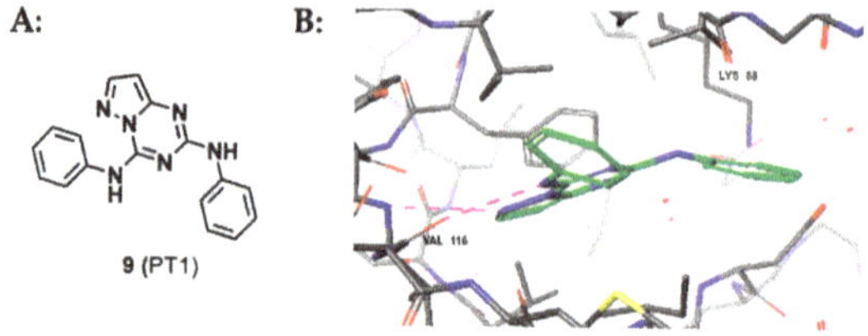

Figure 7. (**A**) Structure of CK2α inhibitor PT1 **9**; (**B**) crystal structure of PT1 bound to CK2α; bonding interactions are shown in magenta; red points indicate presence of a water molecule (PDB 2PVH).

Subsequent structure–activity relationship studies led to the development of three compounds that differed at the phenyl substituent (PT2 **10**, PT3 **11**, and PT4 **12**, Figure 8) [70]. Although all the compounds displayed nanomolar K_i for CK2, they failed to exhibit potent inhibition of cell growth in the human colorectal carcinoma cell line HCT116 and human prostate cancer PC3 cell lines when tested using an MTT assay. Therefore, further improvement in physicochemical properties was required, resulting in the development of a second generation of pyrazolo-triazines, for example, PT5 **13** [71]. Efforts to increase cell permeability resulted in a reduction in planarity in the second generation through macrocyclization with an alkyl side chain. Although this successfully increased cell permeability, a 10-fold increase in K_i was observed and PT5 had comparable cell growth inhibition to the first-generation derivatives. Pyrazolo-triazines have the potential to be developed into successful CK2 inhibitors; however, binding affinity must first be optimized. To date, no such optimization of pyrazolo-triazines has been published, and there are no data detailing the selectivity of this class of compounds.

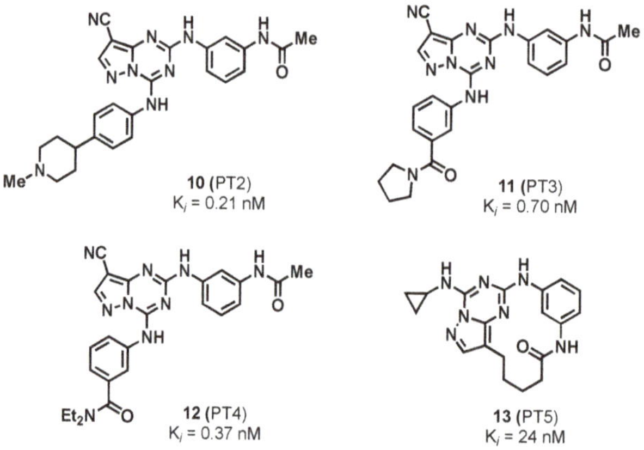

Figure 8. Structures of CK2α inhibitors PT2 **10**, PT3 **11**, PT4 **12**, and PT5 **13**.

Dowling et al. identified a related group of compounds known as pyrazolo-pyrimidines. In their work, kinase-focused subset screening methods, structure–activity relationship studies, and crystallography were employed [72]. Using these methods ultimately led to the identification of a lead compound AZ-7h **14**, Figure 9, which has picomolar binding affinity to CK2 (K_d = 6.33 pM), and nanomolar growth inhibition activity in HCT116 (GI_{50} = 10 nM, HCT116) [73]. The compound's selectivity was tested at 0.1 μM against a panel of 402 kinases, which showed only 12 kinases being inhibited by more than 50%, of which all were CMGC family members. Although limited off-target activity was observed, AZ-7h showed nanomolar activity for death-associated protein kinase 2 (DAPK2) and DAPK3 (IC_{50} = 8.0 nM and IC50 = 18 nM, respectively). In vivo mouse PK studies showed poor oral bioavailability of AZ-7h [73]. However, dose-dependent tumor growth inhibition was achieved through intravenous and intraperitoneal injection. This suggests that further optimization of AZ-7h could yield a promising CK2 inhibitor; however, activity against DAPK2 and DAPK3 should be reduced.

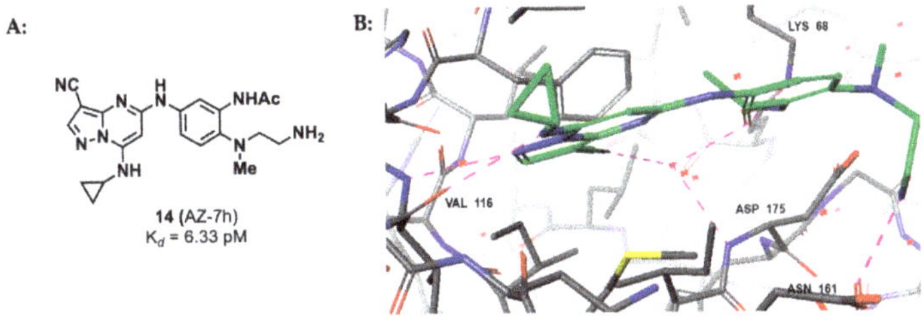

Figure 9. (**A**) Structure of CK2α inhibitor AZ-7h **14**; (**B**) crystal structure of AZ-7h bound to CK2α; residues that are involved in binding are labelled; red points indicate presence of water molecule (PDB 5H8E).

Through optimization of the pyrazolopyrimidine scaffold of AZ-7h, the Structural Genomics Consortium (SGC-UNC) developed SGC-CK2-1 **15**, Figure 10, (IC_{50} = 4.2 nM, and IC_{50} = 2.3 nM for CK2α and CK2α′, respectively) [74]. Sub-micromolar target engagement of CK2 was determined using nanoBRET assays in human embryonic kidney 293 (HEK-239) cells (IC_{50} = 36 nM and IC_{50} = 16 nM for CK2α and CK2α′, respectively), and, when tested against a panel of 403 wild-type human protein kinases at 1 μM, only three kinases were found to be inhibited by more than 90%. The authors claim that, unexpectedly, SGC-CK2-1 "does not demonstrate significant antiproliferative activity against a panel of 140 different cancer cell lines". This claim sparked premature conclusions that the broad cancer essentiality of CK2 had therefore been disproved [75]. However, further investigation is needed to determine the potential effects of SGC-CK2-1 on cancer given that CK2 is implicated in all the recognized cancer hallmarks [44] beyond just influencing cell proliferation. The reader is directed towards a comprehensive review regarding this argument [76]. It is important to note that SGC-CK2-1 is an exceptional tool and represents the most selective CK2 inhibitor to date and would therefore be a first-choice compound for the exploration of CK2 cellular functions. A further review, which provides further details on the development and uses of SGC-CK2-1, is brought to the attention of the reader [77].

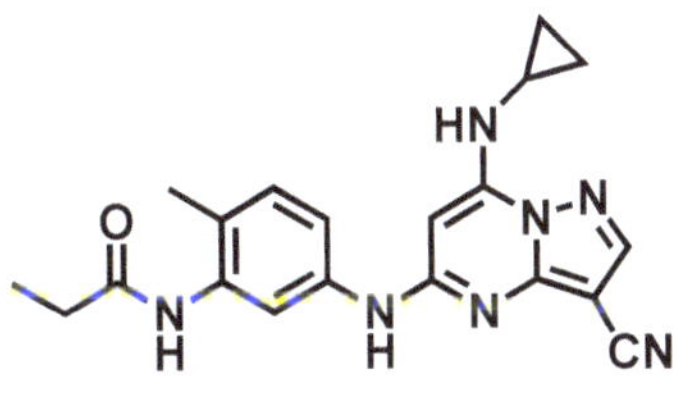

15 (SGC-CK2-1)
IC_{50} CK2α = 4.2 nM
CK2α′ = 2.3 nM

Figure 10. Structure of CK2α/α′ inhibitor SGC-CK2-1 **15**.

2.1.4. Indoloquinazolines Such as CX-4945

CX-4945 **16**, Figure 11, an indoloquinazoline, also known as silmitasertib, was developed by Siddiqui-Jain et al. in 2010 and is a potent orally bioavailable ATP-competitive inhibitor of CK2 (IC_{50} = 1 nM, K_i = 0.38 nM) [78]. CX-4945 is characterized by its comparatively small polar surface area, few rotatable bonds, and low aqueous solubility. It possesses a single carboxylic acid and two aromatic nitrogen heterocycles, which are both weakly basic. CX-4945′s potent binding affinity is attributed to the formation of an ionic bridge with Lys68, in addition to hydrophobic interactions and hydrogen bonding with the hinge region of the ATP site [27,28,73].

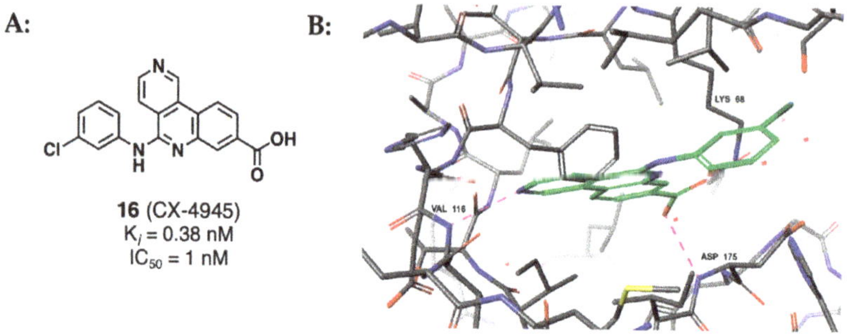

Figure 11. (**A**) Structure of CK2α inhibitor CX-4945 **16**; (**B**) crystal structure of CX-4945 bound to CK2α; bonding interactions are shown in magenta; red points indicate presence of a water molecule (PDB 3NGA).

CX-4945 was granted orphan drug designation by the FDA for advanced cholangiocarcinoma in 2017 [79]. In 2021, CX-4945 demonstrated excellent preclinical anti-tumor activity and strong synergism with gemcitabine and cisplatin in phase Ib/II clinical studies (ClinicalTrials.gov identifier: NCT02128282) [80,81]. This combined therapeutic approach has the potential to be a promising first-line treatment against locally advanced and metastatic cholangiocarcinoma.

When screened in a selectivity panel of 238 kinases, CX-4945 was shown to inhibit a further seven kinases by over 90% at a concentration of 500 nM. The most significant inhibition was against dual-specificity tyrosine regulated kinases DRYK1A and DRYK1B; proviral integration site for Moloney murine leukemia virus kinase 1 (PIM-1), and CLK2 [27]. Despite suboptimal selectivity, CX-4945 is currently viewed as the gold standard of CK2 inhibitors due to its strong inhibitory activity and oral bioavailability. This illustrates a potential shift in perspective regarding off-target kinase activity as only moderate adverse side effects have been observed in CX-4945 clinical trials, and targeting multiple kinases with related substrate phosphorylation patterns could be considered advantageous [82]. Nonetheless, the development of more selective inhibitors is crucial for the advancement of CK2 chemical probes.

Recently, Menyhart et al. evaluated the selectivity of CX-4945 and SGC-CK2-1 via triple SILAC quantitative phosphoproteomics using human osteosarcoma U2OS cells expressing exogenous wild-type CSNK2A1 or an inhibitor-resistant triple mutant (TM, V66A/H160D/I174A) [83]. Only a minority of the phosphosites that were downregulated in response to CX-4945 treatment (15% at 4 h and 5% at 24 h) were found to be CSNK2A1-dependent. However, the majority of the phosphosites downregulated in response to SGC-CK2-1 treatment (more than 55% after 4 h and 24 h) were found to be CSNK2A1-dependent. Thus, SGC-CK2-1 is significantly more selective for CK2 than CX-4945.

Following the development of CX-4945 **16**, structure–activity relationship studies led to the development of CX-5011 **17** and CX-5279 **18**, (K_i = 0.18 nM and K_i = 0.22 nM for CX-5011 and CX-5279, respectively) [84], Figure 12. Both new derivatives contain a pyrimidine ring instead of pyridine and showed better specificity for CK2 than CX-4945 (the Gini coefficients were 0.735, 0.755, and 0.615 for CX-5011, CX-5279, and CX-4945, respectively [85]), which improves upon one of the main downfalls of CX-4945 [69,84].

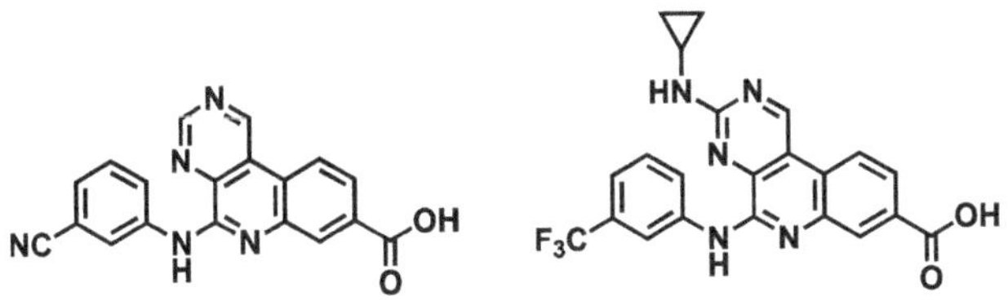

17 CX-5011
K_i = 0.18 nM

18 CX-5279
K_i = 0.22 nM

Figure 12. Structures of CX-4945 **16** derivatives CX-5011 **17** and CX-5279 **18**.

3. Extending beyond the ATP Site

3.1. Dual-Binding Ligands

The development of dual-binding therapeutics, especially those that inhibit synergistic targets, has received increasing attention in anticancer drug development. Many dual-binding bromodomain and extra-terminal domain (BET)/kinase inhibitors have been described, which simultaneously regulate multiple targets in disease pathways and have synergistic anti-tumor effects [86–88]. A dual-binding ligand approach could be a more effective therapeutic strategy than single-target therapeutics. To date, several CK2-based dual-binding ligands have been reported in the literature that have the potential to be successful clinical candidates.

3.1.1. CK2/PIM Dual-Binding Ligands

Proviral integration site for Moloney murine leukemia virus (PIM) kinases are serine/threonine kinases, much like CK2, which interact with c-Myc [89,90]. PIM kinases are attractive targets in diseases that have high PIM expression, such as leukemia and prostate cancer [91,92]. CK2 and PIM both act on similar pathways, which, when dysregulated, result in tumorigenesis [93,94]. Off-target PIM inhibition has been observed in selectivity studies of CK2 inhibitors, making dual-binding CK2/PIM kinases a feasible therapeutic strategy [27].

CK2/PIM dual-binding inhibitors were first reported in the literature by Lopez-Ramos et al. in 2010 [95]. A series of CK2/PIM inhibitors (CPA **19**, CPB **20**, and AMR **21**, Figure 13), which had nanomolar IC_{50} values for CK2 and PIM kinases, were developed through automated in vitro screening and hit expansion techniques. Unfortunately, these CK2/PIM dual-binding inhibitors are not suitable for use in the clinic due to poor cell permeability.

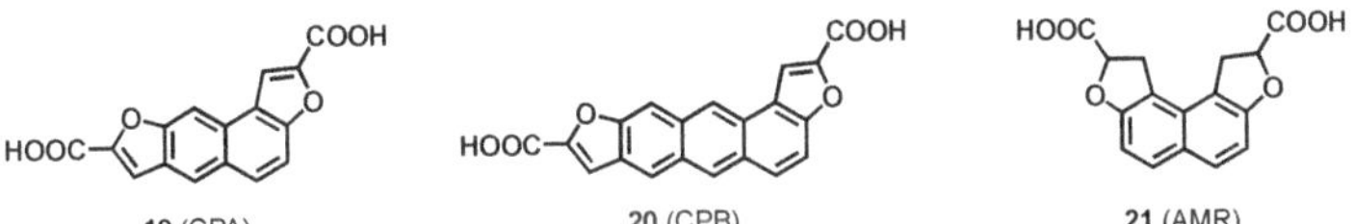

19 (CPA)
CK2 IC_{50} = 100 nM
PIM-1 IC_{50} = 60 nM

20 (CPB)
CK2 IC_{50} = 63 nM
PIM-1 IC_{50} = 20 nM

21 (AMR)
CK2 IC_{50} = 200 nM
PIM-1 IC_{50} = 31 nM

Figure 13. Structures of CK2/PIM dual-binding inhibitors CPA **19**, CPB **20**, and AMR **21**.

NBC **22**, Figure 14, was initially developed as a CK2 inhibitor alongside anthraquinone derivative MNX **6** by Meggio et al. in 2004 [65]. NBC displayed potent inhibitory activity against CK2 (IC_{50} = 0.37 μM, K_i = 0.22 μM) but was found to inhibit PIM kinases, particularly PIM-1 and PIM-3 (IC_{50} = 3.1 μM and 0.34 μM, respectively). Furthermore, NBC induced apoptosis in Jurkat cells and displayed DC_{50} values around 15 μM, making NBC a promising CK2/PIM dual-binding ligand [96].

The inhibitory potential of the known CK2α inhibitor TBI **23**, Figure 14, was explored by Cozza at al., where significant off-target activity against PIM-1 was identified [97]. The selectivity of TBI was then tuned towards CK2 and PIM-1 via inclusion of a deoxyribose to yield TDB (CK2 IC_{50} = 32 nM, PIM-1 IC_{50} = 86 nM) [98]. TDB **24**, Figure 14, was found to show permanent inhibition of cell survival and migration of U2OS cells to a greater extent than "single-target" CK2 inhibitors, such as CX-4945, which is thought to be attributed to the synergistic effect of simultaneous CK2 and PIM-1 inhibition. However, CX-4945 displayed greater in vitro potency than TBI despite lower cytotoxicity [99].

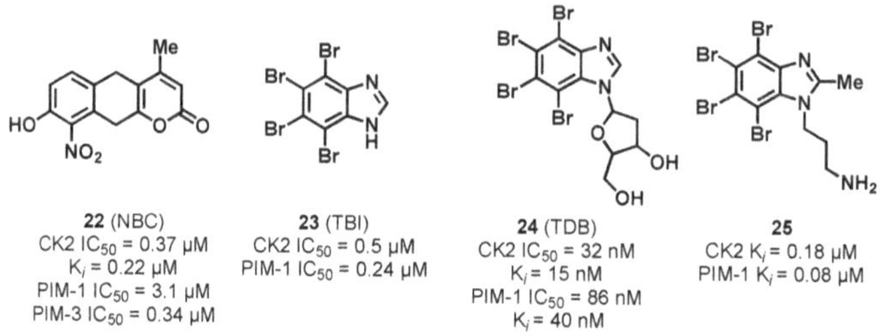

Figure 14. Structures of CK2/PIM dual-binding inhibitors NBC **22**, TBI **23**, TDB **24**, and **25**.

Further analogues of CK2/PIM-1 dual-binding inhibitors were developed by Chojnaki et al. in 2018 based on the structure of TBI [100]. Aminopropyl-substituted derivative **25** was identified, which exhibits potent inhibition of CK2 and PIM-1 (K_i = 0.18 and 0.08 μM for CK2 and PIM-1, respectively). In vitro studies showed that **25**, Figure 14, inhibited cell proliferation in human T-lymphoblasts CCRF-CEM, human breast cancer MCF-7, and PC3 cancer cell lines, and cell viability was reduced more significantly when compared with TBI and CX-4945, proving the synergistic effect of CK2/PIM-1 that dual-binding inhibitors could have in terms of a clinical benefit over 'single-target' CK2 inhibition.

3.1.2. CK2/BRD4 Dual-Binding Ligands

Bromodomain-containing protein 4 (BRD4), a member of BET family, is a histone acetyltransferase (HAT) that plays a pivotal role in embryogenesis and cancer development [101,102]. Studies show that CK2 is responsible for the phosphorylation of BRD4 [101,103,104]. Hyperphosphorylation of BRD4 by CK2 is associated with drug resistance in triple-negative breast cancer (TNBC), making CK2/BRD4 dual-binding ligands a feasible therapeutic approach in breast cancer treatment [14,44,105,106].

Moreover, **26**, Figure 15, is a CK2/BRD4 dual-binding inhibitor, first described by Zhang et al. in 2021, and was developed via rational drug design and structure–activity relationship studies [107]. Furthermore, **26** was found to possess potent and similar inhibition against CK2 (IC_{50} = 230 nM) and BRD4 (IC_{50} = 180 nM). In in vitro experiments, **26** was shown to inhibit proliferation and induce dose-dependent apoptosis and autophagy-related cell death in human TNBC MDA-MB-231 and MDA-MB-468 cells. In vivo experiments further validated a therapeutic effect, with potent anticancer activity being observed without any obvious toxicities. Hence, CK2/BRD4 dual-binding ligands have emerged as an appealing strategy for treating TNBC.

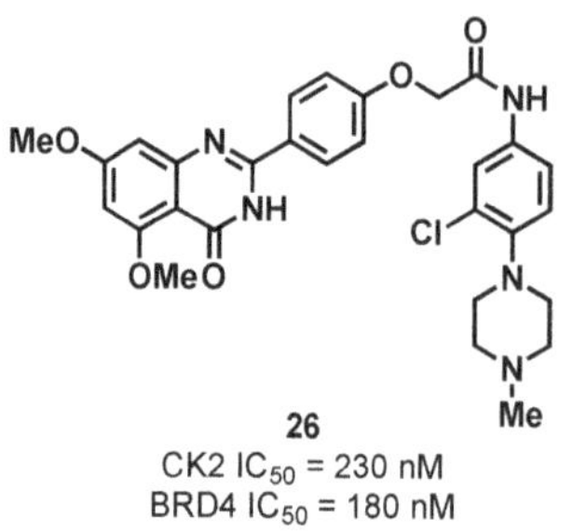

Figure 15. Structure of CK2/BRD4 dual-binding ligand **26**.

3.1.3. CK2/SRPK1 Dual Inhibitor

Serine-arginine protein kinase 1 (SRPK1) is an oncoprotein that plays a key role in the epidermal growth factor (EGFR)/Akt pathway, contributing to tumorigenesis [108]. SRPK1 is involved in angiogenesis and is overexpressed in numerous cancer types, such as prostate, breast and lung cancers, and glioma [109,110]. Furthermore, CK2 has been found to be the main kinase that phosphorylates SRPK1 [111]. Therefore, CK2/SRPK1 dual inhibitors could be used as anti-angiogenic therapies.

SRPIN803 **27**, Figure 16, was identified by Morooka et al. as a CK2/SRPK1 dual inhibitor (IC_{50} = 2.4 μM and 203 nM for CK2 and SRPK1, respectively) through pharmacophore docking models followed by in vitro kinase assays [112]. Exposure of SRPIN803 to Jurkat cells resulted in a significant reduction in cell viability, and suppression of vascular endothelial growth factor (VEGF) production was observed in a dose- and time-dependent manner in human retinal pigment epithelial ARPE-19 cells. Furthermore, genes, including *IL8*, *HMOX1*, and *HK2*, involved in angiogenesis were downregulated according to gene-expression array data. In an in vivo mouse model of age-related macular degeneration (AMD), SRPIN803, administered in the form of topical eye ointment, significantly inhibited choroidal neovascularization. Thus, SRPIN803 merits further investigation as an inhibitor of VEGF and as a topical ointment for ocular neovascularization in a clinical setting.

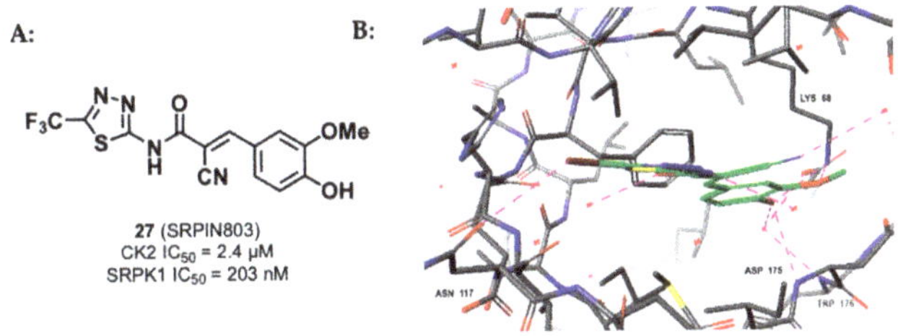

Figure 16. (**A**) Structure of CK2/SRPK1 dual inhibitor SRPIN803 **27**; (**B**) crystal structure of SRPIN803 bound to CK2α; bonding interactions are shown in magenta; red points indicate the presence of a water molecule (PDB 6RFE).

In 2021, Leonidis et al. developed a series of c(RGDyK) peptide conjugates of SRPIN803, of which geo35 **28**, Figure 17, was the most cytotoxic against MC7 and MRC5 cell lines (IC_{50} = 61 and 63 μM, respectively) [113]. Furthermore, the most active compound, geo35 (CK2 IC_{50} = 85.2 μM and SRPK1 IC_{50} = >100 μM), induced antiangiogenic activity in zebrafish embryos in a dose-dependent fashion. However, SRPIN803 alone was found to be more potent than geo35. Furthermore, geo35 displayed weak binding affinity to SRPK1, and it is unknown whether the observed cytotoxicity can be attributed to inhibition of both CK2 and SRPK1 or just CK2 alone. However, the development of an active peptide conjugate suggests that this approach could be adopted to develop a new class of antiangiogenic therapeutics.

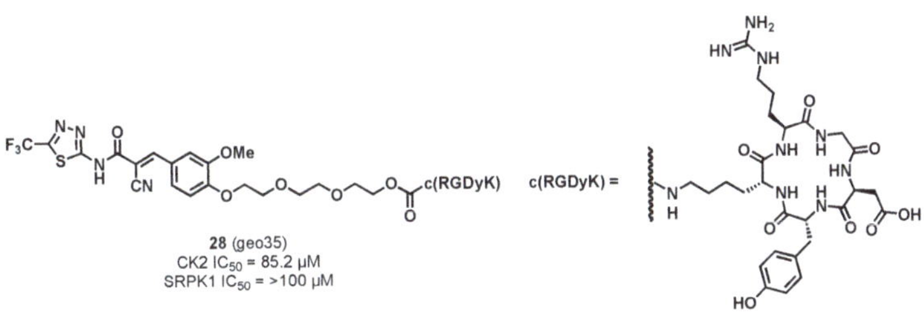

Figure 17. Structure of CK2/SRPK1 dual inhibitor geo35 **28** and peptide c(RGDyK).

3.1.4. CK2/HDAC1 Dual Inhibitor

Histone deacetylases (HDACs) are a family of epigenetic proteins that control gene transcription and regulation, alongside cell proliferation, differentiation, migration, death, and angiogenesis [114]. As CK2 and HDAC are both related in similar cancer-related biological pathways, it is speculated that simultaneous inhibition of these targets by a dual inhibitor should improve efficacy compared to single-target therapeutics [115].

Recently, the Ramos group developed a series of CK2/HDAC1 inhibitors through combining the structures of vorinostat **29**, Figure 18, a known HDAC1 inhibitor, and TBB or DMAT, known CK2 inhibitors [116–119]. The series, to which compound **30**, Figure 18, belongs, had low micromolar activity in enzymatic assays and low micromolar LC_{50} values across numerous cell lines. In 2020, the Ramos group reported another series of CK2/HDAC1 dual-binding inhibitors in which CX-4945 replaced the DMAT-derived portion [120]. The lead compound, **31**, Figure 19, displayed 3.0- and 3.5-times higher activity against recombinant CK2 and HDAC1 than CX-4945 and vorinostat, respectively. However, the in vitro inhibition observed with **31** in human lymph node carcinoma of the prostate (LNCaP) cells (IC_{50} = 16.31 μM) was lower than the individual parent compounds, which could be attributed to poorer cell permeability of the lead compound. Therefore, further optimization of the pharmacokinetic properties of **31** is needed before it could be a potential therapeutic.

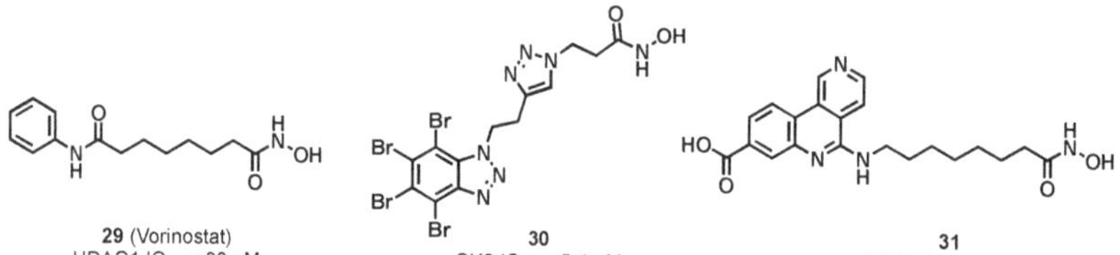

29 (Vorinostat)
HDAC1 IC_{50} = 33 nM

30
CK2 IC_{50} = 5.4 μM
HDAC1 IC_{50} = 5.0 μM

31
CK2 IC_{50} = 1.7 nM
HDAC1 IC_{50} = 3.3 nM

Figure 18. Structures of HDAC1 inhibitor vorinostat **29** and CK2/HDAC1 dual inhibitors **30** and **31**.

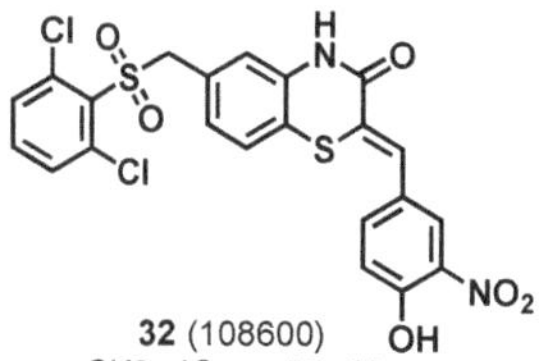

32 (108600)
CK2α IC_{50} = 50 nM
CK2α' IC_{50} = 5 nM
TNIK IC_{50} = 5 nM
DYRK1A IC_{50} = 16 nM
DYRK1B IC_{50} = 7 nM

Figure 19. Structure of CK2/TNIK/DYRK1 multiple inhibitor 108600 **32**.

3.1.5. CK2/TNIK/DYRK1 Multiple Inhibitor

Dual-specificity tyrosine-regulated class 1 kinases (DYRK1) have multiple implications in cell differentiation and proliferation pathways via phosphorylation of key cell cycle regulators, such as CYCLIN D1 and p21, and regulate their degradation [98,121]. DYRK1 kinases also regulate chromatin modification and gene expression [122]. TRAF2- and NCK-interacting kinase (TNIK) has emerged as a kinase that is critical in the regulation of Wnt/β-catenin cell signaling pathway [123]. Collectively, CK2, DYRK1, and TNIK kinases activate STAT3, Wnt/β-catenin, PI3K/Akt, Hedgehog, and Notch 1 signaling molecules. Therefore, simultaneous inhibition of these three kinases, and their associated cancer-promoting pathways, could sensitize malignant drug-resistant cancer cells to standard-of-care chemotherapy.

A novel multi-kinase inhibitor, 108600 **32**, Figure 19, inhibited CK2, TNIK, and DYRK1 activity in a dose-dependent manner in triple-negative breast cancer cell lines [124]. Moreover, 108600 displayed IC_{50} values for CK2α, CK2α', TNIK, DYRK1A, and DYRK1B of 50, 5, 5, 16, and 7 nM. Surprisingly, 108600's inhibitory activity against the CK2α isoform is 10-fold higher than the CK2α' isoform, indicating potential for isoform-selective derivatives to be developed. An unfavorable conformational change in CK2α was observed upon binding of 108600, which is not conductive with holoenzyme formation [124]. 108600 could, therefore, be acting as an ATP-competitive inhibitor and as an allosteric inhibitor. Treatment of LM2-4 cells, a highly metastatic variant of MDA-MB-231, showed that 108600 was an effective suppressor of established metastases when used in combination with paclitaxel. In an in vivo patient-derived xenograft (PDX) mouse model, 108600 successfully acted synergistically with paclitaxel, even when tumors were non-responsive to paclitaxel as a single agent. This may prove to be highly advantageous in a clinical setting and could lead to improvements in morbidity and mortality rates associated with advanced TNBC, and those that are resistant to chemotherapy [125].

3.2. Substrate Binding Site Inhibition

An alternative approach for CK2 inhibition is to target the substrate binding site and therefore inhibit the binding of CK2 substrates. One defining feature of CK2 is that it solely phosphorylates acidophilic substrates [10]. Therefore substrate-competitive inhibitors with great selectivity could be developed to regulate CK2's activity.

Polyglutamyl peptides were first identified as substrate-competitive inhibitors by Meggio et al. in 1983 [126]. $(Glu)_{70}$ was found to inhibit CK2 in vitro (K_i = 0.11 µM) and did not have activity against closely related proteins, such as CK1. This highlighted that naturally occurring polypeptides that contain long stretches of acidic units could act as substrate-competitive CK2 inhibitors.

Perea et al. identified peptide P15 (WMSPRHLGT) through screening of a random cyclic peptide phage display library [127]. P15 was found to inhibit CK2 substrate phosphorylation in vitro in a competitive manner. The known cell-penetrating peptide TAT was attached to the N-terminus of P15, along with two cysteine residues attached to either end of P15. Cyclization of the modified peptide via a disulfide bridge afforded the cell-permeable peptide CIGB-325 (formerly known as P15-TAT and CIGB-300), which displayed moderate inhibition of cell viability across different cancerous cell lines. Additionally, intra-tumoral administration of CIGB-325 into TC-1 lung epithelial tumors in C57BL6 mice led to a significant reduction in tumor growth [127].

In 2008, CIGB-325 was administered to patients with cervical cancer in its first-in-man clinical trial [128]. It was observed that 75% of the patients had significant lesion reduction, and 19% of the patients showed full histological regression. In 2020, a preclinical trail was conducted to evaluate the potential of CIGB-325 as a treatment for breast cancer [14]. CIGB-325 demonstrated reduced breast cancer cell growth across the MDA-MB-231, MCF-7, and sarcomatoid mammary carcinoma F3II cell lines, and exhibited apoptosis and cell cycle arrest in vitro. In malignant cells, cell adhesion, migration, and clonogenic capacity were reduced. Promisingly, in an orthotopic model, treatment of CIGB-325 resulted in the inhibition of breast cancer colonization of the lung as the size and number of metastatic lesions was reduced. These encouraging results propose CIGB-325 as an adjuvant therapy post-surgery to limit tumor metastasis and recurrence.

In 2020, an exploratory clinical trial of CIGB-325 was conducted to investigate the use of the synthetic peptide against COVID-19 [129]. CIGB-325 was administered intravenously to COVID-19 patients, along with standard-of-care treatment, over a period of 15 days. Significantly fewer pulmonary lesions were observed at day 7 in patients who had received CIGB-325 and standard-of-care treatment, indicating that CK2 inhibitors could be used in combinatorial therapy against COVID-19.

3.3. Bi-Specific ATP/Substrate Competitive Inhibition

The substrate binding channel of CK2 has been defined based on the substrate binding channels identified in other kinases [130]. However, to date, there are no published crystal structure data to show a substrate of CK2α, or substrate channel inhibitor, bound in this channel. Bi-specific ATP/substrate-competitive inhibitors have emerged as a therapeutic strategy for selective CK2 inhibitors. These inhibitors incorporate both an ATP-competitive binder and an acidophilic peptide to bind in an ATP- and substrate-competitive manner. Due to the lack of crystal structure data, it is difficult to predict how much binding in the substrate channel contributes to the overall binding affinity of these inhibitors.

The first bi-specific ATP/substrate-competitive inhibitor was ARC-1502 **33**, Figure 20, developed by Enkvist et al. in 2012 [131]. ARC-1502 (K_i = 0.5 nM) contained the ATP-competitive inhibitor TBI conjugated to an aspartic acid-rich peptide. Alongside a strong binding affinity for CK2α, ARC-1502 exhibited good selectivity: when tested at 1 μM against a panel of one-hundred-forty kinases, only nine other kinases were inhibited at more than 50%. Unfortunately, ARC-1502 is not cell-permeable and is susceptible to proteolytic degradation; therefore, its uses as a chemical probe are limited.

A:

B:

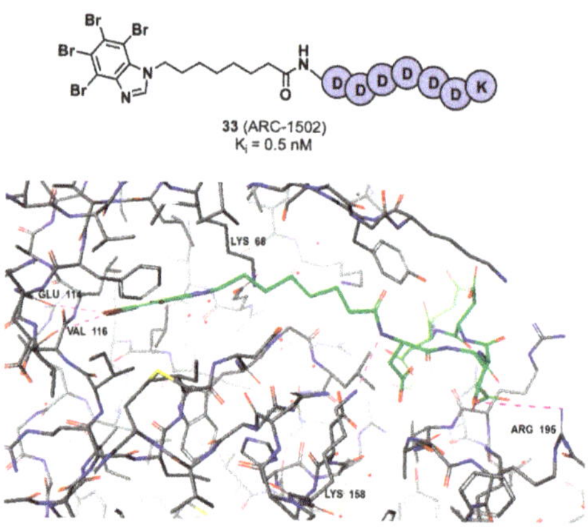

Figure 20. (**A**) Structure of the first bi-specific ATP/substrate competitive inhibitor ARC-1502 **33**; (**B**) crystal structure of ARC-1502 bound to CK2α; bonding interactions are shown in magenta; red points indicate the presence of a water molecule (PDB 6SPX).

Following ARC-1502, Viht et al. developed a cell-permeable and stable derivative of ARC-1502, named ARC-1859 [132]. This improved bi-specific inhibitor was designed as a pro-drug: the acidic aspartic acid side chains were 'masked' with cell-cleavable acetoxymethyl esters. The stability of the peptide was also improved through the replacement of amino acids with a poly-N-substituted glycine peptoid chain. In vitro, ARC-1502 was found to inhibit the phosphorylation of CK2α substrates Cdc37 and NFκB in a concentration-dependent manner.

In 2017, Vahter et al. developed a series of bi-specific ATP/substrate-competitive inhibitors using CX-4945 as the ATP site binder [133]. The most promising inhibitors of the series, ARC-1424-50 and its fluorescently labelled counterpart ARC-1513-50 **34**, Figure 21, showed outstanding binding affinity for CK2 (K_d = 37 and 16 pM, respectively). When tested at 1 μM in a panel of one-hundred-forty kinases, twenty-three kinases were inhibited at more than 50% and six were strongly inhibited at more than 90%. Therefore, ARC-1424-50 is one of the best chemical tools for competition experiments to measure binding affinities of other CK2α inhibitors due to its picomolar activity.

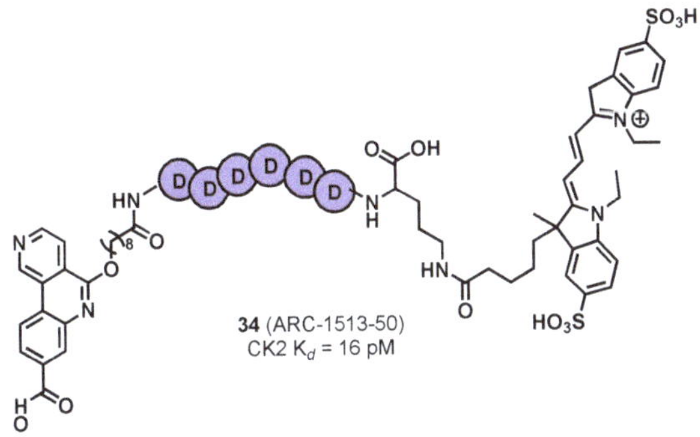

Figure 21. Structure of ARC-1513-50 **34**, the fluorescently labelled counterpart of CK2α inhibitor ARC-1424-50.

3.4. Inhibitors Acting in the αD Site

A pocket adjacent to the ATP site, named the αD site, was discovered by Brear et al. in 2016 [134]. The site was found through high-concentration fragment screening and is unique to CK2α/α′. Therefore, targeting this site could possibly lead to the creation of highly selective CK2 inhibitors. Most reported inhibitors that bind to the αD site simultaneously bind to the ATP site. There is one reported compound that is proposed to bind to the αD site and allosterically inhibit CK2; however, there are no structural data to support this hypothesis, and it remains unclear whether the αD site can act as an allosteric site alone [135].

Through crystallographic fragment screening efforts, De Fusco et al. successfully identified fragments **35** and **36** that bind to the ATP site, shown in Figure 22 [32]. Remarkably, several cell-permeable small molecules with picomolar affinity to the ATP site have been discovered. These fragments are ATP-competitive as they compete with endogenous ATP and thus prevent phosphorylation of CK2's substrates.

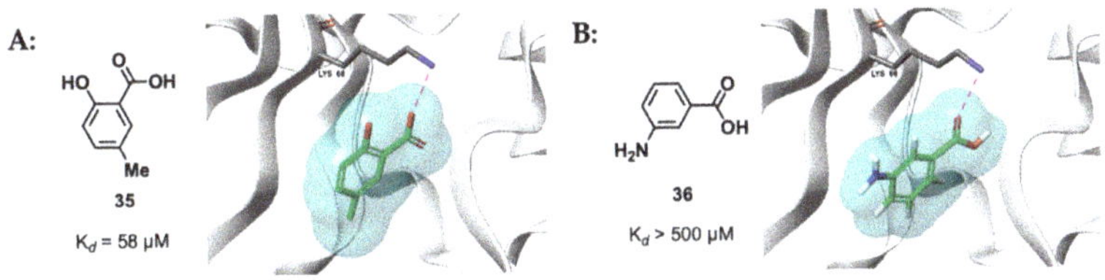

Figure 22. Structures of ATP site fragments **35** and **36**; adjacent are their respective ribbon crystal structures; residues involved in binding are labelled ((**A**): PDB 5CSP and (**B**): PDB 5CSV).

A fragment-based drug discovery approach, via collaboration of the Spring and Hyvönen groups, resulted in a series of benzylamine biaryl molecules that bind in the αD site [32,134]. Due to the proximity of the ATP and αD sites, a weak ATP site fragment **36**, Figure 22, was linked to an αD fragment. It was hypothesized that linking fragments that bind either the αD or ATP site would result in a selective CK2 inhibitor; selectivity would be driven by binding to the αD pocket. This proved true for the resulting inhibitor CAM4066 **37**, Figure 23, which exhibited subnanomolar affinity in enzymatic assays and low micromolar cellular activity (K_d = 320 nM, IC_{50} = 370 nM, GI_{50} = 8.8 μM for pro-CAM4066). Excitingly, CAM4066 possessed a Gini coefficient of 0.82 (52 kinase panel, 2 μM CAM4066), making CAM4066 the most selective CK2 inhibitor to date. The promising selectivity and biological data suggest that the unique binding mode of CAM4066 serves as an effective strategy for achieving potent selectivity and good inhibition when developing kinase inhibitors.

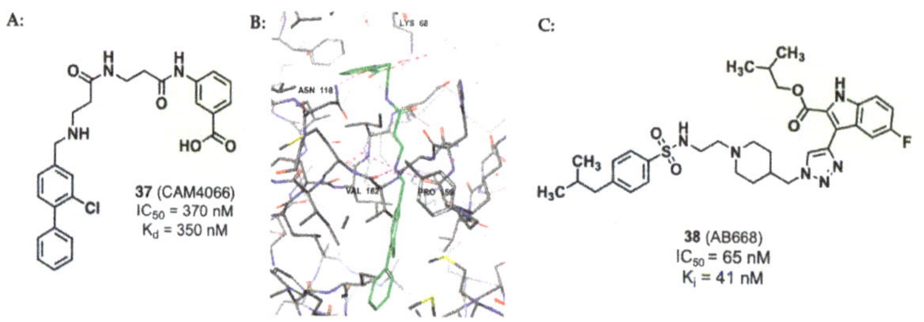

Figure 23. (**A**) Structure of CAM4066 **37**; the ATP site binder is highlighted in green and the αD site binder is highlighted in blue; (**B**) crystal structure of CAM4066 bound to CK2α ATP and αD sites; bonding interactions are shown in magenta; red points indicate the presence of a water molecule (PDB 5CU3); (**C**) structure of AB668 **38**; the ATP site binder is highlighted in green and the αD site binder is highlighted in blue.

Bancet et al. recently discovered AB668 **38** (K_i = 41 nM, IC_{50} = 65 nM), Figure 23, which also binds to the αD pocket and ATP site [136]. AB668 was screened against a panel of 468 kinases at a concentration of 2 μM, and only one other kinase (RPS6KA5) displayed a percentage inhibition above 50%. Additionally, AB668 was found to induce apoptotic cell death in 786-O renal carcinoma (at a concentration of 4 μM) and A375 melanoma (at a concentration of 5 μM) cell lines after 48 h, detected via live cell imaging. Interestingly, AB668 was better at inducing apoptosis in both cell lines than CX-4945 and SGC-CK2-1. Furthermore, AB668 did not induce cytotoxicity in extracts of non-cancerous HEK-293 cells, and the viability of normal human breast epithelial cells (MCF10A) was unchanged at high concentrations of AB668. These results suggest that only cancerous cell lines are sensitive to AB668. However, further in vitro and in vivo studies would be needed to better understand this anticancer effect.

3.5. Holoenzyme Assembly Inhibition

Targeting the CK2α/β interface is an alternative strategy of CK2 inhibition and disrupts formation of the holoenzyme complex.

One notable peptide that targets the CK2α/β protein-protein interaction (PPI) is CAM7117 **39**, Figure 24, developed by the Spring and Hyvönen groups [137]. CAM7117 was developed through the optimization of peptide Pc (IC_{50} = 3.0 μM, K_d = 1 μM), previously identified by Laudet et al. [138]. Pc contains the central interacting region of the CK2β C-terminal loop cyclized via a disulfide bridge. In the development of CAM7117, a structure-based approach was adopted to determine which covalent constraint would hold the peptide in an optimal conformation. Additionally, molecular modeling and X-ray crystallography of the peptide sequence revealed a single point mutation within the central region of Pc, namely Ile192 to Trp. Using copper-catalyzed azide-alkyne cycloaddition (CUAAC) chemistry and the movement of one of the cyclizing residues by one position yielded CAM7117 (K_d = 0.2 μM, GI_{50} = 33 μM). Unfortunately, CAM7117 contains unnatural amino acids, and its size limits any further optimization attempts.

In 2022, the Spring group developed another peptide-based CK2α/β PPI inhibitor, P8C9 **40**, Figure 25, through an iterative cycle of enzymatic assays, X-ray crystallography, molecular modelling, and cellular assays [139]. The peptide successfully binds CK2α at the CK2α/β PPI interaction site and is easily functionalized, highly stable in serum, and small enough to be further optimized. Cell-permeable analogues were synthesized, TAT-P8C9 and R3-P8C9, which successfully inhibited cell proliferation. These analogues can serve as chemical probes to aid the development of novel CK2α/β PPI inhibitors that can be used as therapeutics.

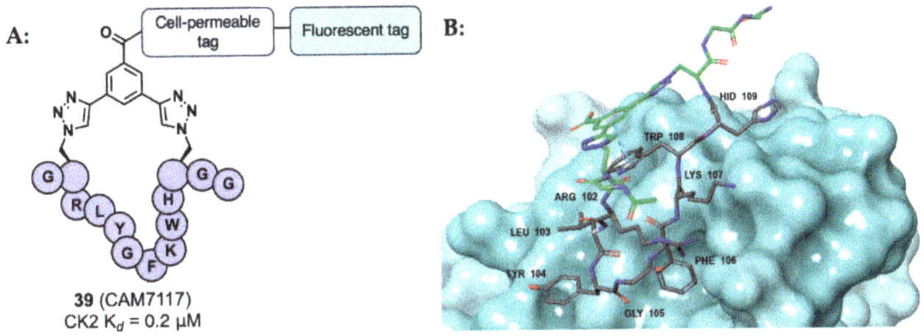

Figure 24. (**A**) Structure of CK2α/β interface binder CAM7117 **39**; (**B**) crystal structure of CAM7117 bound to CK2α/β interface (PDB 6Q4Q).

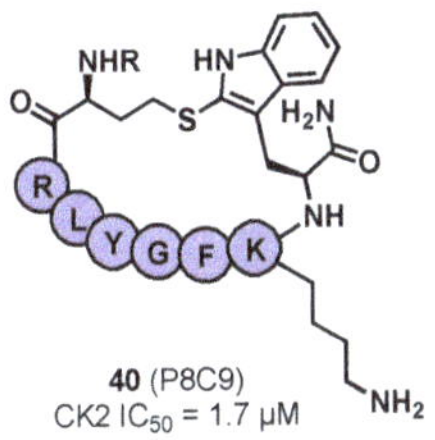

Figure 25. Structure of CK2α/β PPI inhibitor P8C9 **40**, where R = cell-penetrating peptide.

In addition to peptides targeting the CK2α/β interface, Kufareva et al. developed a small molecule probe **41**, Figure 26, that suppressed subunit association in vitro [140]. The procedure of fumigation was applied to the CK2β-binding interface of CK2α, followed by the ICM PocketFinder algorithm, which identified druggable conformations of the target pocket. The best conformations were then subjected to virtual screening, which evaluated **40** as a hit compound. Compound **41** was found to selectively inhibit the phosphorylation of a CK2β-dependent peptide, with an estimated IC_{50} of 50 μM. Additionally, 50 μM of **41** selectively inhibited phosphorylation of a CK2β-dependent protein, namely Olig-2 transcription factor, by ~50% as compared to the same experiment without the inhibitor. An in vitro CK2α/β interaction assay showed that **41** inhibited the CK2α/β subunit interaction in a dose-dependent manner. Finally, 100 μM of **41** was screened against a panel of 45 Ser/Thr kinases and only one other kinase was inhibited, namely PIM-1 at 36%. Furthermore, the Gini coefficient was calculated to be 0.81, comparable with the Gini coefficient of CAM4066, which is 0.82. These results highlight the promise of targeting the CK2α/β interface in the development of highly selective CK2 inhibitors.

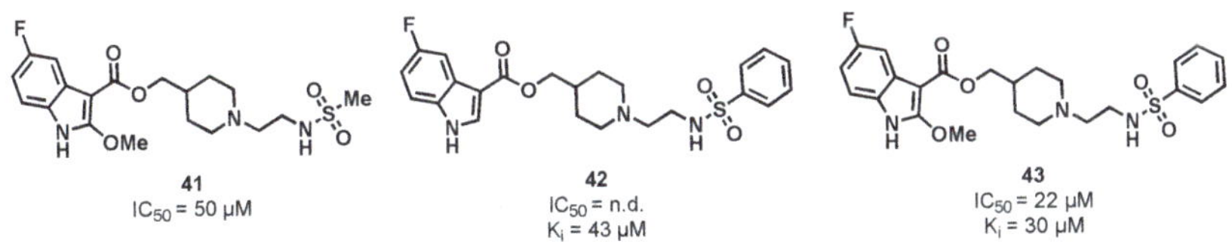

Figure 26. Structures of CK2α/β interface inhibitors **41**, **42**, and **43**.

Compound **41** was used as a starting point in subsequent structure–activity relationship studies, which resulted in the development of compounds **42** (K_d = 43 μM) and **43** (K_d = 30 μM, IC_{50} = 22 μM), Figure 26, which inhibited phosphorylation of Olgio-2 by 66% and 80%, respectively [141]. In addition to interaction with the CK2α/β interface, an allosteric effect was observed: the electron density of ATP in crystal structures that have **42** or **43** bound is very weak compared to that observed in the apo form. This suggests that

ATP is being destabilized by the binding of **42** or **43**. Unfortunately, these inhibitors were not subjected to the 45-kinase selectivity panel and their inhibitory activities against other kinases is currently unknown.

3.6. CK2 Proteolysis-Targeting Chimeras

Proteolysis-targeting chimeras (PROTACs) are heterobifunctional molecules that have emerged as an alternative therapeutic strategy to overcome limitations often encountered when using small molecule inhibitors [141,142]. PROTACs consist of an E3-ubiquitin ligase binder and a protein of interest binder (in this case CK2), connected by a linker. PROTACs hijack the cell's ubiquitin–proteasome system (UPS) to induce proteasomal degradation of the target protein. This occurs via formation of a ternary complex, consisting of an E3-ubiquitin ligase, PROTAC, and the protein of interest, which holds the E3-ubiquitin ligase and protein of interest in proximity for the transfer of ubiquitin to the protein of interest [143]. After several iterations of ubiquitin transfer, a polyubiquitin chain forms on the protein of interest, which is recognized by the 26S proteasome and results in degradation of the protein of interest.

In 2018, Chen et al. incorporated known small-molecule CK2α inhibitor CX-4945 into a series of cereblon (CRBN)-recruiting PROTACs, using pomalidomide as the E3-ubiquitin ligase binder [144]. Degradation of CK2 in a time-dependent manner was found with 10 μM of one PROTAC **44**, Figure 27, (IC_{50} = 17 μM) in MDA-MB-231 cells after 24 h. It remains unclear whether the α, α′ and/or β subunits were equally degraded. Promisingly, the PROTAC also upregulated p53 and inhibited phosphorylation of Akt, a known CK2α substrate. Furthermore, apoptotic analysis of MDA-MB-231 cells showed the rate of apoptosis of the PROTAC (26.2%, 17.3 μM) was higher than that of CX-4945 (16.8%, 15.7 μM) after 24 h. After a 24 h incubation with 35 μM of both compounds, the rate of apoptosis was still higher with the PROTAC (31.0%) than compared with CX-4945 (19.3%). The faster rate of apoptosis with the PROTAC could be advantageous over the original binder; however, more in vitro and in vivo studies are needed to determine any potential clinical advantages.

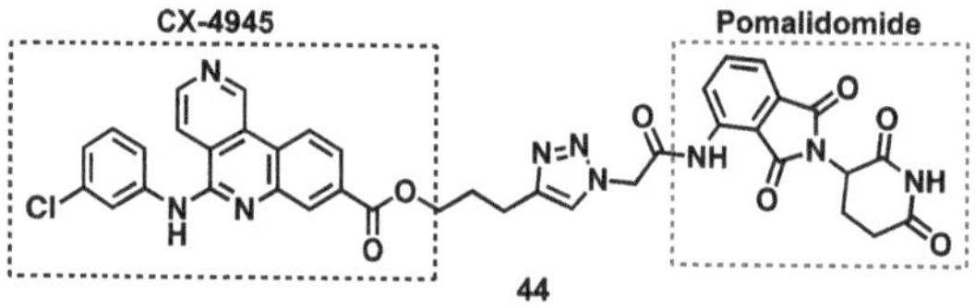

44

Figure 27. Structure of CK2/CRBN recruiting PROTAC **44**, which contains CX-4945 as the CK2 binder and pomalidomide as the CRBN binder.

4. Conclusions

The main aim of this review was to provide an update regarding CK2 inhibition strategies. In this review, we have discussed important features of the protein kinase CK2 and its role in numerous diseases, particularly cancer. We hope to have provided the reader with an overview of different ATP-competitive therapeutics, as well as their limitations. Furthermore, we hope to have provided insight into the main developments of inhibitors that act outside the ATP site.

There have been numerous efforts to develop effective and clinically useful CK2 inhibitors, and one small molecule, CX-4945, and one peptide, CIGB-325, have entered clinical trials. However, due to selectivity issues associated with CX-4945 and poor oral bioavailability encountered with peptides, we are still a long way from seeing CK2 as an established target in clinical oncology. Therefore, there is emphasis on developing selective CK2 inhibitors, which has driven researchers to explore CK2 beyond the ATP site. Two sites external to the ATP site have emerged, namely the αD site and the CK2α/β PPI interface, as valid sites for selective inhibition. Furthermore, new strategies have emerged to develop selective CK2 therapeutics: dual-functional inhibitors, bi-substrate inhibitors, and PROTACs. It is reasonable to hypothesize that continued research in this field will result in the development of potent, selective, and cell-permeable chemical probes that could be optimized to yield a clinically useful CK2 therapeutic. It is possible to also foresee, with continued chemical and biochemical developments, development of covalent inhibitors and small molecule/peptide hybrids that target multiple sites simultaneously.

Due to significant developments in CK2 inhibition, especially those discussed in this review, one can speculate that CK2 inhibition will remain at the forefront of kinase research over the coming years, especially in the pursuit of selective kinase inhibitors. The development of selective CK2 inhibitors will have major implications in a multitude of disease types, especially cancer and COVID-19.

Author Contributions: Conceptualization, S.D.-R.; software, R.M.W.; formal analysis, R.M.W. and S.D.-R.; investigation, S.D.-R.; data curation, S.D.-R.; writing—original draft preparation, S.D.-R.; writing—review and editing, S.D.-R., R.M.W., P.D.B., M.H. and D.R.S.; visualization, S.D.-R.; supervision, D.R.S. and M.H.; funding acquisition D.R.S. All authors have read and agreed to the published version of the manuscript.

Funding: S.D.-R. thanks AstraZeneca (AZ) for a studentship and financial support. D.R.S acknowledges support from the EPSRC, BBSRC, MRC, AZ, and the Cystic Fibrosis Trust UK.

Conflicts of Interest: The authors declare no conflicts of interest.

References

1. Hou, Z.; Liu, H. Mapping the Protein Kinome: Current Strategy and Future Direction. *Cells* **2023**, *12*, 925. [CrossRef]
2. Obsilova, V.; Obsil, T. The 14-3-3 Proteins as Important Allosteric Regulators of Protein Kinases. *Int. J. Mol. Sci.* **2020**, *21*, 8824. [CrossRef]
3. Roskoski, R., Jr. Small Molecule Protein Kinase Inhibitors Approved by Regulatory Agencies Outside of the United States. *Pharmacol. Res.* **2023**, *194*, 106847. [CrossRef] [PubMed]
4. Montenarh, M. Cellular Regulators of Protein Kinase CK2. *Cell Tissue Res.* **2010**, *342*, 139. [CrossRef]
5. Kannan, N.; Neuwald, A.F. Evolutionary Constraints Associated with Functional Specificity of the CMGC Protein Kinases MAPK, CDK, GSK, SRPK, DYRK, and CK2α. *Protein Sci.* **2004**, *13*, 2059. [CrossRef]
6. Burnett, G.; Kennedy, E.P. The Enzymatic Phosphorylation of Proteins. *J. Biol. Chem.* **1954**, *211*, 969. [CrossRef]
7. Venerando, A.; Ruzzene, M.; Pinna, L.A. Casein Kinase: The Triple Meaning of a Misnomer. *Biochem. J.* **2014**, *460*, 141. [CrossRef] [PubMed]
8. Niefind, K.; Guerra, B.; Ermakowa, I.; Issinger, O.G. Crystal structure of human protein kinase CK2: Insights into basic properties of the CK2 holoenzyme. *EMBO J.* **2001**, *20*, 5320. [CrossRef]
9. Pinna, L.A. Protein Kinase CK2: A Challenge to Canons. *J. Cell Sci.* **2002**, *115*, 3873. [CrossRef]
10. Roffey, S.E.; Litchfield, D.W. CK2 Regulation: Perspectives in 2021. *Biomedicines* **2021**, *9*, 1361. [CrossRef]
11. Chen, Y.; Wang, Y.; Wang, J.; Zhou, Z.; Cao, S.; Zhang, J. Strategies of Targeting CK2 in Drug Discovery: Challenges, Opportunities, and Emerging Prospects. *J. Med. Chem.* **2023**, *66*, 2257. [CrossRef] [PubMed]
12. Sarno, S.; Ghisellini, P.; Pinna, L.A. Unique activation mechanism of protein kinase CK2. *J. Biol. Chem.* **2002**, *277*, 22509. [CrossRef] [PubMed]
13. Núñez de Villavicencio Díaz, T.; Mazola, Y.; Perera Negrín, Y.; Cruz García, Y.; Guirola Cruz, O.; Perea Rodríguez, S.E. Predicting CK2 Beta-Dependent Substrates Using Linear Patterns. *Biochem. Biophys. Rep.* **2015**, *4*, 20. [CrossRef] [PubMed]
14. Gottardo, M.F.; Capobianco, C.S.; Sidabra, J.E.; Garona, J.; Perera, Y.; Perea, S.E.; Alonso, D.F.; Farina, H.G. Preclinical Efficacy of CIGB-300, an Anti-CK2 Peptide, on Breast Cancer Metastasic Colonization. *Sci. Rep.* **2020**, *10*, 14689. [CrossRef] [PubMed]
15. Guerra, B. Protein Kinase CK2 Subunits Are Positive Regulators of AKT Kinase. *Int. J. Oncol.* **2006**, *28*, 685. [CrossRef] [PubMed]
16. Yu, M.; Yeh, J.; Van Waes, C. Protein Kinase CK2 Mediates Inhibitor-Kappa B Kinase and Aberrant Nuclear Factor-κB Activation by Serum Factor(s) in Head and Neck Squamous Carcinoma Cells. *Cancer Res.* **2006**, *66*, 6722. [CrossRef] [PubMed]
17. Zheng, Y.; Qin, H.; Frank, S.J.; Deng, L.; Litchfield, D.W.; Tefferi, A.; Pardanani, A.; Lin, F.-T.; Li, J.; Sha, B.; et al. A CK2-Dependent Mechanism for Activation of the JAK-STAT Signaling Pathway. *Blood* **2011**, *118*, 156. [CrossRef] [PubMed]
18. Gao, Y.; Wang, H. Casein Kinase 2 Is Activated and Essential for Wnt/β-Catenin Signaling. *J. Biol. Chem.* **2006**, *281*, 18394. [CrossRef] [PubMed]
19. Jia, H.; Liu, Y.; Xia, R.; Tong, C.; Yue, T.; Jiang, J.; Jia, J. Casein Kinase 2 Promotes Hedgehog Signaling by Regulating Both Smoothened and Cubitus Interruptus. *J. Biol. Chem.* **2010**, *285*, 37218. [CrossRef]
20. Zhang, S.; Long, H.; Yang, Y.-L.; Wang, Y.; Hsieh, D.; Li, W.; Au, A.; Stoppler, H.J.; Xu, Z.; Jablons, D.M.; et al. Inhibition of CK2α Down-Regulates Notch1 Signalling in Lung Cancer Cells. *J. Cell. Mol. Med.* **2013**, *17*, 854. [CrossRef]

21. Borgo, C.; D'Amore, C.; Sarno, S.; Salvi, M.; Ruzzene, M. Protein kinase CK2: A potential therapeutic target for diverse human diseases. *Sig. Transduct. Target Ther.* **2021**, *6*, 183. [CrossRef] [PubMed]
22. Ruzzene, M.; Pinna, L.A. Addiction to Protein Kinase CK2: A Common Denominator of Diverse Cancer Cells? *Biochim. Biophys. Acta BBA—Proteins Proteom.* **2010**, *1804*, 499. [CrossRef]
23. Faust, M.; Montenarch, M. Subcellular localisation of protein kinase CK2. A key to its function? *Cell Tissue Res.* **2000**, *301*, 329. [CrossRef] [PubMed]
24. Trembley, J.H.; Li, B.; Kren, B.T.; Gravely, A.A.; Caicedo-Granados, E.; Klein, M.A.; Ahmed, K. CX-4945 and siRNA-Mediated Knockdown of CK2 Improves Cisplatin Response in HPV(+) and HPV(−) HNSCC Cell Lines. *Biomedicines* **2021**, *9*, 571. [CrossRef] [PubMed]
25. Meza, C.P.Q.; Ruzeene, M. Protein Kinase CK2 and SARS-CoV-2: An Expected Interplay Story. *Kinases Phosphatases* **2023**, *1*, 141. [CrossRef]
26. Breen, M.E.; Soellner, M.B. Small Molecule Substrate Phosphorylation Site Inhibitors of Protein Kinases: Approaches and Challenges. *ACS Chem. Biol.* **2015**, *10*, 175. [CrossRef]
27. Grygier, P.; Pustelny, K.; Nowak, J.; Golik, P.; Popowicz, G.M.; Plettenburg, O.; Dubin, G.; Menezes, F.; Czarna, A. Silmitasertib (CX-4945), a Clinically Used CK2-Kinase Inhibitor with Additional Effects on GSK3β and DYRK1A Kinases: A Structural Perspective. *J. Med. Chem.* **2023**, *66*, 4009. [CrossRef] [PubMed]
28. Lee, J.Y.; Yun, J.-S.; Kim, W.-K.; Chun, H.-S.; Jin, H.; Cho, S.; Chang, J.H. Structural Basis for the Selective Inhibition of Cdc2-Like Kinases by CX-4945. *BioMed Res. Int.* **2019**, *2019*, 6125068. [CrossRef]
29. Iegre, J.; Atkinson, E.L.; Brear, P.D.; Cooper, B.M.; Hyvönen, M.; Spring, D.R. Chemical Probes Targeting the Kinase CK2: A Journey Outside the Catalytic Box. *Org. Biomol. Chem.* **2021**, *19*, 4380. [CrossRef]
30. Schwartz, P.A.; Murray, B.W. Protein Kinase Biochemistry and Drug Discovery. *Bioorg. Chem.* **2011**, *39*, 192. [CrossRef]
31. Nuñez de Villavicencio-Diaz, T.; Rabalski, A.J.; Litchfield, D.W. Protein Kinase CK2: Intricate Relationships within Regulatory Cellular Networks. *Pharmaceuticals* **2017**, *10*, 27. [CrossRef] [PubMed]
32. De Fusco, C.; Brear, P.; Iegre, J.; Georgiou, K.H.; Sore, H.F.; Hyvönen, M.; Spring, D.R. A Fragment-Based Approach Leading to the Discovery of a Novel Binding Site and the Selective CK2 Inhibitor CAM4066. *Bioorg. Med. Chem.* **2017**, *25*, 3471. [CrossRef]
33. Niefind, K.; Guerra, B.; Pinna, L.A.; Issinger, O.-G.; Schomburg, D. Crystal Structure of the Catalytic Subunit of Protein Kinase CK2 from Zea Mays at 2.1 Å Resolution. *EMBO J.* **1998**, *17*, 2451. [CrossRef] [PubMed]
34. Papinutto, E.; Ranchio, A.; Lolli, G.; Pinna, L.A.; Battistutta, R. Structural and Functional Analysis of the Flexible Regions of the Catalytic α-Subunit of Protein Kinase CK2. *J. Struct. Biol.* **2012**, *177*, 382. [CrossRef] [PubMed]
35. Niefind, K.; Raaf, J.; Issinger, O.-G. Protein kinase CK2 in health and disease: Protein kinase CK2: From structures to insights. *Cell Mol. Life Sci.* **2009**, *66*, 1800. [CrossRef] [PubMed]
36. Lettieri, A.; Borgo, C.; Zanieri, L.; D'Amore, C.; Oleari, R.; Paganoni, A.; Pinna, L.A.; Cariboni, A.; Salvi, M. Protein Kinase CK2 Subunits Differentially Perturb the Adhesion and Migration of GN11 Cells: A Model of Immature Migrating Neurons. *Int. J. Mol. Sci.* **2019**, *20*, 5951. [CrossRef] [PubMed]
37. Bibby, A.C.; Litchfield, D.W. The Multiple Personalities of the Regulatory Subunit of Protein Kinase CK2: CK2 Dependent and CK2 Independent Roles Reveal a Secret Identity for CK2beta. *Int. J. Biol. Sci.* **2005**, *1*, 67. [CrossRef] [PubMed]
38. Litchfield, D.W. Protein kinase CK2: Structure, regulation, and role in cellular decisions of life and death. *Biochem. J.* **2003**, *369*, 1–5. [CrossRef]
39. Filhol, O.; Martiel, J.-L.; Cochet, C. Protein Kinase CK2: A New View of an Old Molecular Complex. *EMBO Rep.* **2004**, *5*, 351. [CrossRef]
40. Trembley, J.H.; Wang, G.; Unger, G.; Slaton, J.; Ahmed, K. Protein Kinase CK2 in Health and Disease. *Cell. Mol. Life Sci.* **2009**, *66*, 1858. [CrossRef]
41. Chua, M.M.J.; Ortega, C.E.; Sheikh, A.; Lee, M.; Abdul-Rassoul, H.; Hartshorn, K.L.; Dominguez, I. CK2 in Cancer: Cellular and Biochemical Mechanisms and Potential Therapeutic Target. *Pharmaceuticals* **2017**, *10*, 18. [CrossRef] [PubMed]
42. Hanahan, D.; Weinberg, R.A. The Hallmarks of Cancer. *Cell* **2000**, *100*, 57. [CrossRef] [PubMed]
43. Hanahan, D.; Weinberg, R.A. Hallmarks of Cancer: The next Generation. *Cell* **2011**, *144*, 646. [CrossRef] [PubMed]
44. Trembley, J.H.; Kren, B.T.; Afzal, M.; Scaria, G.A.; Klein, M.A.; Ahmed, K. Protein Kinase CK2—Diverse Roles in Cancer Cell Biology and Therapeutic Promise. *Mol. Cell. Biochem.* **2023**, *478*, 899. [CrossRef]
45. Faust, R.A.; Gapany, M.; Tristani, P.; Davis, A.; Adams, G.L.; Ahmed, K. Elevated Protein Kinase CK2 Activity in Chromatin of Head and Neck Tumors: Association with Malignant Transformation. *Cancer Lett.* **1996**, *101*, 31. [CrossRef]
46. Yenice, S.; Davis, A.T.; Goueli, S.A.; Akdas, A.; Limas, C.; Ahmed, K. Nuclear casein kinase 2 (CK-2) activity in human normal, benign hyperplastic, and cancerous prostate. *Prostate* **1994**, *24*, 11–16. [CrossRef] [PubMed]
47. Mandato, E.; Manni, S.; Zaffino, F.; Semenzato, G.; Piazza, F. Targeting CK2-Driven Non-Oncogene Addiction in B-Cell Tumors. *Oncogene* **2016**, *35*, 6045. [CrossRef]
48. Zou, J.; Luo, H.; Zeng, Q.; Dong, Z.; Wu, D.; Liu, L. Protein Kinase CK2α Is Overexpressed in Colorectal Cancer and Modulates Cell Proliferation and Invasion via Regulating EMT-Related Genes. *J. Transl. Med.* **2011**, *9*, 97. [CrossRef]
49. Zhang, H.-X.; Jiang, S.-S.; Zhang, X.-F.; Zhou, Z.-Q.; Pan, Q.-Z.; Chen, C.-L.; Zhao, J.-J.; Tang, Y.; Xia, J.-C.; Weng, D.-S. Protein Kinase CK2α Catalytic Subunit Is Overexpressed and Serves as an Unfavorable Prognostic Marker in Primary Hepatocellular Carcinoma. *Oncotarget* **2015**, *6*, 34800. [CrossRef]

50. Turowec, J.P.; Vilk, G.; Gabriel, M.; Litchfield, D.W. Characterizing the Convergence of Protein Kinase CK2 and Caspase-3 Reveals Isoform-Specific Phosphorylation of Caspase-3 by CK2α': Implications for Pathological Roles of CK2 in Promoting Cancer Cell Survival. *Oncotarget* **2013**, *4*, 560. [CrossRef]
51. Zhou, B.; Ritt, D.A.; Morrison, D.K.; Der, C.J.; Cox, A.D. Protein Kinase CK2α Maintains Extracellular Signal-Regulated Kinase (ERK) Activity in a CK2α Kinase-Independent Manner to Promote Resistance to Inhibitors of RAF and MEK but Not ERK in BRAF Mutant Melanoma. *J. Biol. Chem.* **2016**, *291*, 17804. [CrossRef] [PubMed]
52. Takahashi, K.; Setoguchi, T.; Tsuru, A. Inhibition of casein kinase 2 prevents growth of human osteosarcoma. *Oncol. Rep.* **2017**, *37*, 1141. [CrossRef] [PubMed]
53. Atkinson, E.L.; Iegre, J.; Brear, P.D.; Zhabina, E.A.; Hyvönen, M.; Spring, D.R. Downfalls of Chemical Probes Acting at the Kinase ATP-Site: CK2 as a Case Study. *Molecules* **2021**, *26*, 1977. [CrossRef] [PubMed]
54. Tamm, I.; Folkers, K.; Shunk, C.H.; Horsfall, F.L. Inhibition of Influenza Virus Multiplication by N-Glycosides of Benzimidazoles. *J. Exp. Med.* **1954**, *99*, 227. [CrossRef] [PubMed]
55. Zandomeni, R.; Zandomeni, M.C.; Shugar, D.; Weinmann, R. Casein Kinase Type II Is Involved in the Inhibition by 5,6-Dichloro-1-Beta-D-Ribofuranosylbenzimidazole of Specific RNA Polymerase II Transcription. *J. Biol. Chem.* **1986**, *261*, 3414. [CrossRef]
56. Szyszka, R.; Grankowski, N.; Felczak, K.; Shugar, D. Halogenated Benzimidazoles and Benzotriazoles as Selective Inhibitors of Protein Kinases CK-I and CK-II from Saccharomyces Cerevisiae and Other Sources. *Biochem. Biophys. Res. Commun.* **1995**, *208*, 418. [CrossRef]
57. Wiley, R.H.; Hussung, K.F. Halogenated Benzotriazoles. *J. Am. Chem. Soc.* **1957**, *79*, 4395. [CrossRef]
58. Pagano, M.A.; Meggio, F.; Ruzzene, M.; Andrzejewska, M.; Kazimierczuk, Z.; Pinna, L.A. 2-Dimethylamino-4,5,6,7-Tetrabromo-1H-Benzimidazole: A Novel Powerful and Selective Inhibitor of Protein Kinase CK2. *Biochem. Biophys. Res. Commun.* **2004**, *321*, 1040. [CrossRef] [PubMed]
59. Pagano, M.A.; Bain, J.; Kazimierczuk, Z.; Sarno, S.; Ruzzene, M.; Di Maira, G.; Elliott, M.; Orzeszko, A.; Cozza, G.; Meggio, F.; et al. The Selectivity of Inhibitors of Protein Kinase CK2: An Update. *Biochem. J.* **2008**, *415*, 353. [CrossRef]
60. Mishra, S.; Pertz, V.; Zhang, B.; Kaur, P.; Shimada, H.; Groffen, J.; Kazimierczuk, Z.; Pinna, L.A.; Heisterkamp, N. Treatment of P190 Bcr/Abl Lymphoblastic Leukemia Cells with Inhibitors of the Serine/Threonine Kinase CK2. *Leukemia* **2007**, *21*, 178. [CrossRef]
61. Siddiqui, Y.H.; Kershaw, R.M.; Humphreys, E.H.; Assis Junior, E.M.; Chaudhri, S.; Jayaraman, P.-S.; Gaston, K. CK2 Abrogates the Inhibitory Effects of PRH/HHEX on Prostate Cancer Cell Migration and Invasion and Acts through PRH to Control Cell Proliferation. *Oncogenesis* **2017**, *6*, e293. [CrossRef]
62. Ulges, A.; Witsch, E.J.; Pramanik, G.; Klein, M.; Birkner, K.; Bühler, U.; Wasser, B.; Luessi, F.; Stergiou, N.; Dietzen, S.; et al. Protein Kinase CK2 Governs the Molecular Decision between Encephalitogenic TH17 Cell and Treg Cell Development. *Proc. Natl. Acad. Sci. USA* **2016**, *113*, 10145. [CrossRef]
63. Gartman, J.A.; Tambar, U.K. Recent Total Syntheses of Anthraquinone-Based Natural Products. *Tetrahedron* **2022**, *105*, 132501. [CrossRef] [PubMed]
64. Janeczko, M.; Masłyk, M.; Kubiński, K.; Golczyk, H. Emodin, a Natural Inhibitor of Protein Kinase CK2, Suppresses Growth, Hyphal Development, and Biofilm Formation of Candida Albicans. *Yeast* **2017**, *34*, 253. [CrossRef]
65. Meggio, F.; Pagano, M.A.; Moro, S.; Zagotto, G.; Ruzzene, M.; Sarno, S.; Cozza, G.; Bain, J.; Elliott, M.; Deana, A.D.; et al. Inhibition of Protein Kinase CK2 by Condensed Polyphenolic Derivatives: An In Vitro and In Vivo Study. *Biochemistry* **2004**, *43*, 12931. [CrossRef] [PubMed]
66. Cozza, G. The Development of CK2 Inhibitors: From Traditional Pharmacology to in Silico Rational Drug Design. *Pharmaceuticals* **2017**, *10*, 26. [CrossRef] [PubMed]
67. De Moliner, E.; Moro, S.; Sarno, S.; Zagotto, G.; Zanotti, G.; Pinna, L.A.; Battistutta, R. Inhibition of Protein Kinase CK2 by Anthraquinone-Related Compounds: A Structural Insight. *J. Biol. Chem.* **2003**, *278*, 1831. [CrossRef]
68. Cozza, G.; Mazzorana, M.; Papinutto, E.; Bain, J.; Elliott, M.; di Maira, G.; Gianoncelli, A.; Pagano, M.A.; Sarno, S.; Ruzzene, M.; et al. Quinalizarin as a Potent, Selective and Cell-Permeable Inhibitor of Protein Kinase CK2. *Biochem. J.* **2009**, *421*, 387. [CrossRef]
69. Cozza, G.; Venerando, A.; Sarno, S.; Pinna, L.A. The Selectivity of CK2 Inhibitor Quinalizarin: A Reevaluation. *BioMed Res. Int.* **2015**, *2015*, e734127. [CrossRef]
70. Nie, Z.; Perretta, C.; Erickson, P.; Margosiak, S.; Almassy, R.; Lu, J.; Averill, A.; Yager, K.M.; Chu, S. Structure-Based Design, Synthesis, and Study of Pyrazolo[1,5-a][1,3,5]Triazine Derivatives as Potent Inhibitors of Protein Kinase CK2. *Bioorg. Med. Chem. Lett.* **2007**, *17*, 4191. [CrossRef]
71. Nie, Z.; Perretta, C.; Erickson, P.; Margosiak, S.; Lu, J.; Averill, A.; Almassy, R.; Chu, S. Structure-Based Design and Synthesis of Novel Macrocyclic Pyrazolo[1,5-a] [1,3,5]Triazine Compounds as Potent Inhibitors of Protein Kinase CK2 and Their Anticancer Activities. *Bioorg. Med. Chem. Lett.* **2008**, *18*, 619. [CrossRef]
72. Dowling, J.E.; Chuaqui, C.; Pontz, T.W.; Lyne, P.D.; Larsen, N.A.; Block, M.H.; Chen, H.; Su, N.; Wu, A.; Russell, D.; et al. Potent and Selective Inhibitors of CK2 Kinase Identified through Structure-Guided Hybridization. *ACS Med. Chem. Lett.* **2012**, *3*, 278. [CrossRef]

73. Dowling, J.E.; Alimzhanov, M.; Bao, L.; Chuaqui, C.; Denz, C.R.; Jenkins, E.; Larsen, N.A.; Lyne, P.D.; Pontz, T.; Ye, Q.; et al. Potent and Selective CK2 Kinase Inhibitors with Effects on Wnt Pathway Signaling in Vivo. *ACS Med. Chem. Lett.* **2016**, *7*, 300. [CrossRef] [PubMed]
74. Wells, C.I.; Drewry, D.H.; Pickett, J.E.; Tjaden, A.; Krämer, A.; Müller, S.; Gyenis, L.; Menyhart, D., Litchfield, D.W.; Knapp, S.; et al. Development of a Potent and Selective Chemical Probe for the Pleiotropic Kinase CK2. *Cell Chem. Biol.* **2021**, *28*, 546.e10. [CrossRef] [PubMed]
75. Licciardello, M.P.; Workman, P. A New Chemical Probe Challenges the Broad Cancer Essentiality of CK2. *Trends Pharmacol. Sci.* **2021**, *42*, 313. [CrossRef]
76. Salvi, M.; Borgo, C.; Pinna, L.A.; Ruzzene, M. Targeting CK2 in Cancer: A Valuable Strategy or a Waste of Time? *Cell Death Discov.* **2021**, *7*, 1. [CrossRef] [PubMed]
77. Ong, H.W.; Drewry, D.H.; Axtman, A.D. CK2 Chemical Probes: Past, Present, and Future. *Kinases Phosphatases* **2023**, *1*, 288. [CrossRef]
78. Siddiqui-Jain, A.; Drygin, D.; Streiner, N.; Chua, P.; Pierre, F.; O'Brien, S.E.; Bliesath, J.; Omori, M.; Huser, N.; Ho, C.; et al. CX-4945, an orally bioavailable selective inhibitor of protein kinase CK2, inhibits prosurvival and angiogenic signaling and exhibits antitumor efficacy. *Cancer Res.* **2010**, *70*, 10288. [CrossRef]
79. Senhwa Biosciences CX-4945 Granted Orphan Drug Designation by the US FDA in Cholangiocarcinoma. News Release. Senhwa Biosciences, Inc. January 4 2017. Available online: https://www.prnewswire.com/news-releases/senhwa-biosciences-cx-4945-granted-orphan-drug-designation-by-the-us-fda-in-cholangiocarcinoma-300385278.html (accessed on 14 February 2024).
80. D'Amore, C.; Borgo, C.; Sarno, S.; Salvi, M. Role of CK2 Inhibitor CX-4945 in Anti-Cancer Combination Therapy—Potential Clinical Relevance. *Cell. Oncol. Dordr.* **2020**, *43*, 1003. [CrossRef]
81. Chon, H.J.; Bae, K.J.; Lee, Y.; Kim, J. The Casein Kinase 2 Inhibitor, CX-4945, as an Anti-Cancer Drug in Treatment of Human Hematological Malignancies. *Front. Pharmacol.* **2015**, *6*, 70. [CrossRef]
82. Garuti, L.; Roberti, M.; Bottegoni, G. Multi-Kinase Inhibitors. *Curr. Med. Chem.* **2015**, *22*, 695. [CrossRef]
83. Menyhart, D.; Gyenis, L.; Jurcic, K.; Roffey, S.E.; Puri, A.; Jovanovic, P.; Szkop, K.J.; Pittock, P.; Lajoie, G.; Axtman, A.D.; et al. Comparison of CX-4945 and SGC-CK2-1 as Inhibitors of CSNK2 Using Quantitative Phosphoproteomics: Triple SILAC in Combination with Inhibitor-Resistant CSNK2. *Curr. Res. Chem. Biol.* **2023**, *3*, 100041. [CrossRef]
84. Battistutta, R.; Cozza, G.; Pierre, F.; Papinutto, E.; Lolli, G.; Sarno, S.; O'Brien, S.E.; Siddiqui-Jain, A.; Haddach, M.; Anderes, K.; et al. Unprecedented Selectivity and Structural Determinants of a New Class of Protein Kinase CK2 Inhibitors in Clinical Trials for the Treatment of Cancer. *Biochemistry* **2011**, *50*, 8478. [CrossRef]
85. Ursu, A.; Childs-Disney, J.L.; Angelbello, A.J.; Costales, M.G.; Meyer, S.M.; Disney, M.D. Gini Coefficients as a Single Value Metric to Define Chemical Probe Selectivity. *ACS Chem. Biol.* **2020**, *15*, 2031. [CrossRef]
86. Ember, S.W.; Lambert, Q.T.; Berndt, N.; Gunawan, S.; Ayaz, M.; Tauro, M.; Zhu, J.-Y.; Cranfill, P.J.; Greninger, P.; Lynch, C.C.; et al. Potent Dual BET Bromodomain-Kinase Inhibitors as Value Added Multi-Targeted Chemical Probes and Cancer Therapeutics. *Mol. Cancer Ther.* **2017**, *16*, 1054. [CrossRef]
87. Ciceri, P.; Müller, S.; O'Mahony, A.; Fedorov, O.; Filippakopoulos, P.; Hunt, J.P.; Lasater, E.A.; Pallares, G.; Picaud, S.; Wells, C.; et al. Dual Kinase-Bromodomain Inhibitors for Rationally Designed Polypharmacology. *Nat. Chem. Biol.* **2014**, *10*, 305. [CrossRef] [PubMed]
88. Karim, R.M.; Bikowitz, M.J.; Chan, A.; Zhu, J.-Y.; Grassie, D.; Becker, A.; Berndt, N.; Gunawan, S.; Lawrence, N.J.; Schönbrunn, E. Differential BET Bromodomain Inhibition by Dihydropteridinone and Pyrimidodiazepinone Kinase Inhibitors. *J. Med. Chem.* **2021**, *64*, 15772. [CrossRef]
89. Zhang, Y.; Wang, Z.; Li, X.; Magnuson, N.S. Pim kinase-dependent inhibition of c-Myc degradation. *Oncogene* **2008**, *27*, 4809. [CrossRef] [PubMed]
90. Panchal, N.K.; Sabina, E.P. A Serine/Threonine Protein PIM Kinase as a Biomarker of Cancer and a Target for Anti-Tumor Therapy. *Life Sci.* **2020**, *255*, 117866. [CrossRef] [PubMed]
91. Decker, S.; Finter, J.; Forde, A.J.; Kissel, S.; Schwaller, J.; Mack, T.S.; Kuhn, A.; Gray, N.; Follo, M.; Jumaa, H.; et al. PIM Kinases Are Essential for Chronic Lymphocytic Leukemia Cell Survival (PIM2/3) and CXCR4-Mediated Microenvironmental Interactions (PIM1). *Mol. Cancer Ther.* **2014**, *13*, 1231. [CrossRef]
92. Luszczak, S.; Kumar, C.; Sathyadevan, V.K.; Simpson, B.S.; Gately, K.A.; Whitaker, H.C.; Heavey, S. PIM Kinase Inhibition: Co-Targeted Therapeutic Approaches in Prostate Cancer. *Signal Transduct. Target. Ther.* **2020**, *5*, 7. [CrossRef] [PubMed]
93. Blanco-Aparicio, C.; Carnero, A. Pim Kinases in Cancer: Diagnostic, Prognostic and Treatment Opportunities. *Biochem. Pharmacol.* **2013**, *85*, 629. [CrossRef] [PubMed]
94. Arrouchi, H.; Lakhlili, W.; Ibrahimi, A. A Review on PIM Kinases in Tumors. *Bioinformation* **2019**, *15*, 40. [CrossRef] [PubMed]
95. López-Ramos, M.; Prudent, R.; Moucadel, V.; Sautel, C.; Barette, C.; Lafanechère, L.; Mouawad, L.; Grierson, D.; Schmidt, F.; Florent, J.; et al. New Potent Dual Inhibitors of CK2 and Pim Kinases: Discovery and Structural Insights. *FASEB J.* **2010**, *24*, 3171. [CrossRef] [PubMed]
96. Sarno, S.; Mazzorana, M.; Traynor, R.; Ruzzene, M.; Cozza, G.; Pagano, M.A.; Meggio, F.; Zagotto, G.; Battistutta, R.; Pinna, L.A. Structural Features Underlying the Selectivity of the Kinase Inhibitors NBC and dNBC: Role of a Nitro Group That Discriminates between CK2 and DYRK1A. *Cell. Mol. Life Sci.* **2012**, *69*, 449. [CrossRef] [PubMed]

97. Cozza, G.; Sarno, S.; Ruzzene, M.; Girardi, C.; Orzeszko, A.; Kazimierczuk, Z.; Zagotto, G.; Bonaiuto, E.; Di Paolo, M.L.; Pinna, L.A. Exploiting the Repertoire of CK2 Inhibitors to Target DYRK and PIM Kinases. *Biochim. Biophys. Acta BBA—Proteins Proteom.* **2013**, *1834*, 1402. [CrossRef] [PubMed]
98. Cozza, G.; Girardi, C.; Ranchio, A.; Lolli, G.; Sarno, S.; Orzeszko, A.; Kazimierczuk, Z.; Battistutta, R.; Ruzzene, M.; Pinna, L.A. Cell-Permeable Dual Inhibitors of Protein Kinases CK2 and PIM-1: Structural Features and Pharmacological Potential. *Cell. Mol. Life Sci.* **2014**, *71*, 3173. [CrossRef]
99. Girardi, C.; Ottaviani, D.; Pinna, L.A.; Ruzzene, M. Different Persistence of the Cellular Effects Promoted by Protein Kinase CK2 Inhibitors CX-4945 and TDB. *BioMed Res. Int.* **2015**, *2015*, 185736. [CrossRef]
100. Chojnacki, K.; Wińska, P.; Wielechowska, M.; Łukowska-Chojnacka, E.; Tölzer, C.; Niefind, K.; Bretner, M. Biological Properties and Structural Study of New Aminoalkyl Derivatives of Benzimidazole and Benzotriazole, Dual Inhibitors of CK2 and PIM1 Kinases. *Bioorg. Chem.* **2018**, *80*, 266. [CrossRef]
101. Donati, B.; Lorenzini, E.; Ciarrocchi, A. BRD4 and Cancer: Going beyond Transcriptional Regulation. *Mol. Cancer* **2018**, *17*, 164. [CrossRef]
102. Di Micco, R.; Fontanals-Cirera, B.; Low, V.; Ntziachristos, P.; Yuen, S.K.; Lovell, C.D.; Dolgalev, I.; Yonekubo, Y.; Zhang, G.; Rusinova, E.; et al. Control of Embryonic Stem Cell Identity by BRD4-Dependent Transcriptional Elongation of Super-Enhancer-Associated Pluripotency Genes. *Cell Rep.* **2014**, *9*, 234. [CrossRef] [PubMed]
103. Wu, S.-Y.; Lee, A.-Y.; Lai, H.-T.; Zhang, H.; Chiang, C.-M. Phospho Switch Triggers BRD4 Chromatin Binding and Activator Recruitment for Gene-Specific Targeting. *Mol. Cell* **2013**, *49*, 843. [CrossRef]
104. Malvezzi, F.; Stubbs, C.J.; Jowitt, T.A.; Dale, I.L.; Guo, X.; DeGnore, J.P.; Degliesposti, G.; Skehel, J.M.; Bannister, A.J.; McAlister, M.S. Phosphorylation-Dependent BRD4 Dimerization and Implications for Therapeutic Inhibition of BET Family Proteins. *Commun. Biol.* **2021**, *4*, 1. [CrossRef]
105. Wu, S.-Y.; Lee, C.-F.; Lai, H.-T.; Yu, C.-T.; Lee, J.-E.; Zuo, H.; Tsai, S.Y.; Tsai, M.-J.; Ge, K.; Wan, Y.; et al. Opposing Functions of BRD4 Isoforms in Breast Cancer. *Mol. Cell* **2020**, *78*, 1114.e10. [CrossRef]
106. Sanz-Alvarez, M.; Cristobal, I.; Luque, M.; Santos, A.; Zazo, S.; Madoz-Gurpide, J.; Carames, C.; Chiang, C.M.; Garcia-Foncillas, J.; Eroles, P.; et al. Expression of Phosphorylated BRD4 is Markedly Associated with the Activation Status of the PP2A Pathway and Shows a Strong Prognostic Value in Triple Negative Breast Cancer Patients. *Cancers* **2021**, *31*, 1246. [CrossRef]
107. Zhang, J.; Tang, P.; Zou, L.; Zhang, J.; Chen, J.; Yang, C.; He, G.; Liu, B.; Liu, J.; Chiang, C.-M.; et al. Discovery of Novel Dual-Target Inhibitor of Bromodomain-Containing Protein 4/Casein Kinase 2 Inducing Apoptosis and Autophagy-Associated Cell Death for Triple-Negative Breast Cancer Therapy. *J. Med. Chem.* **2021**, *64*, 18025. [CrossRef]
108. Huang, J.-Q.; Duan, L.-X.; Liu, Q.-Y.; Li, H.-F.; Hu, A.-P.; Song, J.-W.; Lin, C.; Huang, B.; Yao, D.; Peng, B.; et al. Serine-Arginine Protein Kinase 1 (SRPK1) Promotes EGFR-TKI Resistance by Enhancing GSK3β Ser9 Autophosphorylation Independent of Its Kinase Activity in Non-Small-Cell Lung Cancer. *Oncogene* **2023**, *42*, 1233. [CrossRef] [PubMed]
109. Nikas, I.P.; Themistocleous, S.C.; Paschou, S.A.; Tsamis, K.I.; Ryu, H.S. Serine-Arginine Protein Kinase 1 (SRPK1) as a Prognostic Factor and Potential Therapeutic Target in Cancer: Current Evidence and Future Perspectives. *Cells* **2019**, *9*, 19. [CrossRef]
110. Yi, N.; Xiao, M.; Jiang, F.; Liu, Z.; Ni, W.; Lu, C.; Ni, R.; Chen, W. SRPK1 Is a Poor Prognostic Indicator and a Novel Potential Therapeutic Target for Human Colorectal Cancer. *OncoTargets Ther.* **2018**, *11*, 5359. [CrossRef]
111. Mylonis, I.; Giannakouros, T. Protein kinase CK2 phosphorylates and activates the SR protein-specific kinase 1. *Biochem. Biophys. Res. Commun.* **2003**, *301*, 650. [CrossRef]
112. Morooka, S.; Hoshina, M.; Kii, I.; Okabe, T.; Kojima, H.; Inoue, N.; Okuno, Y.; Denawa, M.; Yoshida, S.; Fukuhara, J.; et al. Identification of a Dual Inhibitor of SRPK1 and CK2 That Attenuates Pathological Angiogenesis of Macular Degeneration in Mice. *Mol. Pharmacol.* **2015**, *88*, 316. [CrossRef] [PubMed]
113. Leonidis, G.; Dalezis, P.; Trafalis, D.; Beis, D.; Giardoglou, P.; Koukiali, A.; Sigala, I.; Nikolakaki, E.; Sarli, V. Synthesis and Biological Evaluation of a c(RGDyK) Peptide Conjugate of SRPIN803. *ACS Omega* **2021**, *6*, 28379. [CrossRef] [PubMed]
114. Seto, E.; Yoshida, M. Erasers of Histone Acetylation: The Histone Deacetylase Enzymes. *Cold Spring Harb. Perspect. Biol.* **2014**, *6*, a018713. [CrossRef] [PubMed]
115. Tsai, S.C.; Seto, E. Regulation of histone deacetylase 2 by protein kinase CK2. *J. Biol. Chem.* **2002**, *277*, 31826. [CrossRef] [PubMed]
116. Bubna, A.K. Vorinostat—An Overview. *Indian J. Dermatol.* **2015**, *60*, 419. [CrossRef]
117. Ruzzene, M.; Penzo, D.; Pinna, L.A. Protein Kinase CK2 Inhibitor 4,5,6,7-Tetrabromobenzotriazole (TBB) Induces Apoptosis and Caspase-Dependent Degradation of Haematopoietic Lineage Cell-Specific Protein 1 (HS1) in Jurkat Cells. *Biochem. J.* **2002**, *364*, 41. [CrossRef] [PubMed]
118. Schneider, C.C.; Hessenauer, A.; Götz, C.; Montenarh, M. DMAT, an Inhibitor of Protein Kinase CK2 Induces Reactive Oxygen Species and DNA Double Strand Breaks. *Oncol. Rep.* **2009**, *21*, 1593. [CrossRef] [PubMed]
119. Purwin, M.; Hernández-Toribio, J.; Coderch, C.; Panchuk, R.; Skorokhyd, N.; Filipiak, K.; de Pascual-Teresa, B.; Ramos, A. Design and Synthesis of Novel Dual-Target Agents for HDAC1 and CK2 Inhibition. *RSC Adv.* **2016**, *6*, 66595. [CrossRef]
120. Rangasamy, L.; Ortín, I.; Zapico, J.M.; Coderch, C.; Ramos, A.; de Pascual-Teresa, B. New Dual CK2/HDAC1 Inhibitors with Nanomolar Inhibitory Activity against Both Enzymes. *ACS Med. Chem. Lett.* **2020**, *11*, 713. [CrossRef]
121. Deboever, E.; Fistrovich, A.; Hulme, C.; Dunckley, T. The Omnipresence of DYRK1A in Human Diseases. *Int. J. Mol. Sci.* **2022**, *23*, 9355. [CrossRef]

122. Di Vona, C.; Daniela Bezdan, D.; Islam, A.; Salichs, E.; López-Bigas, N.; Ossowski, S.; de la Luna, S. Chromatin-wide Profiling of DYRK1A Reveals a Role as a Gene-Specific RNA Polymerase II CTD Kinase. *Mol. Cell* **2015**, *57*, 506. [CrossRef] [PubMed]
123. Mahmoudi, T.; Li, V.S.; Ng, S.S.; Taouatas, N.; Vries, R.G.; Mohammed, S.; Heck, A.J.; Clevers, H. The kinase TNIK is an essential activator of Wnt target genes. *EMBO J.* **2009**, *28*, 3329. [CrossRef] [PubMed]
124. Sato, K.; Padgaonkar, A.A.; Baker, S.J.; Cosenza, S.C.; Rechkoblit, O.; Subbaiah, D.V.; Domingo-Domenech, J.; Bartkowski, A.; Port, E.R.; Aggarwal, A.K.; et al. Simultaneous CK2/TNIK/DYRK1 inhibition by 108600 suppresses triple negative breast cancer stem cells and chemotherapy-resistant disease. *Nat. Commun.* **2021**, *12*, 4671. [CrossRef]
125. Sato, K.; Baker, S.J.; Reddy, E.P.; Irie, H.Y. Abstract 308: Novel Cancer Stem Cell Inhibitor 108600 Modulates Tumor Immunomicroenvironment of Triple Negative Breast Cancer (TNBC). *Cancer Res.* **2022**, *82*, PD3-08. [CrossRef]
126. Meggio, F.; Pinna, L.A.; Marchiori, F.; Borin, G. Polyglutamyl Peptides: A New Class of Inhibitors of Type-2 Casein Kinases. *FEBS Lett.* **1983**, *162*, 235. [CrossRef] [PubMed]
127. Perea, S.E.; Reyes, O.; Puchades, Y.; Mendoza, O.; Vispo, N.S.; Torrens, I.; Santos, A.; Silva, R.; Acevedo, B.; López, E.; et al. Antitumor Effect of a Novel Proapoptotic Peptide that Impairs the Phosphorylation by the Protein Kinase 2 (Casein Kinase 2). *Cancer Res.* **2004**, *64*, 7127. [CrossRef] [PubMed]
128. Perea, S.E.; Baladron, I.; Garcia, Y.; Perera, Y.; Lopez, A.; Soriano, J.L.; Batista, N.; Palau, A.; Hernández, I.; Farina, H.; et al. CIGB-300, a Synthetic Peptide-Based Drug That Targets the CK2 Phosphoaceptor Domain. Translational and Clinical Research. *Mol. Cell. Biochem.* **2011**, *356*, 45. [CrossRef]
129. Cruz, L.R.; Baladrón, I.; Rittoles, A.; Díaz, P.A.; Valenzuela, C.; Santana, R.; Vázquez, M.M.; García, A.; Chacón, D.; Thompson, D.; et al. Treatment with an Anti-CK2 Synthetic Peptide Improves Clinical Response in COVID-19 Patients with Pneumonia. A Randomized and Controlled Clinical Trial. *ACS Pharmacol. Transl. Sci.* **2020**, *4*, 206. [CrossRef] [PubMed]
130. Cozza, G.; Zanin, S.; Sarno, S.; Costa, E.; Girardi, C.; Ribaudo, G.; Salvi, M.; Zagotto, G.; Ruzzene, M.; Pinna, L.A. Design, Validation and Efficacy of Bisubstrate Inhibitors Specifically Affecting Ecto-CK2 Kinase Activity. *Biochem. J.* **2015**, *471*, 415. [CrossRef]
131. Enkvist, E.; Viht, K.; Bischoff, N.; Vahter, J.; Saaver, S.; Raidaru, G.; Issinger, O.-G.; Niefind, K.; Uri, A. A Subnanomolar Fluorescent Probe for Protein Kinase CK2 Interaction Studies. *Org. Biomol. Chem.* **2012**, *10*, 8645. [CrossRef]
132. Viht, K.; Saaver, S.; Vahter, J.; Enkvist, E.; Lavogina, D.; Sinijärv, H.; Raidaru, G.; Guerra, B.; Issinger, O.-G.; Uri, A. Acetoxymethyl Ester of Tetrabromobenzimidazole-Peptoid Conjugate for Inhibition of Protein Kinase CK2 in Living Cells. *Bioconjug. Chem.* **2015**, *26*, 2324. [CrossRef]
133. Vahter, J.; Viht, K.; Uri, A.; Enkvist, E. Oligo-Aspartic Acid Conjugates with Benzo[c][2,6]Naphthyridine-8-Carboxylic Acid Scaffold as Picomolar Inhibitors of CK2. *Bioorg. Med. Chem.* **2017**, *25*, 2277. [CrossRef] [PubMed]
134. Brear, P.; De Fusco, C.; Hadje Georgiou, K.; Francis-Newton, N.J.; Stubbs, C.J.; Sore, H.F.; Venkitaraman, A.R.; Abell, C.; Spring, D.R.; Hyvönen, M. Specific Inhibition of CK2α from an Anchor Outside the Active Site. *Chem. Sci.* **2016**, *7*, 6839. [CrossRef]
135. Li, C.; Zhang, X.; Zhang, N.; Zhou, Y.; Sun, G.; Zhao, L.; Zhong, R. Identification and Biological Evaluation of CK2 Allosteric Fragments through Structure-Based Virtual Screening. *Molecules* **2020**, *25*, 237. [CrossRef]
136. Bancet, A.; Frem, R.; Jeanneret, F.; Mularoni, A.; Bazelle, P.; Roelants, C.; Delcros, J.G.; Guichou, J.F.; Pillet, C.; Coste, I.; et al. Cancer Selective Cell Death Induction by a Bivalent CK2 Inhibitor Targeting the ATP Site and the Allosteric αD Pocket. *iScience.* **2024**, *27*, 108903. [CrossRef] [PubMed]
137. Iegre, J.; Brear, P.; Baker, D.J.; Tan, Y.S.; Atkinson, E.L.; Sore, H.F.; Donovan, D.H.O.; Verma, C.S.; Hyvönen, M.; Spring, D.R. Efficient Development of Stable and Highly Functionalised Peptides Targeting the CK2α/CK2β Protein–Protein Interaction. *Chem. Sci.* **2019**, *10*, 5056. [CrossRef]
138. Laudet, B.; Barette, C.; Dulery, V.; Renaudet, O.; Dumy, P.; Metz, A.; Prudent, R.; Deshiere, A.; Dideberg, O.; Filhol, O.; et al. Structure-Based Design of Small Peptide Inhibitors of Protein Kinase CK2 Subunit Interaction. *Biochem. J.* **2007**, *408*, 363. [CrossRef] [PubMed]
139. Atkinson, E.; Iegre, J.; D'Amore, C.; Brear, P.; Salvi, M.; Hyvonen, M.; Spring, D. Development of Small Cyclic Peptides Targeting the CK2α/β Interface. *ChemRxiv* **2022**. [CrossRef]
140. Kufareva, I.; Bestgen, B.; Brear, P.; Prudent, R.; Laudet, B.; Moucadel, V.; Ettaoussi, M.; Sautel, C.F.; Krimm, I.; Engel, M.; et al. Discovery of Holoenzyme-Disrupting Chemicals as Substrate-Selective CK2 Inhibitors. *Sci. Rep.* **2019**, *9*, 15893. [CrossRef]
141. Békés, M.; Langley, D.R.; Crews, C.M. PROTAC Targeted Protein Degraders: The Past Is Prologue. *Nat. Rev. Drug Discov.* **2022**, *21*, 181. [CrossRef]
142. Sun, X.; Gao, H.; Yang, Y.; He, M.; Wu, Y.; Song, Y.; Tong, Y.; Rao, Y. PROTACs: Great Opportunities for Academia and Industry. *Signal Transduct. Target. Ther.* **2019**, *4*, 1. [CrossRef] [PubMed]
143. Ciechanover, A.; Schwartz, A.L. The Ubiquitin-Proteasome Pathway: The Complexity and Myriad Functions of Proteins Death. *Proc. Natl. Acad. Sci. USA* **1998**, *95*, 2727. [CrossRef] [PubMed]
144. Chen, H.; Chen, F.; Liu, N.; Wang, X.; Gou, S. Chemically Induced Degradation of CK2 by Proteolysis Targeting Chimeras Based on a Ubiquitin–Proteasome Pathway. *Bioorg. Chem.* **2018**, *81*, 536. [CrossRef] [PubMed]

kinases and phosphatases

MDPI

Article

Regulation of Mouse CK2α (*Csnk2a1*) Promoter Expression In Vitro and in Cell Lines

Gregory A. Imbrie [†], Nicholas G. Wilson, David C. Seldin [‡] and Isabel Dominguez [*,‡]

Department of Medicine, School of Medicine, Boston University, Boston, MA 02118, USA; gimbrie@mgb.org (G.A.I.); nwilson9@bu.edu (N.G.W.)

* Correspondence: isdoming@bu.edu

† Current address: Heart Vascular Institute, Wentworth-Douglass Hospital, Mass General Brigham, Dover, NH 03820, USA.

‡ These authors contributed equally to this work.

Abstract: CK2α is a kinase important for essential cellular and biological processes. CK2α is ubiquitously expressed, albeit at different tissue levels, and its transcript levels are dysregulated in disease. However, there is limited knowledge on the regulation of CK2α gene expression. The best one studied, the human *CSNK2A1* (CK2α) gene promoter, contains uncharacterized binding motifs for NF-κB. Our goal was to investigate the role of NF-κB in *Csnk2a1* promoter regulation. We cloned the mouse *Csnk2a1* promoter which had significant sequence homology with the human *CSNK2A1* promoter. Using promoter deletions, we identified a minimal promoter region containing transcription factor motifs (NF-κB, Ets-1, Sp1) consistent with those published for the *CSNK2A1* promoter. Electrophoretic mobility shift assays demonstrated specific NF-κB subunit binding to the minimal promoter. NF-κB subunit transfection and extracellular NF-κB stimulation in non-tumor cell lines led to increased transactivation of the mouse minimal promoter. These data, together with data on the regulation of NF-κB by CK2 kinase activity, suggest a positive-feedback loop between CK2α and NF-κB. Non-tumor cell line re-plating and increased percent confluence upregulated *Csnk2a1* transcript levels which differed from tumor cell line published data. In summary, *Csnk2a1* promoter is regulated by NF-κB signaling and during cellular proliferation.

Keywords: *csnk2a1*; protein kinase CK2, CK2α; promoter; transcription factor motifs; NF-κB; p50; cell confluence; transcripts

1. Introduction

Protein kinase CK2 is a highly-conserved holoenzyme composed of catalytic subunits (CK2α and CK2α′) and a regulatory subunit (CK2β) [1–3]. There is also an intronless CK2α pseudogene (*CSNK2A3*) whose function is not well understood. There is significant literature showing the involvement of protein kinase CK2 proteins in various cellular and biological processes and in diseases. These include cell survival [4,5] and proliferation [6], viability of yeast [7], mammalian development [8,9], *Xenopus* dorsal axis formation [10] and oncogenesis [11–14]. Due to the importance of CK2 proteins, a number of studies investigated their endogenous expression. CK2 proteins are ubiquitously expressed however the protein levels differ between tissues [6,15–17]. There is also elevated *CK2* gene expression and protein kinase CK2 activity levels in a variety of different cancer types (reviewed in Chua et al. [14]). Despite their importance, the mechanism(s) controlling expression of CK2 genes and their dysregulation in diseases are not yet understood.

 https://doi.org/10.3390/kinasesphosphatases3030015

Of the CK2 genes, the *CK2α* gene (*CSNK2A1*) has the most data on promoter regulation. The Pyerin laboratory has significantly contributed to the understanding of its genomic structure and expression. The human *CSNK2A1* gene has features consistent with a housekeeping gene: TATA box-less, presence of GC boxes, and a CpG island around exon 1 [18]. The human minimal promoter region contains potential binding sites for the transcription factors Sp1, Ets-1, and NF-κB. These transcription factors play important roles in expression of cytokine and chemokine genes, cellular functions of lymphoid cells and angiogenesis (Ets-1), in the control of genes regulating cell growth, apoptosis, differentiation and immune responses (Sp1), and in the control of genes involved in inflammation, immunity, differentiation, cell growth, tumorigenesis, and apoptosis (NF-κB). Protein kinase CK2 also has roles in many of these cellular and biological processes.

The Sp1, Ets-1, and NF-κ B sites may be functional, as electrophoretic mobility shift assay (EMSA) analysis shows that proteins present in HeLa nuclear extracts bind specifically to *CSNK2A1* gene promoter segments [19]. Importantly, mutation of these binding sites has a significant negative impact on promoter segment activity [19–21]. From their binding site mutation experiments, the Pyerin laboratory proposed a model where Sp1 and Ets-1 are part of a negative feed-back loop to regulate the promoter and proposed that NF-κB serves to fine tune *CSNK2A1* expression. Nevertheless, the significance of NF-κB in *CSNK2A1* promoter regulation has not been studied in vivo. In addition, we lack studies of *CSNK2A1* promoter regulation in a species besides humans, studies utilizing non-cancer cell lines, and the effect of signaling pathways on promoter regulation.

The relationship between protein kinase CK2 and NF-κB is of particular interest to our research team as NF-κB is a well-known proto-oncogene understood to be involved in numerous cell functions, including cell growth, proliferation, anti-apoptosis, and metastasis [22]. Two distinct and interrelated signaling pathways have been proposed for NF-κB signaling activation. One is stimulated by developmental signals which leads to immune cell differentiation and maturation and secondary lymphoid organogenesis (non-canonical), and another is stimulated by inflammatory signals that leads to inflammation (canonical) [23]. Both require the inactivation of the NF-κB inhibitor IκBδ by degradation. The family of NF-κB transcriptional factors is comprised of different members: NF-κB1 (p50) and RelA (p65) which participate in both canonical and not canonical signaling, NF-κB2 (p52) and RelB which participate in non-canonical signaling, and c-Rel which participates in canonical signaling [24]. These five NF-κB monomers can yield up to 15 NF-κB family protein complexes, of which the most common is a p50/p65 heterodimer to induce or repress transcriptional activity [25,26]. In addition to its normal functions, NF-κB signaling is constitutively activated in some cancers which leads to increased proliferation, anti-apoptosis, angiogenesis, epithelial to mesenchymal transition, and metastasis [27].

The data presented here provide information regarding the regulation of mouse *Csnk2a1* promoter regulation in NIH-3T3 (embryonic fibroblast cell line). We identified the gene promoter, a minimal promoter, and transcription binding motifs, and showed the binding of p50 in competitive binding assays. We determined the role of NF-κB signaling in *Csnk2a1* transactivation utilizing NF-κB subunit transfections in NIH-3T3 and standard and physiological NF-κB signaling pathway agonists in mouse peripheral B lymphocytes. We propose a positive regulatory loop between CK2 and NF-κB. In contrast to studies in human cancer cell lines [20,21], *Csnk2a1* transcripts increased shortly after re-plating and in conditions of increasing cell confluence in NIH-3T3 and C57MG (mouse mammary epithelia) cell lines.

2. Results and Discussion

2.1. Characterization of the Mouse *Csnk2a1* Promoter

We utilized the Genome Reference Consortium Mouse Build 39 (GRCm39) to identify the *Mus musculus Csnk2a1* gene. *Csnk2a1* is placed at bases 152,068,468 to 152,123,772 of chromosome 2. We first compared the mouse and human sequence homology upstream of mouse and human exon 1. The *Homo sapiens CSNK2A1* is placed at bases 472,498 to 543,790 (complement) on chromosome 20 in the Genome Reference Consortium Human Build 38 patch release 14 (GRCh38.p14). We used mVISTA to visualize the sequence homology of 1000 bp sequences upstream and including mouse and human exon 1 (Figure 1A). In this 1000 bp sequence alignment, there were several regions with significant sequence homology. Using SIM, the overall similarity of the two sequences was found to be 62.7%. Note that exon 1 is untranslated in both species (153 bp in mice and 119 bp in humans).

A

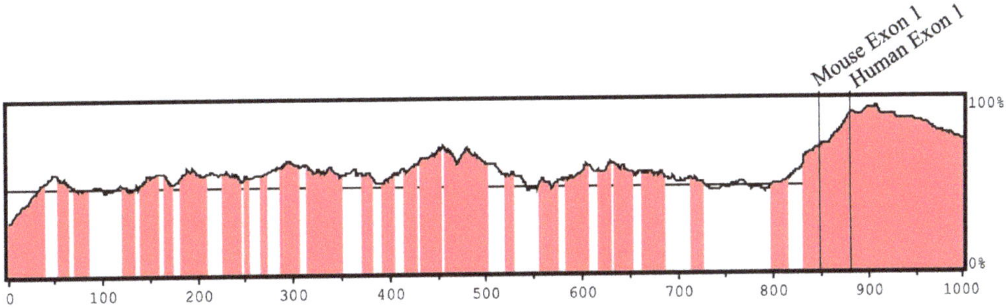

B

```
Mus Musculus   1  AGCCTCGCTCTGGTCCCTGCGGCTGGCGGCCGAGCCGTGTGTCTCCTCCTCCGCCGCCGC
Homo Sapiens   1  AGCCTCGCTCTGGTCCCTGCGGCTGGCGGCCGAGCCGTGTGTCTCCTCCTCCATCGCCGC
                  ****************************************************  ******

Mus Musculus  61  CATATTGTCTGTGTGAAGCTAGGGGAGCGCGGCTATTGCCGCTGCCGCTTCCACCGCAG
Homo Sapiens  61  CATATTGTCTGTGTGAGCAGAGGGGAGAGCGGCCGCCGCCGCTGCCGCTTCCACCACAG
                  ****************    ******* *****    ****************** ***
```

Figure 1. Mouse *Csnk2a1* and human *CSNK2A1* sequence alignment. (**A**) 1000 bp sequence comparison upstream and through exon 1 of mouse *Csnk2a1* and human *CSNK2A1*. Areas in red indicate regions of at least 70% similarity which are at least 10 bp long. Noted on this figure are the start positions of mouse *Csnk2a1* exon 1 and human *CSNK2A1* exon 1. This figure was generated using mVista. (**B**) Sequence alignment of the last 119 bp of the 153 bp mouse *Csnk2a1* exon 1 and all of human *CSNK2A1* exon 1 (119 bp). This alignment was generated using SIM. Asterisks (*) indicate positions conserved.

We analyzed the promoter sequences to identify similarities between both species. Exon 1, the transcriptional start site1 (TSS1), is untranslated in both species (153 bp in mice and 119 bp in humans). Sequence alignment showed that the last 119 bp of the mouse *Csnk2a1* exon 1 has an 89.9% similarity with the 119 bp human *CSNK2A1* exon 1 (Figure 1B). The sequence of the first 34 bp of mouse exon 1 has a 91.2% similarity to the sequence upstream of the TSS1 in humans (Figure 1B).

Review of mouse *Csnk2a1* transcript variants listed in NCBI found that the transcriptional start site (TSS) was variable. Eight of the 13 transcript variants contained the 153 bp exon 1, which we utilized in this study. Two more variants contained the same exon 1 start, however with extended exon 1 sequences. The other three variants did not contain any portion of our selected exon 1, and two of these were significantly truncated transcript variants.

In mice, a putative TATA box with the sequence 5′-TATAA-3′ is found at position −90, which is likely non-functional, as most TATA-box motifs are located between positions −20 to −35 [28]. The human *CSNK2A1* promoter was reported not to include a TATA box or CAAT box [18,29]. Using the last human genome compilation, we confirmed that there were no TATA box sequences upstream of human *CSNK2A1* exon 1. Similarly, there is no CAAT box upstream of the mouse promoter. There is a CAAT box in the human promoter found at −117, most likely not functional, as CAAT box motifs are between −75 to −80 [28].

Taken together, the *CSNK2A1* mouse and human promoters have similar characteristics indicating conservation of regulation cross-species.

2.2. Identification of the Mouse Csnk2a1 Minimal Promoter

To understand the regulation of the mouse *Csnk2a1* gene, we next identified its minimal promoter region using similar methods to Krehan et al. [19]. To determine the mouse minimal promoter, we generated plasmids pLuc1 (−3955 to +153), pLuc2 (−735 to +153), pLuc3 (−453 to +153), pLuc4 (−273 to +153), pLuc5 (−273 to +31), pLuc6 (−183 to +153), pLuc7 (−135 to +153), pLuc8 (−95 to +153), and pLuc9 (−273 to −80) (Figure 2A). We transfected these plasmids into subconfluent NIH-3T3 cells along with Renilla to control transfection efficiency. The luciferase activity of the *Csnk2a1* promoter deletion variants was then normalized to the activity of the full-length *Csnk2a1* promoter, pLuc1 (Figure 2B). pLuc2-4 and pLuc6-8 maintain complete activity, suggesting that the region upstream from −735 is not essential for promoter activity. Welch's *t*-test was performed on all pLuc constructs against pLuc1 and it was found that luciferase activity for pLuc4 ($p = 0.002$) and pLuc7 ($p = 0.011$) were significantly different from that of pLuc1. pLuc5 (−273 to +31) construct retains full activity, therefore the +31 to +153 (the majority of exon 1) region is not required for *Csnk2a1* promoter activity. pLuc9 (−273 to −81), containing a deletion of the entire region downstream of the putative TATA sequence, exhibits a total loss of activity. With Welch's *t*-test it was found that the activity of pLuc5 ($p = 0.015$) and pLuc9 ($p = < 0.001$) was significantly different from that of pLuc1. This suggests that the minimal functional mouse *Csnk2a1* promoter must span or be contained within −95 to +31. Further studies could use additional deletion constructs to investigate whether smaller sequences upstream of exon 1 retain promoter function. The results also suggest that the region upstream of the minimal promoter (−3955 to −735) may contain a transcriptional silencer(s), as pLuc1 has less activity than the 5′ deletions, although this needs to be investigated. The region upstream of the minimal promoter (−735 to −95) may also contain a transcriptional silencer(s) given that pLuc1 through pLuc7 have decreased luciferase activity relative to pLuc8. However, it should be noted that this observation is not significant when we compared the activity of all pLuc constructs to that of pLuc8 using Welch's *t*-test.

Next, we investigated the homology between the mouse and human minimal promoters. We performed sequence alignment using our identified mouse *Csnk2a1* minimal promoter and the Krehan et al. human *CSNK2A1* minimal promoter (Figure 3). Krehan et al. identified the human *CSNK2A1* minimal promoter in a region comprising positions −89 to 15 using the current position for exon 1, with a region of maximal promoter activity located from positions −59 to −4 (Note: Krehan et al. identified two transcription start sites (TSS1 and TSS2); in this work, we use the current start of human *CSNK2A1* exon 1 which is TSS2 by Krehan et al.) [19]. The 126 bp mouse *Csnk2a1* minimal promoter and 104 bp human *CSNK2A1* minimal promoter, when aligned, have a region of overlap of 85 bp with 79.2% similarity as determined by SIM. Contained in this 85 bp region of overlap is 55 bp of the 56 bp region of maximal activity identified by Krehan et al [19]. Looking just at this region of maximal activity, there is 80.7% similarity between the mouse and human promoter sequences.

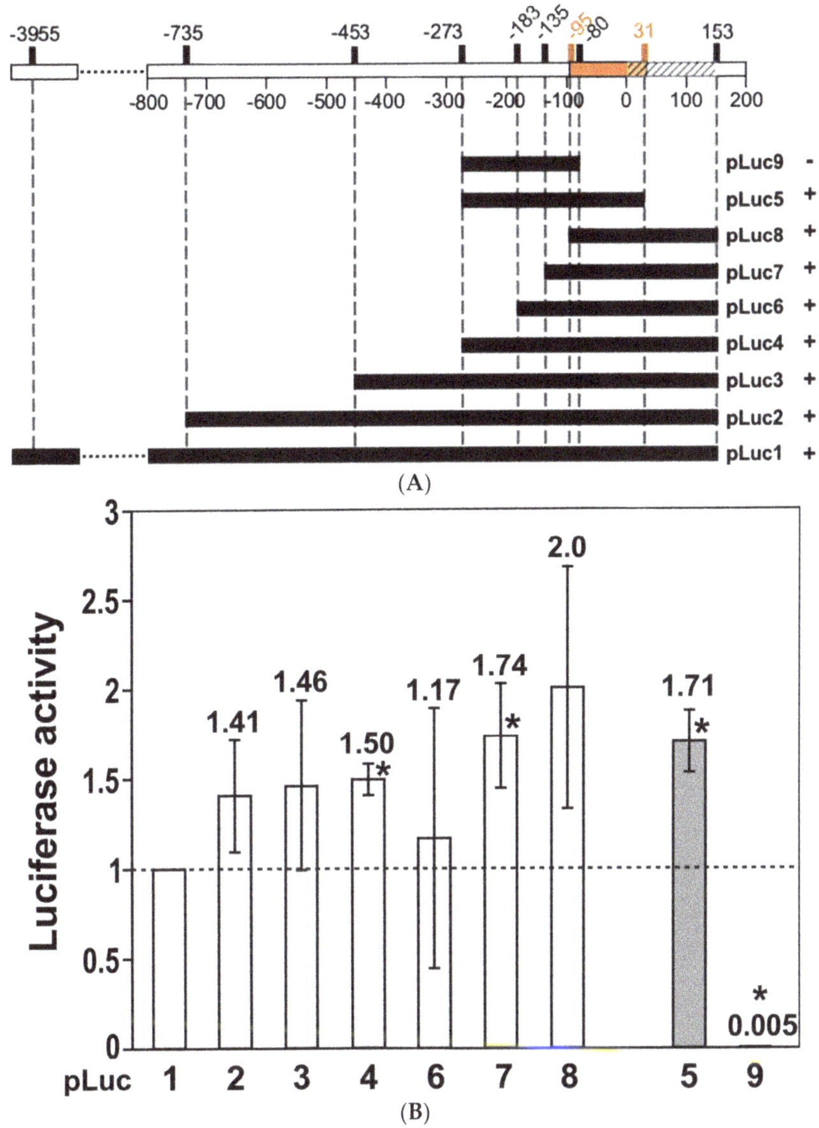

Figure 2. Mouse *Csnk2a1* promoter deletion constructs and luciferase assays. (**A**) Schematic mouse *Csnk2a1* promoter and the generated promoter–luciferase deletion clones. The start of exon 1 is labeled as position 1 (dashed box). The minimal promoter spans from −95 to +31 (orange box). (**B**) Luciferase assay results for the promoter–luciferase deletion clones normalized to Renilla activity. Luciferase activity is normalized to pLuc1 activity. Each plasmid construct underwent two independent transfections performed in duplicate. Bars represent average normalized luciferase activity and error bars represent confidence intervals. The pLuc9 construct showed no luciferase activity. Asterisks represent values which are significantly different from pLuc1 (*) indicates statistically significant ($p < 0.05$).

```
                                -95
MusMusculus     1 -----CAGATGATATAA-AG------CCAG--TCGGCGGGGGCTGCGCTA   36
                       |..|.|.||.|| ||      ||||  |       |||.||
HomoSapiens     1 AATCCCTAAGGTTACAATAGGACATCCCAGCAT-------GGCCGC----   39

MusMusculus    37 AGTCAGAG-----CCTCCGAGGGCGGGGCGCCTCCGCCTTTTCCG--GCT   79
                  |.||||||     ||||.|.||||||.|              ||.|  |||
HomoSapiens    40 ATTCAGAGAGATTCCTCTGGGGGCGGAG------------TCGGAAGCT   76
                     -89
                     SP1             0 (TS)        ELK1          NRF2
MusMusculus    80 ---CCGCCCCGCCT-CTGGTTGGGAGGGGGCTTCCGCTTCCGGCAGCGGA  125
                     .|||||||||| |||| |.||||||||.||||||||||||||||.|.
HomoSapiens    77 GTCTCGCCCCGCCTCCTGG-TAGGAGGGGGTTTCCGCTTCCGGCAGCAGC  125
                                               NF-κB            ETS-
                     30                 (p50, p65, c-Rel)         1
MusMusculus   126 GGCTGCAGCCTCGCTCTGGTCCCTGCGGCTGGCGGCCGAGCCGTGTGTCT  175
                  ||||||||||||||||||||||||||||||||||||||||||||||||||
HomoSapiens   126 GGCTGCAGCCTCGCTCTGGTCCCTGCGGCTGGCGGCCGAGCCGTGTGTCT  175
                      0 (TS)          15

MusMusculus   176 CCTCCTCCGCCGCCGCCATATTGTCTGTGTGA--AGCTAGGGGAGCGCGG  223
                  ||||||||..||||||||||||||||||||||  ||  |||||||.||||
HomoSapiens   176 CCTCCTCCATCGCCGCCATATTGTCTGTGTGAGCAG--AGGGGAGAGCGG  223

MusMusculus   224 CTATTGCCGCTGCCGCTTCCACCGCAG     250
                  |....||||||||||||||||||.|||
HomoSapiens   224 CCGCCGCCGCTGCCGCTTCCACCACAG     250
```

Figure 3. Putative transcription factor binding sites in the mouse *Csnk2a1* and human *CSNK2A1* promoters. Both the mouse and human have the position between the start of their respective exon 1 and upstream regions as position zero (0). The green region (−89 to 15) represents the *Mus musculus Csnk2a1* minimal promoter identified in this paper. The yellow region (−59 to 15) represents the *Homo sapiens CSNK2A1* minimal promoter identified by Krehan et al. [19]. The red region (−59 to −4) represents the *Homo sapiens CSNK2A1* region of maximal activity within the minimal promoter identified by Krehan et al [19]. Putative binding sites for the transcription factors SP1, NFKB1 (p50), REL-A (p65), CREL, Ets-1, ELK1, and NRF2 were predicted within this promoter region of maximal activity using TFBIND. This alignment was generated using EMBOSS Needle.

2.3. Transcription Factor Binding Analysis of the Minimal Csnk2a1 Promoter

The mouse *Csnk2a1* and human *CSNK2A1* minimal promoter sequences were analyzed to predict transcription factor binding via the TRANSFAC R3.4 database utilizing TFBIND. The analysis generated the similarity to the consensus binding sequence, and we used 0.8 as the similarity cut-off to generate the list of potential transcription binding sites. This analysis identified potential binding sites for SP1 (91.4% similarity in mice, 95.1% similarity in humans), NF-κB p50 (83.9%, 91.4%), NF-κB p65 (85.4%, 96.2%), C-Rel (92.1%, 98.1%), Elk1 (93.0%, 85.3%), Ets-1 (96.4%, 96.4%), and Nrf2 (93.7%, 93.7%) (Figure 3). These findings largely agree with the transcription factors identified by Pyerin et al. (NF-κB, Ets-1, Sp1) as having a potential role in the human *CSNK2A1* promoter [19]. Supporting the role of Ets-1, a study in hepatocellular carcinoma cells showed that the histone deacetylase inhibitors AR42 and MS-275 increased *CK2α* transcription and enhanced the recruitment of Ets-1 to the CK2α promoter. This occurred without altering the expression of Ets-1 [30]. Future studies could investigate whether Sp1 and NF-κB are also recruited to the *Csnk2a1* promoter under these and other conditions.

In addition, the TFBIND analysis showed the potential for additional regulation of the *Csnk2a1* promoter by Elk1 and Nrf2. Elk1, a subclass of the Ets family, is involved in cell proliferation, differentiation and survival, hematopoiesis, angiogenesis, cognition, neurodegeneration, and cancer. Elk1 is ubiquitously expressed and highly expressed in cortex and lymphoblasts [31]. Nrf2 is also ubiquitously expressed with highest expression in blood cells, thyroid, smooth muscle, and bronchial epithelial cells. Activation of Nrf2 transactivates cytoprotective proteins [32].

In summary, the observation that the consensus sites for these transcription factors (NF-κB, Ets-1, Sp1) are preserved in the minimal promoters of both mouse and human further strengthens the importance of these transcription factors as regulators for *Csnk2a1*.

2.4. NF-κB Subunits Bind the Csnk2a1 Promoter

Here we focus on NF-κB interaction with the *Csnk2a1* promoter as it is understudied. The NF-κB (c-Rel) site is preserved in both mouse and human minimal promoters; however, the mouse sequence has a one base difference within the consensus (Figure 3). This is noteworthy as the consensus binding site for NF-κB (c-Rel) is loose (SGGRNWTTCC, where S = C or G, W = A or T, R = A or G, Y = C or T, K = G or T, M = A or C, N = any base pair) [33].

To test a direct interaction between NF-κB and the mouse *Csnk2a1* minimal promoter, EMSA was performed with a double-stranded oligonucleotide probe overlapping the putative NF-κB in the *Csnk2a1* minimal promoter. Nuclear extracts were prepared from NIH-3T3 untransfected cells and cells transfected with p50 and c-Rel subunits. Potential specific bands, denoted by arrowheads, were observed (Figure 4). To assess the specificity of these bands, a competitor NF-κB-specific oligonucleotide encoding the c-myc upstream response element (URE) was introduced at concentrations of 5× and 50×. An excess of the URE should outcompete specific binding of the *Csnk2a1* promoter oligonucleotide to genuine NF-κB transcription factors resulting in eliminating bands in the EMSA. Furthermore, as NF-κB signaling often involves a p50 homodimer or heterodimer, a supershift analysis was conducted using a p50 antibody. Any shift up to a slower mobility complex or alterations in the density of the shifted bands would indicate the presence of p50 in the transcriptional complex.

The band designated by the black arrowhead intensifies in the presence of the p50 supershifting antibody and disappears when challenged with a 50× competing URE oligonucleotide, indicating its specificity for NF-κB. The band designated by the white arrowhead disappears with the p50 antibody and is eliminated with both 5× and 50× competitor URE oligonucleotide. This suggests that the bands marked by the white and black arrowheads could potentially be p50 homodimers or heterodimers. The band designated by the gray arrowhead exhibits a shift with the p50 antibody, confirming the presence of p50. However, this band darkens with the competitor URE oligonucleotide and is not competed away. This observation could be attributed to p50 binding in a complex with another transcription factor and/or possibly acting on a non-canonical NF-κB site [34]. Here, we demonstrate for the first time that p50 interacted with the *Csnk2a1* minimal promoter, potentially forming different NF-κB complexes. Based on the mouse and human minimal promoter homology we hypothesize that p50 is likely to interact with the human *CSNK2A1* minimal promoter as well. This fits well with data from the Pyerin laboratory on the *CSNK2A1* minimal promoter [19]. Oligonucleotides containing the *CSNK2A1* gene promoter segment that contains the NF-κB binding sequence can bind p65 (an NF-κB subunit)) found in HeLa nuclear extracts. Electrophoretic mobility shift assay (EMSA) analysis show that proteins present in HeLa nuclear extracts bind specifically (reduced protein binding in the presence of oligonucleotides with the consensus motif mutated) to the *CSNK2A1* gene promoter segment that contains the NF-κB binding sequence [19–21].

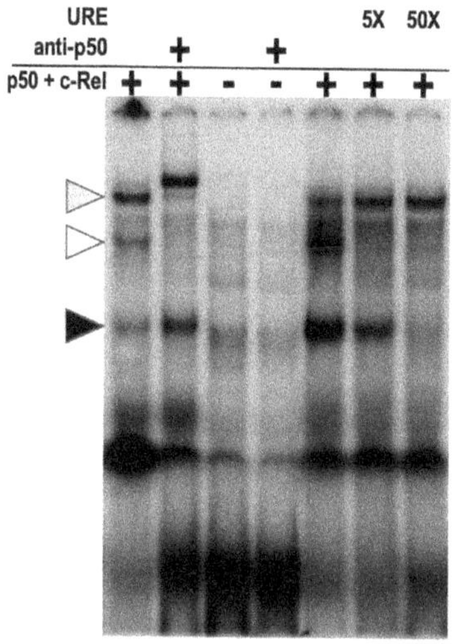

Figure 4. Electrophoretic mobility shift assay utilizing an oligonucleotide containing the putative NF-κB site in the mouse *Csnk2a1* promoter. Nuclear extracts of p50 and c-Rel transfected or untransfected NIH-3T3 cells were used as indicated by + and − over the lanes. Samples where antibody anti-p50 and URE were added are indicated by + over the lanes. The shift assay detected two distinctive bands associated with p50 (black and white arrowheads) and a third band that could potentially involve the formation of a complex between p50 and an unidentified transcription factor or binding to a non-canonical NF-κB site (gray arrowhead).

2.5. *Csnk2a1 Transcription Is Upregulated by NF-κB Subunit Expression*

The Pyerin studies, which proposed NF-κB to have a role in transcriptional regulation of the human *CSNK2A1* minimal promoter, also demonstrated that point mutations (3 bases at a time) of the NF-κB consensus sequence reduced promoter activity. Our laboratory and others have previously studied biological relationships between protein CK2 and NF-κB in cancer, which together indicate that protein kinase CK2 and NF-κB interact in several signaling pathways [13]; therefore, we investigated the role of NF-κB in regulating the *Csnk2a1* promoter.

We first tested whether NF-κB regulates the transcription of the *Csnk2a1* promoter by transfecting NIH-3T3 with NF-κB subunits and analyzed the changes in luciferase activity of *Csnk2a1* promoter constructs. For this, plasmid pLuc8, containing only the mouse minimal promoter and exon 1, was co-transfected with different combinations of NF-κB subunits (p50, p65, RelB) into NIH-3T3 cells at 30% confluence and subsequently harvested 48 h later. Bcl3 was added to some of these transfections as it has been shown to decrease repressive p50 and p52 homodimers and allow transcriptional activation from other NF-κB family complexes [35,36]. For these experiments, Renilla proved to be an inadequate control as we observed that NF-κB subunit transfection enhanced pRL-SV40 Renilla expression, potentially through NF-κB binding sites in its promoter. Therefore, luciferase activity was normalized to the respective protein concentration in each lysate. Cells were co-transfected with GFP to confirm equal transfection efficiency.

For the first series of co-transfections, 200 ng of pLuc8, was co-transfected in duplicate with 4 μg of each the NF-κB subunits (p50 + RelB, p50 + p65, p50 + Bcl3), and pCDNA3 was used as a negative control. When normalized to the activity of the pCDNA3 control, the luciferase activity of each co-transfection was as follows: p50 + RelB, 2.97-fold; p50 + p65, 2.20-fold; p50 + Bcl3, 2.40-fold.

A second series of co-transfections was performed by co-transfecting 200 ng pLuc8 in triplicate with 3 µg of the following NF-κB subunit combinations: p50 alone, p50 + cRel, p50 + RelB, p50 + p65, p50 + Bcl3, Bcl3 + p52 (Figure 5). Relative to the activity of pCDNA3, the luciferase activity of all co-transfection increased. It is interesting that the p50+p50 transfections led to increased activity of the *Csnk2a1* promoter construct, as the p50 homodimer is thought to repress transcription. However, we did not confirm that the p50+p50 transfections actually led to formation of p50 homodimers. It is possible that these p50 subunits instead formed heterodimers with other members of the NF-κB family which induce transcription. Indeed, it was demonstrated in the past that p50 preferentially forms heterodimers [37,38]. In summary, diverse combinations of NF-κB subunits increased transactivation of the *Csnk2a1* promoter construct. This is an important new finding, suggesting that NF-κB has a positive effect on *Csnk2a1* transcriptional regulation.

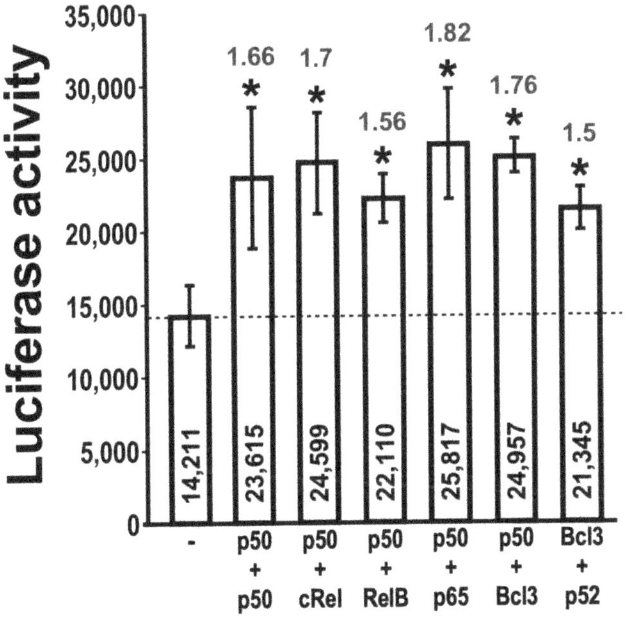

Figure 5. *Csnk2a1* minimal promoter (pLuc8) expression is upregulated by NF-κB. Luciferase activity of pLuc8 after co-transfection with NF-κB subunits (p50 + p50, p50 + cRel, p50 + RelB, p50 + p65, p50 + Bcl3, and Bcl3 + p52), or pCDNA3. Columns represent average luciferase activity (average number included in the bar), and error bars are standard deviations. The number above the columns represents the fold increase over the control. (*) indicates statistically significant ($p < 0.05$).

The levels of *Csnk2a1* promoter activation by NF-κB shown here (1.5 to 1.8×) are larger than the levels of *CSNK2A1* promoter activation by transfection of Ets-1 in HeLa cells (1.25×) [20]. This was unexpected, as Pyerin demonstrated that mutations of Sp1 and Ets-1 binding sites reduced *CSNK2A1* transactivation to a much larger extent (70–75%) than mutation of NF-κB binding sites (40%), and from this posited that NF-κB may serve to fine-tune *CSNK2A1* expression [19]. Nonetheless, our data here indicated that NF-κB could be a significant driver of *Csnk2A1*. Conservation of NF-κB motifs between the mouse and human *CSNK2A1* minimal promoter further suggests its importance in regulation. The difference between the degree of upregulation between our NF-κB data and Pyerin's Ets-1 data could be explained by differences in the cells used (non-cancer vs. cancer cells) [19]. Human cancer cells may have almost maximal expression of *CSNK2A1*, diminishing the effect of Ets-1 on promoter upregulation, whereas NIH-3T3, a non-cancer cell line, may have low basal *Csnk2a1* expression, allowing NF-κB subunit transfection to induce stronger *Csnk2a1* promoter activation. The difference may be also due to differences in the length of the promoter sequences utilized (minimal versus or not) or in transfection efficiency. Future experiments could compare the activation of the different promoters in parallel using diverse cell lines to address the contribution of the different transcription factors in promoter regulation.

2.6. Regulation of Endogenous Mouse Csnk2a1 Promoter by Extracellular NF-κB Agonists

Our experiments so far showed that NF-κB subunits bound and increased transcription of the mouse *Csnk2a1* minimal promoter. We next determined whether activation of NF-κB signaling by extracellular agonists could upregulate endogenous *Csnk2a1* promoter. The expectation is that if NF-κB upregulates *Csnk2a1* promoter transcription, then activation of NF-κB signaling should lead to increased levels of endogenous *Csnk2a1* mRNA transcripts. NF-κB signaling pathway stimulants (i.e., they signal via NF-κB family protein complexes) include phorbol myristic acid + ionomycin, IgM, CD40 and CD8a, and lipopolysaccharide which we use in this study [39–42].

For this study, mouse peripheral B lymphocytes were chosen for their ability to activate the NF-κB signaling pathway in a stimulable manner [39]. To stimulate the NF-κB signaling pathway, the following chemical and physiological growth stimulants were chosen: PMA (phorbol myristic acid) + I (ionomycin) at two different concentrations (Snow protocol and Roth protocols described in the Methods Section) [39,43], lipopolysaccharide [42,44,45], anti-mouse IgM [40,41,46], and CD40 ligand + CD8a [47]. Following B lymphocyte stimulation, RT-qPCR analysis was used to measure *Csnk2a1* copy number which was normalized to endogenous β-actin *(Actb)*.

For the first series of B lymphocyte stimulation experiments, PMA + I was used to stimulate rested B lymphocytes and samples processed after addition (0) and after 4, 20, 32, and 48 h. PMA + I resulted in significant early upregulation of *Csnk2a1* mRNA at the four-hour time point (three-fold over time 0) (Figure 6A). From 24 h onwards, *Csnk2a1* copy number was significantly downregulated, suggesting negative feedback.

Next, physiological agonists anti-IgM, LPS, and CD40 ligand + CD8a were used and compared with two different PMA + I stimulation protocols (Snow and Roth). Cells were collected immediately after stimulation or after 2.5 or 5 h (Figure 6B). One "P + I Snow" five-hour time point was found to have poor dissociation curves and unusable qPCR data and therefore is not included. All the agonists increased *Csnk2a1* mRNA levels at 2.5 h which was maintained at 5 h. The increase in *Csnk2a1* mRNA levels associated with each stimulus at 2.5 h ranged from a 1.5- to almost 4-fold increase, with the greatest increase found in PMA + I and anti-IgM. Lastly, we confirmed that our chosen chemical or physiological stimulants increased NF-κB signaling by evaluating their stimulation of IκBα transcription (*Nfkiba*) (Figure 6C). *Nfkiba* was chosen as its transcription is upregulated as part of a negative feedback mechanism in the NF-κB signaling pathway [48].

In a previous study, DeBenedette and Snow demonstrated that protein kinase CK2 activity exhibits a biphasic increase (peaking at 18 and 48 h) in primary B cells upon NF-κB signaling pathway stimulation with PMA + I [39]. They determined that the increased protein kinase CK2 activity levels resulted from stimulation with the polyamine ODC. The increase in protein kinase CK2 activity levels that they observed could be due to increased levels of CK2 protein and/or *Csnk2a1* mRNA. Here, we show that the stimulants PMA

+ I, LPS, anti-IgM, and CD40 ligand + CD8a resulted in increased NF-κB signaling and increased *Csnk2a1* mRNA levels. This increase in *Csnk2a1* mRNA levels by NF-κB signaling pathway stimulation provides a possible explanation for the increase in protein kinase CK2 activity shown by DeBenedette and Snow. Future experiments could determine correlations and/or parallels between protein kinase CK2 protein and activity levels and increased mRNA levels upon NF-κB signaling.

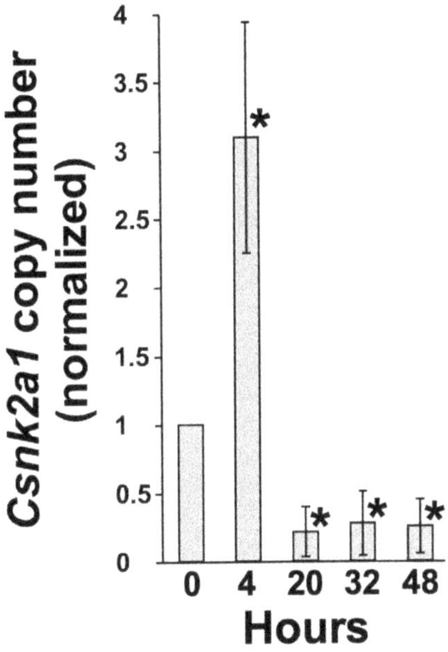

(A)

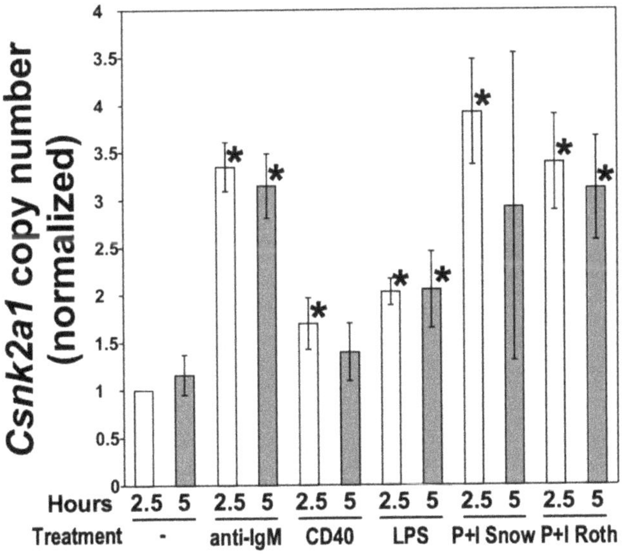

(B)

Figure 6. *Cont.*

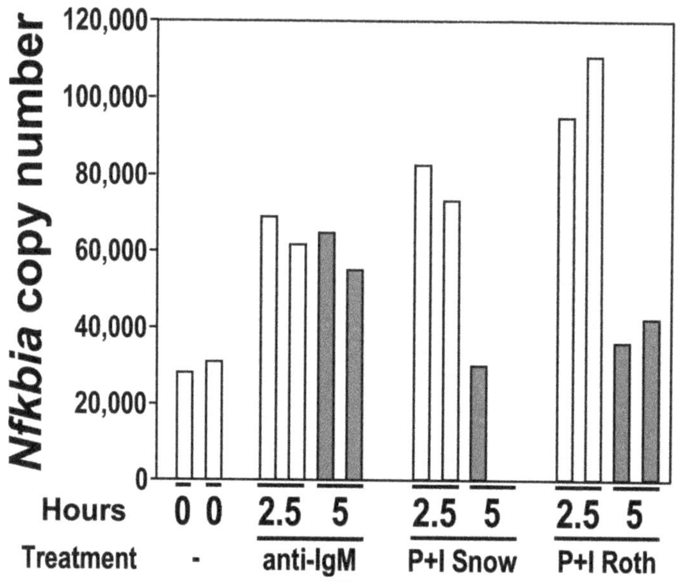

(C)

Figure 6. B cell stimulation resulted in increased *Csnk2a1* mRNA levels and NF-κB signaling. (**A**) qPCR analysis to *Csnk2a1* (primers to exon 9–10) normalized to *Actb* from primary B cells stimulated via addition of PMA + I (20 ng/mL PMA and 0.7 ng ionomycin). This experiment was performed four times in duplicate. Bars represent average normalized Csnk2a1 copy number and error bars represent 95% confidence intervals. (**B**) qPCR analysis to *Csnk2a1* (primers to exon 9–10) normalized to *Actb* from primary B cell stimulation via addition of 15 μg/mL anti-mouse IgM, 1:10 dilution of CD40 ligand + 1:40 dilution of CD8a, 15 μg/mL LPS, or PMA + I (Snow or Roth protocols). This experiment was performed four times in duplicate. Bars represent average normalized *Csnk2a1* copy number and error bars represent 95% confidence intervals. (**C**) qPCR analysis to *Nfkbia* primers and normalized to *Actb* from primary B cell stimulation via addition of 15 μg/mL anti-mouse IgM, or PMA + I (Snow or Roth protocols). This experiment was performed in duplicate and both results are shown. (*) indicates statistically significant ($p < 0.05$).

2.7. *Proposed NF-κB/CK2α Positive Feedback Loop*

In normal B cells, basal NF-κB activity is limited by sequestration in a complex with inhibitor IκBα (Figure 7) [49]. Stimulation of the NF-κB pathway releases NF-κB from this complex to transactivate genes, such as *Csnk2a1*. NF-κB activation also induces the expression of IκBα, thereby resulting in feedback inhibition of the NF-κB pathway. Protein kinase CK2 has been well-established as a positive regulator of NF-κB signaling (Figure 7, blue arrows) [13]. CK2 phosphorylates p65, thereby activating it to enhance NF-κB signaling (Figure 7) [50,51]. CK2 also inactivates IκBα via phosphorylation [50,52,53]. The findings presented in this study suggest a potential positive feedback loop between NF-κB and CK2α, at least in normal B cells. In our proposed model, NF-κB stimulation of CK2α may have a buffering effect through inhibition of IκBα by preventing immediate signaling suppression, thereby sustaining NF-κB signaling (Figure 7).

Additional evidence of a positive self-regulation loop implicating protein kinase CK2 activity in its own expression comes from the study from Lupp et al. demonstrating that expression of CK2α or CK2α′, but not CK2β, are sufficient to transactivate the CK2α and CK2β promoters. In addition, Lupp et al. show that CK2 activity is necessary for CK2α and CK2β promoter activity as 90% inhibition of CK2 kinase activity resulted in a decrease of CK2α and CK2β promoter activity by 50% and 25%, respectively [54]. The mechanism involved in this positive self-regulation loop has not been determined; nonetheless, several recent lines of evidence show that CK2α does not bind to the promoter of CK2α or CK2β, including chromatin immunoprecipitation assays [54] and the yeast-based one-hybrid system [55]. Based on our data, it is plausible that Lupps' positive self-regulation loop is due to the expressed CK2 proteins regulating NF-κB activity.

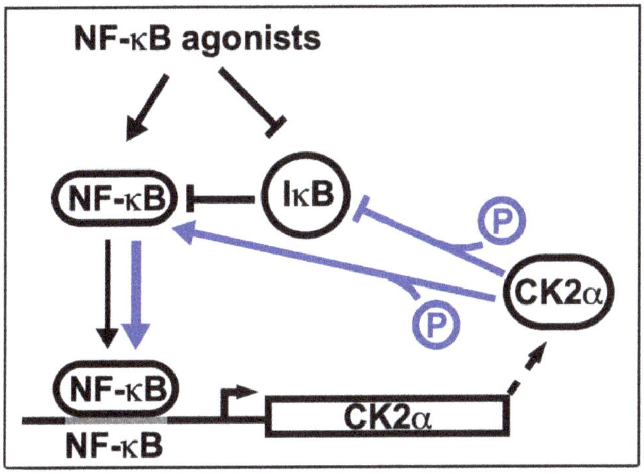

Figure 7. Proposed NF-κB/*Csnk2a1* positive feedback loop.

As CK2α and NF-κB are both known proto-oncogenes that contribute to cellular transformation and the development of cancer, the proposed CK2α-NF-κB positive feedback model has significant implications in cancer biology [13,53,56–58]. Thus, upregulation of *Csnk2a1* or constitutive NF-κB signaling could initiate a perpetually activated positive feedback loop resulting in increased protein kinase CK2 activity and NF-κB signaling. To test this proposed model, future experiments could investigate whether NF-κB signaling activation correlates with increased levels of CK2α transcript, protein, and activity. Additionally, pharmacological blockade of NF-κB or non-degradable IκB super-repressor constructs could be employed to demonstrate that NF-κB signaling is indeed necessary for the early *Csnk2a1* transcriptional increase observed upon NF-κB signaling activation. Lastly, pharmacological blockade of CK2 at different times during NF-κB signaling activation can be used to show that CK2 is needed to inhibit the IκB feedback-loop inhibition.

The proposed sustained elevation of CK2α and NF-κB signaling aligns closely with observations in cancerous cells, where co-overexpression of both CK2α and NF-κB has been observed. For example, mouse mammary gland cancers and human breast cancers that had constitutive NF-κB expression were also found to have elevated protein kinase CK2 levels [52,59,60]. This feedback model could also explain the ability of *Csnk2a1* to induce lymphoma when driven by a μ heavy chain enhancer and promoter in transgenic mice [61]. It is important to note that the resulting lymphomas required a "second hit" to drive cancer proliferation. Similarly, CK2α overexpression in mouse mammary glands leads to late tumor formation, at a median age of almost 2 years [62]. Therefore, alterations in *Csnk2a1* expression may be an important factor in carcinogenesis but may not be sufficient to drive cancer proliferation on its own as reported in other studies for CK2α' [63].

In contrast, a negative feed-back mechanism was proposed for Ets-1 and Sp1 by Pyerin's team. Notably, protein kinase CK2 phosphorylates Sp1, and potential CK2 phosphorylation sites have been identified for Ets-1 [19,50,51,64,65]. Protein kinase phosphorylation of Sp1 decreases its binding to DNA, providing a plausible mechanism for negative self-regulation of CK2 gene transcription [64]. Both the negative and positive feedback mechanism could contribute to precise regulation of the *CK2α* promoter. Other signaling pathways can also regulate the *CSNK2A1* promoter. Indeed, *Csnk2a1* levels are upregulated in mouse mammary gland cells transfected with Wnt-1 [66], and in human breast cancer cells exposed to estrogen [67].

2.8. Re-Plating and Percent Confluence Increased Csnk2a1 Transcript Levels

We examined changes in expression levels of Csnk2a1 transcripts in non-cancer cell lines. For this we investigated *Csnk2a1* transcriptional regulation in NIH-3T3 upon different conditions, such as cell re-plating and cell confluence.

For cell re-plating, NIH-3T3 cells were first grown to 40% confluence. New media was then added, and cells were grown for 10 h. The media was removed, and cells were trypsinized, washed with PBS two times, centrifuged at 1000 rpm for 6 min, and then resuspended in the original media. Cells were collected for RNA analysis both before trypsinization and at 120, 180, 285, 405, and 510 min after re-plating. RT-qPCR was used to evaluate the copy number of *Csnk2a1* mRNA which was normalized to *Actb* mRNA (Figure 8A). Re-plating led to a transient rise in *Csnk2a1* mRNA levels after around 120 min. This transient upregulation of *Csnk2a1* mRNA levels after re-plating suggests that transient upregulation of *Csnk2a1* is beneficial to cells when their adhesion is limited. We can draw parallels between these results and Giusiano's findings of elevated levels of CK2α protein and protein kinase CK2 activity associated with increased metastatic risk [68]. Future re-plating experiments could use CK2 chemical inhibitors, inducible RNAi/siRNA, and inducible CK2 expression to investigate whether the transient upregulation of CK2 is essential for cell survival when adhesion is limited. In addition, parallel studies on cells replated at varying confluences could help determine whether the alterations in *Csnk2a1* mRNA are attributable to the initial adhesion or if they reflect specific confluence levels.

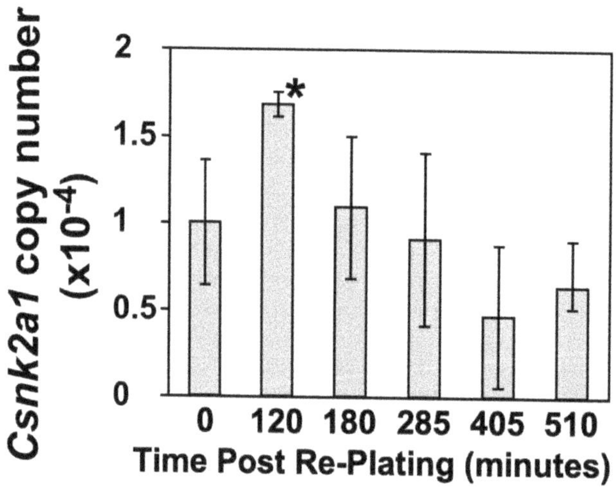

(A)

Figure 8. *Cont.*

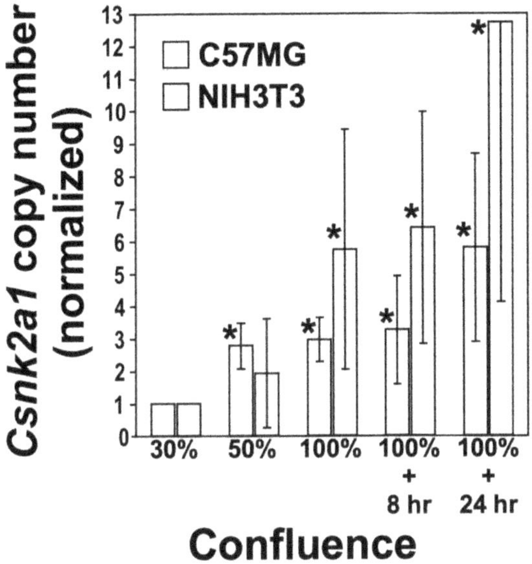

(B)

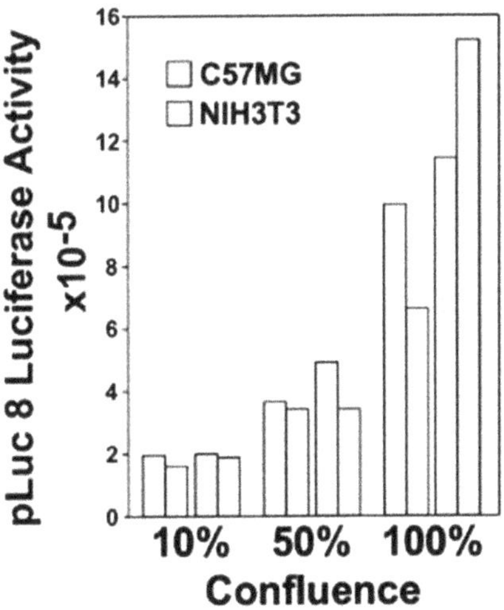

(C)

Figure 8. *Csnk2a1* mRNA levels transiently increased after re-plating and with increased confluence. (**A**) *Csnk2a1* mRNA levels in NIH-3T3 cells were measured via RT-qPCR analysis before trypsinization and at several time points after re-plating. *Csnk2a1* mRNA levels were normalized to *Actb* mRNA. This experiment was performed twice in duplicate. Bars represent average *Csnk2a1* copy number and error bars represent 95% confidence intervals. (**B**) NIH-3T3 and C57MG cells were harvested at increasing levels of confluence. *Csnk2a1* mRNA copy number was analyzed via RT-qPCR and normalized to *Actb* mRNA levels. This experiment was performed four times in duplicate. Bars represent average normalized *Csnk2a1* copy number and error bars represent 95% confidence intervals. (**C**) NIH-3T3 and C57MG cells transfected with pLuc8 were harvested at increasing levels of confluence. pLuc8 transcription was assessed via measurement of luciferase activity normalized to the protein level of the sample. This experiment was performed in duplicate and both results are shown. (*) indicates statistically significant ($p < 0.05$).

To study the effects of increasing cell confluence on *Csnk2a1* transcription, NIH-3T3 and C57MG cells were plated at a very low cell density. These cells were harvested, and the RNA was extracted at increasing levels of confluence: 30%, 50%, 100%, after 8 h at 100% confluence, and after 24 h at 100% confluence. RT-qPCR was used to evaluate the copy number of *Csnk2a1* mRNA which was normalized to *Actb* (Figure 8B). In both NIH-3T3 and C57MG cells, levels of *Csnk2a1* mRNA increased with cell confluence. Next, we investigated whether this effect is mediated by the *Csnk2a1* minimal promoter. For this, the pLuc8 plasmid was transfected into NIH-3T3 at 25% confluence on a plate and allowed to grow 24 h. The cells were then replated at 5–10% confluence. These cells were then harvested for luciferase assay and measurement of protein concentration at increasing levels of confluence: 10%, 50%, and 100% confluence. Due to its 3 h half-life in mammalian cells, the luciferase protein does not accumulate over time. As such, luciferase activity does not reflect an accumulation of protein but rather an increase in *Csnk2a1* minimal promoter activity. Increasing cellular confluence was associated with an increase in *Csnk2a1* minimal promoter activity and resulting luciferase activity (Figure 8C). Both the RT-qPCR and luciferase reporter assays showed that *Csnk2a1* promoter activity increases with increasing cell confluence. This may have implications for cancers in which tumor cells operate at a steady state of "confluence" due to crowded tumor microenvironment. For these "confluent" tumors, *Csnk2a1* transcription may be upregulated, potentially leading to further transformation.

Previous studies showed that the expression levels of *CSNK2A1* transcripts do not change at different confluence percentages in HeLa and JEG-3 cancer cell cultures [21]. The difference with our data, as we discussed above, could be that cancer cells may have almost maximal expression of *CSNK2A1*, diminishing the effect of proliferation on promoter upregulation. Future experiments could address the mechanism underlying this difference. It is plausible that in these proliferation experiments, NF-κB is at least partially responsible for the increase in *Csnk2a1* transcription. In HEK/293 cells, human embryonic kidney fibroblasts, NF-κB-signaling reporter increases with increased confluency [69]. However, once cells are confluent, NF-κB signaling reporter activation decreases in HEK/293 cells. Therefore, it is plausible that NF-κB stimulation of *Csnk2a1* transcription is strongest during proliferation, and at 100% confluence, other transcription factors have greater control on *Csnk2a1* expression in normal cells.

An overall limitation in this study is that CK2α protein levels were not assessed due to the processing of cell lines to test for luciferase levels. Future experiments could build on this study by investigating levels of *Csnk2a1* mRNA, luciferase, CK2α protein levels, and protein kinase CK2 activity at varying degrees of confluence for all the experiments in this work.

3. Materials and Methods

3.1. Bioinformatics Analysis

Ensembl was used to identify the mouse (ENSMUST00000099224.10) and human (ENST00000217244.9, RefSeq Match NM_177559.3) CK2α gene transcripts. To align and visualize the mouse and human promoter sequences, NCBI BLAST+2.15.0 alignment software [70], mVISTA v2.0 (https://genome.lbl.gov/vista/index.shtml), SIM (https://web.expasy.org/sim/, accessed 1 December 2023), and EMBOSS Needle 6.6.0.0 (https://www.ebi.ac.uk/jdispatcher/psa/emboss_needle) were used. To predict potential transcription factor binding sites within the minimal promoter, TFBIND (which queries the transcription factor database TRANSFAC R3.4) was used [71].

3.2. Cloning and Plasmid Constructions

For the plasmid construction described below, all the plasmids and oligonucleotide primers are presented in Supplementary Tables S1 and S2, respectively. All plasmid DNA was isolated from bacteria using the Qiagen Spin Mini Kit or Qiagen Plasmid Maxi Kit. For the isolation of plasmid fragments, as discussed below, restriction digested plasmid DNA was extracted from 1% agarose gel following the manufacturer's instructions of the QIAquick Gel extraction kit protocol.

To generate the mouse *Csnk2a1* promoter–luciferase constructs, a bacterial artificial chromosome (BAC) clone (clone # 34983798473) containing the full mouse *Csnk2a1* genomic region was utilized, and fragments were cloned into pGL3-Basic, a plasmid that contains the luciferase gene *Luc*. We cloned a 4108 bp fragment into pGL3-Basic (construct named pLuc1), which included exon 1 (1 to 153) and 4108 bp upstream from the end of exon 1, as follows. We amplified by a 4108 bp fragment by PCR (−3955 to +153) using elongase enzyme (GibcoBRL Life Technologies, Waltham, MA, USA), a forward primer containing a MluI restriction endonuclease site and a reverse primer containing a NheI restriction endonuclease site. The amplified PCR product was extracted out of an agarose gel and digested with MluI and NheI, which were also used to digest the plasmid pGL3-Basic plasmid (Promega, Madison, WI, USA) which codes for the luciferase enzyme and ampicillin resistance. Following this, calf intestinal phosphatase was used to remove 5′ phosphate groups from the pGL3-Basic and Quick Ligase (New England Biolabs, Ipswich, MA, USA) was used to ligate the resulting linearized plasmid with the 4108 bp promoter fragment. Restriction digestion was used to screen for positives, and the resulting plasmid containing the 4108 bp mouse *Csnk2a1* promoter and luciferase gene was designated pLuc1 (−3955 to +153).

Plasmid deletion variants of pLuc1 were created via additional restriction digests of the pLuc1 plasmid. To create the pLuc2 plasmid, pLuc1 was digested with MluI and EcoRI to remove the first 3221 bp of the promoter. T4 DNA Polymerase was then used to blunt the ends of this linearized plasmid, and it was re-ligated with Quick Ligase resulting in pLuc2 (−735 to +153), a plasmid containing an 888 bp *Csnk2a1* promoter fragment. To create the pLuc3 plasmid, pLuc1 was digested with KpnI to remove the first 3503 bp of the promoter. Re-ligation with Quick Ligase yielded pLuc3 (−453 to +153), a plasmid containing a 606 bp *Csnk2a1* promoter fragment.

To create the pLuc4 plasmid, pLuc3 was amplified via PCR using a single primer which can anneal both downstream (−273) and upstream (base 4801 of pGL3-Basic) of exon 1. The amplified DNA was then treated with methylation sensitive endonuclease DpnI to only digest parental DNA. Transformed *E. coli* colonies were screened by restriction digest with NheI and MluI. The resulting plasmid pLuc4 (−273 to +153) contained a 426 bp *Csnk2a1* promoter fragment. To create the pLuc5 plasmid, pLuc4 was digested with PstI and NheI to remove the region downstream of +31. T4 DNA Polymerase was used to blunt the ends of this linearized plasmid, and it was re-ligated with Quick Ligase. This yielded plasmid pLuc5 (−273 to +31). pLuc5 was transformed into *E. coli* and the resulting colonies were screened by restriction digest with NotI and StyI.

Two-primer deletional PCR was used to create plasmids pLuc6, pLuc7, and pLuc8. To create the pLuc6 plasmid, pLuc1 underwent two-primer deletional PCR with primers. The forward primer binds at −184 and the reverse primer which binds at 4801 bp of pGL3-Basic. To create the pLuc 7 plasmid, pLuc1 underwent two-primer deletional PCR with the forward primer which binds at +47 and the reverse primer which binds at 4801 bp of the pGL3-Basic. To create the pLuc8 plasmid (−95 to +153), pLuc1 underwent two-primer deletional PCR with the forward primer which binds at −95 and the reverse primer which binds at 4801 bp of the pGL3-Basic. Following these amplifications, EcoRI was used to digest the amplified DNA, and it was then ligated with Quick Ligase. These plasmids were then transformed into *E. coli* and the resulting colonies were screened by restriction digest with NotI and StyI.

To create the pLuc9 plasmid (−273 to −80), pLuc4 underwent two-primer deletional PCR on pLuc4 with the forward primer which binds downstream of the primer insert in pLuc4, but upstream of the luciferase open reading frame, at base 55 of pGL3-Basic and the reverse primer which binds at −80. Following amplification, ApaI was used to digest the amplified DNA before ligation with Quick Ligase. pLuc9 was transformed into *E. coli* and the resulting colonies were screened by restriction digest with NotI and StyI.

For the transformations used to create the above plasmid deletion variants, either 1–5 ng of circular DNA or 50 ng of ligated DNA was introduced to competent *E. coli* DH5α or INVαF. The cultures were then incubated on ice for 30 min, heat shocked for 30 s at 42 °C and transferred back to ice to sit for 30 min. Five hundred μL of SOC media or LB broth was then added to the cultures before incubating on shakers at 37 °C for 1 h. Then, 100–300 μL of the transformation was incubated on agar plates supplemented with ampicillin for a period of 12–20 h. Subsequently, colonies were selected and cultured in LB broth with ampicillin.

3.3. Cell Culture and Transfections

All cell work was approved by the Boston University Medical Campus Institutional Safety Committee (protocol 14-1289). All transfections were performed utilizing the Lipofectamine 2000 (Invitrogen, Carlsbad, CA, USA) standard protocol with a few modifications [72]. Adherent NIH-3T3 cells (untransformed mouse fibroblasts, #CRL-1658) were obtained from the American Type Culture Collection (www.atcc.org). C57MG (mouse mammary epithelia) cell line was obtained from Dr. Gail Sonenshein (Cat. # SCC273; Merck/Millipore, Billerica, MA, USA). Cells were cultured in Dulbecco's Modified Eagle's Medium (DMEM) (Cellgro, Manassas, VA, USA) at 37 °C and were seeded in 6-well plates without antibiotics at a concentration of 0.5–0.7 $\times$ 10^4 cells per ml. After a 24-hour incubation period, the cells were suspended in 2 mL of fresh medium without antibiotics and replated. For each transfection sample, 4 μg of plasmid DNA was added to a 250 μL of Opti-MEM. A separate mixture of 250 μL of Opti-MEM and 10 μL of Lipofectamine 2000 was made and then mixed with the DNA mixture before incubating for 20 min to allow DNA-lipid complexes to form. This 500 μL solution was then added to each well containing the NIH-3T3 cells in 2 mL of fresh DMEM. The cells were allowed 24 h for transfection before the media was replaced. To control for transfection efficiency, simultaneous co-transfections of renilla (pRL-SV40, Promega) were performed for each sample using this same transfection protocol.

Following transfections, the Promega Dual Luciferase Reporter Assay System was utilized to quantify the activity of luciferase and renilla. First, the transfected cells were washed with phosphate-buffered saline (PBS) and then lysed with 250 μL of 1× Passive Lysis Buffer. To record luciferase activity, 10 μL of each sample was mixed with 50 μL of Luciferase Assay Reagent II in a polypropylene tube. Luminescence was recorded for 10 s using a luminometer. To record renilla activity, 50 μL of 1× Stop and Glo solution was added to the tube, and a second set of 10 s readings was performed.

3.4. Analysis of Gene Transcription

For the RNA copy number experiments, RNA extraction was performed as follows. Cultured cells were grown as described in the results (e.g., different confluences). Cells were washed with PBS and scraped, before being spun at 1000× g for 5 min at 4 °C. The pellet was resuspended in 1 mL of TRIzol Reagent (Invitrogen, cat # 15596-026) and homogenized by pipetting before incubating for 5–10 min at 15–30 °C. At this stage, cells were often frozen at −80 °C for later extraction. Following incubation, 0.2 mL of RNase-free chloroform was then added to the sample, and it was shaken vigorously for 15 s. The sample was then incubated at room temperature for 5 min before centrifugation at 12,000× *g* for 15 min at 4 °C. The clear RNA-containing supernatant was then pipetted to a new tube and RNase free isopropyl alcohol was added. Samples were then incubated at room temperature for 10 min before centrifugation at 12,000× *g* for 10 min at 4 °C to pellet the RNA. After discarding the supernatant, the RNA pellet was washed with 1 mL of RNase-free 75% ethanol and subsequently centrifuged for 5 min at 75,000× *g* at 4 °C. The supernatant was discarded and the RNA pellet was spun at low speed in a SpeedVac for 5 min before adding 30 µL of DEPC-treated, RNase-free water. RT was performed as described [73]

The PrimerExpress primer analysis program was utilized to select oligonucleotide primers for qPCR which would anneal at 59–61 °C (optimally 60 °C) and spanned an intron, when possible (Table S3). Ensembl mouse (GRCm39) and human (GRC38.p14) genomic sequences were used for primer selection. To verify primer sets, qPCR amplification was performed with the primers on cellular cDNA and plasmid DNA, if applicable. Only primers found to have distinct dissociation curve peaks and linear quantization of cDNA (over 10 two-fold dilutions) and plasmid DNA (over 10 two-fold dilutions) were used for experimental qPCR analysis.

For the qPCR reaction, 25 µL reactions were performed in the presence of 1× BIO-RAD SYBR Green Supermix, 400 nM of each primer, 2 µL of cDNA, and nuclease-free water. qPCR cycling was conducted with a Stratagene mx3000P real-time machine utilizing the SYBR green setting. The parameters for qPCR were: 3 min at 95 °C, followed by 40 cycles of 15 s at 95 °C and 1 minute at 60 °C, followed by 1 cycle of 30 s at 95 °C, 30 s at 60 °C, and an increase to 95 °C for dissociation curve.

Quantification of DNA and RNA was done via UV spectrophotometry at wavelengths of 260 nm and 280 nm with a Bio-Rad SmartSpec Plus spectrophotometer (Bio-Rad Laboratories, Hercules, CA, USA). Conversion ratios of 50 and 40 were applied for DNA and RNA, respectively. The 260/280 ratio served as an indicator for protein contamination (ratio < 1.8).

3.5. Protein Analysis

For protein extraction, cells were washed twice with cold PBS and then centrifuged at 3000 rpm for 4 min. The resulting pellet was washed again with PBS and then lysed in 50 µL of lysis buffer (50 mM Tris–HCl/pH 8.0, 125 mM NaCl, 1% NP-40, 10 mM NaF, 1 mM PMSF, 10 mM Na_3VO_4, 10 mM NaPPi, 5 µg/ml each of leupeptin, aprotinin, antipain and pepstatin) on ice for 10 min. After centrifugation at 12,000× *g*, the protein-containing supernatant separated and stored at −80 °C. To analyze protein concentration, the Pierce BCA Protein Assay Kit (Thermo Fisher Scientific, Waltham, MA, USA) protocol was used. 10 µL of serial dilutions of Bovine Serum Albumin (BSA) in PBS was added to 190 µL of Pierce BCA reagents (solution A to B at a ratio of 50:1). To determine sample protein concentration, the sample absorbance was measured at 570 µm via spectrophotometry (Bio-Rad SmartSpec Plus spectrophotometer) and compared to the BSA dilution standard curve.

3.6. EMSA

Electrophoretic mobility shift assays (EMSA) were performed using a ^{32}P-end-labeled fragment of the *Csnk2a1* mouse promoter containing the c-Rel/NF-κB transcription factor binding site (covering bases 4 to 13 of mouse exon 1). To label the two oligonucleotides (5′ GCATTGGGAGGGGGCTTCCGCTTC 3′ and 5′ GCATGAAGCGGAAGCCCCCTCCCA

3′), 30 to 100 ng of oligonucleotides were boiled in 11 μL of water for 5 min and then rested on ice for 5 min. A mixture of 2 μL of hexanucleotide mix (dATP, dGTP, dTTP; Roche, Cat. No. 11 277 081 001), 3 μL of α^{32}P dCTP, and 1 μL of Klenow enzyme (Roche, Cat. No. 11 008 404 001) were added and the oligonucleotide probe was labeled for 30 min at room temperature. The oligonucleotides were annealed.

The 50 μL annealing reaction contained both primers at a final concentration of 1 mM each in the presence of 20 mM Tris-Cl pH 7.6, 10 mM NaCl, 2 mM $MgCl_2$, and 0.2 mM EDTA. The reaction was performed at 85 °C for 10 min and then at room temperature for 4 h to form the probe listed in Table S3. For isolation of this radiolabeled oligonucleotide probe, STE buffer (0.438 g NaCl in 50 mL TE pH 8.0) was added to the radiolabeling reaction to reach a total volume of 50 μL. One μL of this mixture was taken for sample quantification. The remaining 49 μL was pipetted onto beads in a pre-spun (735× *g* for one minute) ProbeQuant G-50 Micro Column (Amersham Biosciences, Piscataway, NJ, USA). After addition of the probe to the column, it was spun at 735× *g* for 2 min. The flow through volume was assessed and another 1 μL was taken for sample quantification. The pre and post-spin samples were each added to 1 mL of scintillation fluid (Fisher Scientific, Hampton, NH, USA) for measurement in a beta-scintillation counter. The scintillation counts were normalized to volume and compared to assess the incorporation percentage of radiolabeled nucleotide into the oligonucleotide probe.

In the gel shift binding reactions, 1.2 μg of nuclear extract was added to 5 μL of 5× sample buffer (5 μL of Triton X-100, 25 μL of glycerol, 16 μL of 250 M DTT solution, 100 μL of 100 mM HEPES pH 7.5, 845 μL of H_2O) 2.5 μL dIdC, and DR buffer (420 mM KCl, 20 mM HEPES pH 7.9, 1.5 mM $MgCl_2$, 0.2 mM EDTA, 20% glycerol, 1 mM DTT, 0.5 mM PMSF, 10 μg/ml leupeptin, and 1% NP-40). In total, there were 100,000 counts of radiolabeled probe in a total of 25 μL of reaction mixture. For the competition experiments, 1 μL or 5 μL of unlabeled upstream response element (URE) probe (5′ GATCCAAGTCCGGGTT TTCCCCAAC 3′), kindly provided by Dr. Gail Sonenshein, was also added. The binding reaction proceeded for 60 min at room temperature.

A 15 cm acrylamide gel (7.5 mL 37% Acrylamide, 5 mL 10× TBE, 39.8 mL H_20, 35 μL TEMED, and 175 μL of 20% APS) was prepared and pre-run at 100 mV for 30 min. Samples were loaded, including a lane for the 6× loading buffer (also with DR buffer, dIdC, and SB buffer) and a lane for the free probe (also with DR buffer, dIdC, and SB buffer). The loaded gel was run at 200 mV for 3 hours. After, the gels were placed on Whatman paper and wrapped in saran wrap before drying for 1 hour in a gel drier. Gels were then exposed to film overnight at −80 °C.

3.7. Mice B Cell Isolation and Stimulation

All mice were maintained and managed at the Boston University Medical Center Animal Facility in uncrowded cages and husbandry was provided by the ASC (Animal Science Center) personnel. Animal protocol (AN-15183.2015.05) was approved in 2011 by the Boston University Medical Campus IACUC. Balb/c were euthanized using an acceptable method of euthanasia: they were anesthetized with isoflurane followed by cervical dislocation and vital tissue removal. To harvest splenic B cells, spleens were crushed and then cells were treated with anti-thymocyte globulins (gift from Dr. Thomas Rothstein) on ice for 40 min. To lyse any contaminating T cells, the cells were washed and treated with Rabbit complement. The cells were washed again and then layered onto 4 mL of warm Lympholyte-M. The cells were then spun at 1000–1500× *g* at room temperature, and as they spun the B lymphocytes became visible as a fuzzy white layer between the Lympholyte-M layer and the medium. The B lymphocyte layer was removed and washed twice.

To stimulate Balb/c mice splenic B lymphocyte growth, cells were added to RPMI (10% FBS, 2% L-glutamine, 1% penicillin/streptomycin) medium along with various chemical and physiological growth stimulants. For the first series of B lymphocyte stimulation experiments, 20 ng/ml of PMA and 0.7 ng ionomycin/ml were used to stimulate B lymphocytes. For the second series of B lymphocyte stimulation experiments, the following were used: 20 ng/ml and ionomycin at 709 ng/ml (Snow protocol [35]), 200 ng/ml and ionomycin at 600 ng/ml (Roth protocol [43]), 15 μg/ml lipopolysaccharide, 15 μg/ml anti-mouse IgM (AffiniPure (Fab')2 Fragment Goat Anti-Mouse IgM(μ) Chain 1.3 μg/ml, Jackson ImmunoResearch Laboratories), and a 1:10 dilution of CD40 ligand followed by a 1:40 dilution of CD8a 10 min later. The CD40 and CD8a dilutions were provided by Rothstein using their protocol [37]. Notably, it has been thought that the use of anti-IgM to stimulate B lymphocytes may induce apoptosis after 24 hours, but these anti-IgM experiments only used it for 5 hours. Furthermore, trypan blue staining was used to ensure that B lymphocytes remained viable throughout the experiment.

As B cells were stimulated, RNA was collected immediately after stimulation or at other time points. RNA was extracted, RT performed and then qPCR was utilized to generate copy numbers of *Csnk2a1*, *Actb*, and *Nfkbia*. Levels of *Csnk2a1* mRNA and *Nfkbia* mRNA were normalized to *Actb* mRNA. *IκBα* mRNA levels were measured as a positive control for NF-κB signaling pathway activation.

3.8. Statistical Analysis

Statistical analysis was performed for comparison of luciferase activity and gene copy number was performed with Welch's *t*-test in R (4.4.2).

4. Conclusions

In summary, we showed that the mouse *Csnk2a1* promoter sequence contains a minimal promoter sequence in the region 81 bp upstream from the start of exon 1. We showed for the first time that the NF-κB subunit p50 can bind directly to the *Csnk2a1* minimal promoter. We showed for the first time increased *Csnk2a1* transcription upon NF-κB signaling stimulation, either via NF-κB subunit transfection or via stimulation of B lymphocytes with NF-κB signaling agonists. These findings were used to develop a model for NF-κB and *Csnk2a1* positive feedback regulation, one which may have significant implications for cancer biology. Finally, *Csnk2a1* transcriptional regulation was shown to depend on the state of re-plating and confluence, which also may have implications for cancer proliferation and migration.

Supplementary Materials: The following supporting information can be downloaded at: https://www.mdpi.com/article/10.3390/kinasesphosphatases3030015/s1; Table S1. Plasmids; Table S2. Primers used for creation of *Csnk2a1* promoter–luciferase constructs; Table S3. Primers used for RT-qPCR and EMSA; Table S4. Materials List.

Author Contributions: Conceptualization, G.A.I., D.C.S. and I.D.; methodology, G.A.I. and N.G.W.; validation, N.G.W.; formal analysis, G.A.I., D.C.S., I.D. and N.G.W.; investigation, G.A.I. and N.G.W.; writing—original draft preparation, G.A.I. and D.C.S.; writing—review and editing, G.A.I., I.D. and N.G.W.; visualization, G.A.I., I.D. and N.G.W.; supervision, D.C.S. and I.D.; project administration, D.C.S.; funding acquisition, D.C.S. and I.D. All authors have read and agreed to the published version of the manuscript.

Funding: This work was partially supported with funding from the National Institutes of General Medical Sciences (NIGMS)1R01GM098367 and AHA Grant in Aid 10GRNT3010038 (I.D.) and, NIH R01 CA71796 and NIEHS P01 ES11624 (D.C.S.).

Informed Consent Statement: All animals were cared for in accordance with the guidelines of the Animal Welfare Act and experimental procedures had the prior approval of the Boston University Medical Campus Institutional Animal Care and Use Committee (IACUC) (protocol AN-15183.2015.05; Approval date: March 31, 2011). All cell work was approved by the Boston University Medical Campus Institutional Biosafety Committee (protocol 14-1289). Adherent NIH-3T3 cells (untransformed mouse fibroblasts, #CRL-1658) were obtained from the American Type Culture Collection (www.atcc.org). C57MG (mouse mammary epithelia) cell line was obtained from Dr. Gail Sonenshein (Cat. # SCC273; Merck/Millipore). Mouse primary B lymphocytes were obtained as per Materials and Methods.

Data Availability Statement: Experimental protocols and study material are detailed in the article and Supplementary Materials. All data are contained within the article. Further inquiries can be directed to the corresponding author.

Acknowledgments: We would like to thank Johathan Dye for obtaining the mouse splenic B cells for our experiments, Elizabeth Demicco for helping and advising on the NF-κB experiments, Gail Sonenshein and Tom Rothstein for their advice and their laboratories for fruitful discussions. We thank Tom Rothstein for the CD8a and CD40 dilutions used in the experiments. Finally, thanks to the Seldin laboratory for discussions.

Conflicts of Interest: All authors declare that they have no conflicts of interest.

References

1. Guerra, B.; Siemer, S.; Boldyreff, B.; Issinger, O.G. Protein kinase CK2: Evidence for a protein kinase CK2beta subunit fraction, devoid of the catalytic CK2alpha subunit, in mouse brain and testicles. *FEBS Lett.* **1999**, *462*, 353–357. [CrossRef] [PubMed]
2. Niefind, K.; Guerra, B.; Ermakowa, I.; Issinger, O.G. Crystallization and preliminary characterization of crystals of human protein kinase CK2. *Acta. Crystallogr. D. Biol. Crystallogr.* **2000**, *56*, 1680–1684. [CrossRef] [PubMed]
3. Niefind, K.; Guerra, B.; Ermakowa, I.; Issinger, O.G. Crystal structure of human protein kinase CK2: Insights into basic properties of the CK2 holoenzyme. *EMBO J.* **2001**, *20*, 5320–5331. [CrossRef]
4. St-Denis, N.A.; Litchfield, D.W. Protein kinase CK2 in health and disease: From birth to death: The role of protein kinase CK2 in the regulation of cell proliferation and survival. *Cell Mol. Life Sci. CMLS.* **2009**, *66*, 1817–1829. [CrossRef]
5. Ruzzene, M.; Pinna, L.A. Addiction to protein kinase CK2: A common denominator of diverse cancer cells? *Biochim. Biophys. Acta.* **2010**, *1804*, 499–504. [CrossRef]
6. Allende, J.E.; Allende, C.C. Protein kinase CK2: An enzyme with multiple substrates and a puzzling regulation. *FASEB J. Off. Publ. Fed. Am. Soc. Exp. Biol.* **1995**, *9*, 313–323. [CrossRef] [PubMed]
7. Glover, C.V. On the physiological role of casein kinase II in Saccharomyces cerevisiae. *Prog. Nucleic Acid. Res. Mol. Biol.* **1998**, *59*, 95–133.
8. Buchou, T.; Vernet, M.; Blond, O.; Jensen, H.H.; Pointu, H.; Olsen, B.B.; CochetA, C.; Issinger, O.-G.; Boldyreff, B. Disruption of the Regulatory β Subunit of Protein Kinase CK2 in Mice Leads to a Cell-Autonomous Defect and Early Embryonic Lethality. *Mol. Cell Biol.* **2003**, *23*, 908–915. [CrossRef]
9. Xu, X.; Toselli, P.A.; Russell, L.D.; Seldin, D.C. Globozoospermia in mice lacking the casein kinase II alpha' catalytic subunit. *Nat. Genet.* **1999**, *23*, 118–121. [CrossRef]
10. Dominguez, I.; Mizuno, J.; Wu, H.; Imbrie, G.A.; Symes, K.; Seldin, D.C. A role for CK2alpha/beta in Xenopus early embryonic development. *Mol. Cell Biochem.* **2005**, *274*, 125–131. [CrossRef]
11. Trembley, J.H.; Wu, J.; Unger, G.M.; Kren, B.T.; Ahmed, K. *Ck2 Suppression of Apoptosis and Its Implication in Cancer Biology and Therapy*; Wiley-Blackwell: Ames, IA, USA, 2013; pp. 219–343.
12. Seldin, D.C.; Landesman-Bollag, E. *The Oncogenic Potential of CK2*; Wiley-Blackwell: Ames, IA, USA, 2013.
13. Dominguez, I.; Sonenshein, G.E.; Seldin, D.C. CK2 and its role in Wnt and NF-κB signaling: Linking development and cancer. *Cell Mol. Life Sci. CMLS.* **2009**, *66*, 1850–1857. [CrossRef] [PubMed]
14. Chua, M.M.J.; Lee, M.; Dominguez, I. Cancer-type dependent expression of CK2 transcripts. *PLoS ONE* **2017**, *12*, e0188854. [CrossRef] [PubMed]
15. Jakobi, R.; Voss, H.; Pyerin, W. Human phosvitin/casein kinase type II. Molecular cloning and sequencing of full-length cDNA encoding subunit beta. *Eur. J. Biochem.* **1989**, *183*, 227–233. [CrossRef]
16. Litchfield, D.W. Protein kinase CK2: Structure, regulation and role in cellular decisions of life and death. *Biochem. J.* **2003**, *369*, 1–15. [CrossRef]

17. Ahmed, K.; Gerber, D.A.; Cochet, C. Joining the cell survival squad: An emerging role for protein kinase CK2. *Trends Cell Biol.* **2002**, *12*, 226–230. [CrossRef]
18. Wirkner, U.; Voss, H.; Ansorge, W.; Pyerin, W. Genomic organization and promoter identification of the human protein kinase CK2 catalytic subunit alpha (CSNK2A1). *Genomics* **1998**, *48*, 71–78. [CrossRef] [PubMed]
19. Krehan, A.; Ansuini, H.; Bocher, O.; Grein, S.; Wirkner, U.; Pyerin, W. Transcription factors ets1, NF-kappa B, and Sp1 are major determinants of the promoter activity of the human protein kinase CK2alpha gene. *J. Biol. Chem.* **2000**, *275*, 18327–18336. [CrossRef]
20. Krehan, A.; Schmalzbauer, R.; Böcher, O.; Ackermann, K.; Wirkner, U.; Brouwers, S.; Pyerin, W. Ets1 is a common element in directing transcription of the alpha and beta genes of human protein kinase CK2. *Eur. J. Biochem.* **2001**, *268*, 3243–3252. [CrossRef]
21. Pyerin, W.; Ackermann, K. Transcriptional coordination of the genes encoding catalytic (CK2alpha) and regulatory (CK2beta) subunits of human protein kinase CK2. *Mol. Cell. Biochem.* **2001**, *227*, 45–57. [CrossRef]
22. Zinatizadeh, M.R.; Schock, B.; Chalbatani, G.M.; Zarandi, P.K.; Jalali, S.A.; Miri, S.R. The Nuclear Factor Kappa B (NF-kB) signaling in cancer development and immune diseases. *Genes. Dis.* **2020**, *8*, 287–297. [CrossRef]
23. Yu, H.; Lin, L.; Zhang, Z.; Zhang, H.; Hu, H. Targeting NF-κB pathway for the therapy of diseases: Mechanism and clinical study. *Signal Transduct. Target. Ther.* **2020**, *5*, 1–23. [CrossRef] [PubMed]
24. Zhang, Q.; Lenardo, M.J.; Baltimore, D. 30 years of NF-κB: A blossoming of relevance to human pathobiology. *Cell* **2017**, *168*, 37–57. [CrossRef] [PubMed]
25. Smale, S.T. Dimer-specific regulatory mechanisms within the NF-κB family of transcription factors. *Immunol. Rev.* **2012**, *246*, 193–204. [CrossRef]
26. Oeckinghaus, A.; Ghosh, S. The NF-κB Family of Transcription Factors and Its Regulation. *Cold Spring Harb. Perspect. Biol.* **2009**, *1*, a000034. [CrossRef]
27. Khan, A.; Zhang, Y.; Ma, N.; Shi, J.; Hou, Y. NF-κB role on tumor proliferation, migration, invasion and immune escape. *Cancer Gene Ther.* **2024**, *31*, 1599–1610. [CrossRef]
28. Choudhuri, S. (Ed.) Fundamentals of Genes and Genomes. In *Bioinformatics for Beginners*; Oxford Academic Press: Oxford, UK, 2014. Available online: https://www.sciencedirect.com/science/article/pii/B9780124104716000013 (accessed on 21 December 2024).
29. Krehan, A.; Pyerin, W. Intermolecular contact sites in protein kinase CK2. *Mol. Cell Biochem.* **1999**, *191*, 21–28. [CrossRef] [PubMed]
30. Chen, M.-C.; Chen, C.-H.; Chuang, H.-C.; Kulp, S.K.; Teng, C.-M.; Chen, C.-S. A novel mechanism by which histone deacetylase inhibitors facilitate topoisomerase IIα degradation in hepatocellular carcinoma cells. *Hepatology* **2011**, *53*, 148–159. [CrossRef]
31. Besnard, A.; Galan-Rodriguez, B.; Vanhoutte, P.; Caboche, J. Elk-1 a transcription factor with multiple facets in the brain. *Front. Neurosci.* **2011**, *5*, 35. [CrossRef]
32. He, F.; Ru, X.; Wen, T. NRF2, a Transcription Factor for Stress Response and Beyond. *Int. J. Mol. Sci.* **2020**, *21*, 4777. [CrossRef]
33. Shahmuradov, I.A.; Solovyev, V.V. Nsite, NsiteH and NsiteM computer tools for studying transcription regulatory elements. *Bioinformatics* **2015**, *31*, 3544–3545. [CrossRef]
34. Zhao, B.; Barrera, L.A.; Ersing, I.; Willox, B.; Schmidt, S.C.; Greenfeld, H.; Zhou, H.; Mollo, S.B.; Shi, T.T.; Takasaki, K.; et al. The NF-κB Genomic Landscape in Lymphoblastoid B-cells. *Cell Rep.* **2014**, *8*, 1595–1606. [CrossRef]
35. Pan, W.; Deng, L.; Wang, H.; Wang, V.Y.F. Atypical IκB Bcl3 enhances the generation of the NF-κB p52 homodimer. *Front. Cell Dev. Biol.* **2022**, *10*, 930619. [CrossRef]
36. Liu, H.; Zeng, L.; Yang, Y.; Guo, C.; Wang, H. Bcl-3: A Double-Edged Sword in Immune Cells and Inflammation. *Front. Immunol.* **2022**, *13*, 847699. [CrossRef]
37. Fujita, T.; Nolan, G.P.; Ghosh, S.; Baltimore, D. Independent modes of transcriptional activation by the p50 and p65 subunits of NF-kappa B. *Genes. Dev.* **1992**, *6*, 775–787. [CrossRef]
38. Ghosh, G.; Ya-Fan Wang, V.; Huang, D.B.; Fusco, A. NF-κB Regulation: Lessons from Structures. *Immunol. Rev.* **2012**, *246*, 36–58. [CrossRef] [PubMed]
39. DeBenedette, M.; Snow, E.C. Induction and regulation of casein kinase II during B lymphocyte activation. *J. Immunol.* **1991**, *147*, 2839–2845. [CrossRef] [PubMed]
40. Rooney, J.W.; Dubois, P.M.; Sibley, C.H. Cross-linking of surface IgM activates NF-kappa B in B lymphocyte. *Eur. J. Immunol.* **1991**, *21*, 2993–2998. [CrossRef] [PubMed]
41. Francis, D.A.; Karras, J.G.; Ke, X.Y.; Sen, R.; Rothstein, T.L. Induction of the transcription factors NF-kappa B, AP-1 and NF-AT during B cell stimulation through the CD40 receptor. *Int. Immunol.* **1995**, *7*, 151–161. [CrossRef]
42. Covert, M.W.; Leung, T.H.; Gaston, J.E.; Baltimore, D. Achieving stability of lipopolysaccharide-induced NF-kappaB activation. *Science* **2005**, *309*, 1854–1857. [CrossRef]
43. Rothstein, T.L.; Baeker, T.R.; Miller, R.A.; Kolber, D.L. Stimulation of murine B cells by the combination of calcium ionophore plus phorbol ester. *Cell Immunol.* **1986**, *102*, 364–373. [CrossRef]

44. Alexandrov, P.; Zhai, Y.; Li, W.; Lukiw, W. Lipopolysaccharide-stimulated, NF-kB-, miRNA-146a- and miRNA-155-mediated molecular-genetic communication between the human gastrointestinal tract microbiome and the brain. *Folia Neuropathol.* **2019**, *57*, 211–219. [CrossRef] [PubMed]
45. Lukiw, W.J. Bacteroides fragilis Lipopolysaccharide and Inflammatory Signaling in Alzheimer's Disease. *Front. Microbiol.* **2016**, *7*, 1544. [CrossRef] [PubMed]
46. Liu, J.L.; Chiles, T.C.; Sen, R.J.; Rothstein, T.L. Inducible nuclear expression of NF-kappa B in primary B cells stimulated through the surface Ig receptor. *J. Immunol.* **1991**, *146*, 1685–1691. [CrossRef]
47. Mizuno, T.; Rothstein, T.L. B cell receptor (BCR) cross-talk: CD40 engagement creates an alternate pathway for BCR signaling that activates I kappa B kinase/I kappa B alpha/NF-kappa B without the need for PI3K and phospholipase C gamma. *J. Immunol.* **2005**, *174*, 6062–6070. [CrossRef] [PubMed]
48. Sun, S.C.; Ganchi, P.A.; Ballard, D.W.; Greene, W.C. NF-kappa B controls expression of inhibitor I kappa B alpha: Evidence for an inducible autoregulatory pathway. *Science* **1993**, *259*, 1912–1915. [CrossRef]
49. Liu, T.; Zhang, L.; Joo, D.; Sun, S.C. NF-κB signaling in inflammation. *Signal Transduct. Target. Ther.* **2017**, *2*, 17023. [CrossRef]
50. Wang, D.; Westerheide, S.D.; Hanson, J.L.; Baldwin, A.S. Tumor necrosis factor alpha-induced phosphorylation of RelA/p65 on Ser529 is controlled by casein kinase II. *J. Biol. Chem.* **2000**, *275*, 32592–32597. [CrossRef]
51. Bird, T.A.; Schooley, K.; Dower, S.K.; Hagen, H.; Virca, G.D. Activation of nuclear transcription factor NF-kappaB by interleukin-1 is accompanied by casein kinase II-mediated phosphorylation of the p65 subunit. *J. Biol. Chem.* **1997**, *272*, 32606–32612. [CrossRef]
52. Romieu-Mourez, R.; Landesman-Bollag, E.; Seldin, D.C.; Traish, A.M.; Mercurio, F.; Sonenshein, G.E. Roles of IKK kinases and protein kinase CK2 in activation of nuclear factor-kappaB in breast cancer. *Cancer Res.* **2001**, *61*, 3810–3818. [PubMed]
53. Baeuerle, P.A.; Henkel, T. Function and activation of NF-kappa B in the immune system. *Annu. Rev. Immunol.* **1994**, *12*, 141–179. [CrossRef]
54. Lupp, S.; Gumhold, C.; Ampofo, E.; Montenarh, M.; Rother, K. CK2 kinase activity but not its binding to CK2 promoter regions is implicated in the regulation of CK2α and CK2β gene expressions. *Mol. Cell Biochem.* **2013**, *384*, 71–82. [CrossRef] [PubMed]
55. Ackermann, K.; Waxmann, A.; Glover, C.V.; Pyerin, W. Genes targeted by protein kinase CK2: A genome-wide expression array analysis in yeast. *Mol. Cell Biochem.* **2001**, *227*, 59–66. [CrossRef] [PubMed]
56. Xu, X.; Landesman-Bollag, E.; Channavajhala, P.L.; Seldin, D.C. Murine protein kinase CK2: Gene and oncogene. *Mol. Cell Biochem.* **1999**, *191*, 65–74. [CrossRef] [PubMed]
57. Guldenpfennig, C.; Teixeiro, E.; Daniels, M. NF-kB's contribution to B cell fate decisions. *Front. Immunol.* **2023**, *14*, 1214095. [CrossRef]
58. Sovak, M.A.; Bellas, R.E.; Kim, D.W.; Zanieski, G.J.; Rogers, A.E.; Traish, A.M.; Sonenshein, G. Aberrant nuclear factor-kappaB/Rel expression and the pathogenesis of breast cancer. *J. Clin. Investig.* **1997**, *100*, 2952–2960. [CrossRef]
59. Yu, M.; Yeh, J.; Van Waes, C. Protein kinase casein kinase 2 mediates inhibitor-kappaB kinase and aberrant nuclear factor-kappaB activation by serum factor(s) in head and neck squamous carcinoma cells. *Cancer Res.* **2006**, *66*, 6722–6731. [CrossRef]
60. Currier, N.; Solomon, S.E.; Demicco, E.G.; Chang, D.L.F.; Farago, M.; Ying, H.; Dominguez, I.; Sonenshein, G.E.; Cardiff, R.D.; Xiao, Z.-X.J.; et al. Oncogenic signaling pathways activated in DMBA-induced mouse mammary tumors. *Toxicol. Pathol.* **2005**, *33*, 726–737. [CrossRef]
61. Seldin, D.C.; Leder, P. Casein kinase II alpha transgene-induced murine lymphoma: Relation to theileriosis in cattle. *Science.* **1995**, *267*, 894–897. [CrossRef]
62. Protein kinase CK2 in Mammary Gland Tumorigenesis-PubMed. Available online: https://pubmed.ncbi.nlm.nih.gov/11423974/. (accessed on 24 December 2023).
63. Orlandini, M.; Semplici, F.; Ferruzzi, R.; Meggio, F.; Pinna, L.A.; Oliviero, S. Protein kinase CK2alpha' is induced by serum as a delayed early gene and cooperates with Ha-ras in fibroblast transformation. *J. Biol. Chem.* **1998**, *273*, 21291–21297. [CrossRef]
64. Armstrong, S.A.; Barry, D.A.; Leggett, R.W.; Mueller, C.R. Casein kinase II-mediated phosphorylation of the C terminus of Sp1 decreases its DNA binding activity. *J. Biol. Chem.* **1997**, *272*, 13489–13495. [CrossRef]
65. Harris, S.M.; Harvey, E.J.; Hughes, T.R.; Ramji, D.P. The interferon-gamma-mediated inhibition of lipoprotein lipase gene transcription in macrophages involves casein kinase 2- and phosphoinositide-3-kinase-mediated regulation of transcription factors Sp1 and Sp3. *Cell Signal* **2008**, *20*, 2296–2301. [CrossRef] [PubMed]
66. Song, D.H.; Sussman, D.J.; Seldin, D.C. Endogenous protein kinase CK2 participates in Wnt signaling in mammary epithelial cells. *J. Biol. Chem.* **2000**, *275*, 23790–23797. [CrossRef] [PubMed]
67. Das, N.; Datta, N.; Chatterjee, U.; Ghosh, M.K. Estrogen receptor alpha transcriptionally activates casein kinase 2 alpha: A pivotal regulator of promyelocytic leukaemia protein (PML) and AKT in oncogenesis. *Cell Signal.* **2016**, *28*, 675–687. [CrossRef]
68. Giusiano, S.; Cochet, C.; Filhol, O.; Duchemin-Pelletier, E.; Secq, V.; Bonnier, P.; Carcopino, X.; Boubli, L.; Birnbaum, D.; Garcia, S.; et al. Protein kinase CK2α subunit over-expression correlates with metastatic risk in breast carcinomas: Quantitative immunohistochemistry in tissue microarrays. *Eur. J. Cancer* **2011**, *47*, 792–801. [CrossRef]

69. Hellweg, C.E.; Arenz, A.; Bogner, S.; Schmitz, C.; Baumstark-Khan, C. Activation of nuclear factor kappa B by different agents: Influence of culture conditions in a cell-based assay. *Ann. N. Y Acad. Sci.* **2006**, *1091*, 191–204. [CrossRef]
70. Tatusova, T.A.; Madden, T.L. BLAST 2 Sequences, a new tool for comparing protein and nucleotide sequences. *FEMS Microbiol. Lett.* **1999**, *174*, 247–250. [CrossRef] [PubMed]
71. Tsunoda, T.; Takagi, T. Estimating transcription factor bindability on DNA. *Bioinforma Oxf. Engl.* **1999**, *15*, 622–630. [CrossRef]
72. Lipofectamine 2000-US. Available online: https://www.thermofisher.com/us/en/home/references/protocols/cell-culture/transfection-protocol/lipofectamine-2000.html. (accessed on 24 December 2023).
73. Imbrie, G.A.; Wu, H.; Seldin, D.C.; Dominguez, I. Asymmetric Localization of CK2α During Xenopus Oogenesis. *Hum. Genet. Embryol. Curr. Res. Suppl.* **2012**, *S4*, 001. [CrossRef]

MDPI AG
Grosspeteranlage 5
4052 Basel
Switzerland
Tel.: +41 61 683 77 34

Kinases and Phosphatases Editorial Office
E-mail: kinasesphosphatases@mdpi.com
www.mdpi.com/journal/kinasesphosphatases

Mindful Lawyering